Childhood Feeding Disorders

Childhood Feeding Disorders

Biobehavioral Assessment and Intervention

by

Jurgen H. Kedesdy, Ph.D.
University of Massachusetts Medical Center
Worcester

and

Karen S. Budd, Ph.D.
DePaul University
Chicago

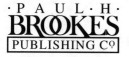
·P A U L·H·
BROOKES
PUBLISHING Cº

Baltimore • London • Toronto • Sydney

Paul H. Brookes Publishing Co., Inc.
Post Office Box 10624
Baltimore, Maryland 21285-0624

www.pbrookes.com

Typeset by Barton Matheson Willse & Worthington, Baltimore, Maryland.
Manufactured in the United States of America by
Versa Press, East Peoria, Illinois.

The cases in this book are composites based on the authors' experiences;
these cases do not represent the lives or experiences of specific individuals; therefore, any similarity to actual individuals or circumstances is co-
incidental, and no implications should be inferred.

Library of Congress Cataloging-in-Publication Data

Kedesdy, Jurgen Horst.
    Childhood feeding disorders : biobehavioral assessment and
  intervention / by Jurgen H. Kedesdy and Karen S. Budd.
      p.   cm.
    Includes bibliographical references and index.
    ISBN 1-55766-316-5
  1. Nutrition disorders in children.   I. Budd, Karen S.   II. Title.
RJ399.N8K43   1998   97-52164
618.92'39—dc21   CIP

British Library Cataloguing in Publication data are available from the
British Library.

Contents

About the Authors

Jurgen H. Kedesdy, Ph.D., Assistant Professor, Division of Developmental and Behavioral Pediatrics, Department of Pediatrics, University of Massachusetts Medical Center, 55 Lake Avenue North, Worcester, Massachusetts 01655. Dr. Kedesdy is Assistant Professor of Pediatrics and Director of the Growth and Nutrition Clinic at the University of Massachusetts Medical Center. Dr. Kedesdy is a pediatric psychologist specializing in the assessment and treatment of children with a wide variety of feeding problems. His interest in this area was cultivated during more than a decade of interdisciplinary practice in pediatric hospitals and pediatric rehabilitation facilities.

Karen S. Budd, Ph.D., Professor, Department of Psychology, DePaul University, 2219 North Kenmore Avenue, Chicago, Illinois 60614. Dr. Budd is Professor of Psychology at DePaul University. She has held academic and hospital positions in clinical psychology and behavioral pediatrics, and she conducts community-based research in the application of behavior analysis to child and family adjustment. She has published innovative research in the treatment of childhood feeding disorders and in related areas of child behavior and parenting competence.

Acknowledgments

We are grateful to many individuals and organizations for their help and support during the writing of this book. Several colleagues provided helpful comments and critical reviews of individual chapters during the course of multiple revisions. These include Diana Arezzo, Evan Charney, Ruth Crowley, Thomas Linscheid, Lynda Ritacco, Bob Thomas, Jody Warner, and Marty Young. We also appreciate the skilled efforts—and the patience—of our editors at Brookes Publishing, who helped guide this book to completion.

We have also learned a great deal from the many colleagues in diverse disciplines who have worked with us in the assessment and treatment of children with feeding and growth problems. Dennis Russo and colleagues in the Behavioral Medicine Clinic at the Children's Hospital in Boston, the members of the Feeding Team at Franciscan Children's Hospital in Boston, the Growth and Nutrition Clinic at the University of Massachusetts Medical Center, feeding specialists at Children's Memorial Hospital in Chicago, Ron Dachman at Behavioral Psychology Associates, and many students and interns with whom we have worked have informed and enriched our thinking about feeding disorders.

Jurgen H. Kedesdy was partially supported by grants from the Massachusetts Department of Public Health and the Share Our Strength Foundation. Karen S. Budd was supported in part by grants from the National Institute of Mental Health (No. R03-MH47539-03) and the University Research Council at DePaul University.

Finally, we are deeply thankful for the patience and countless silent sacrifices of our families. For them, the only recompense may be our *not* writing another book for a while.

To our parents—

Edith and Horst,
to whom I owe a healthy appetite for learning

JHK

and Gladys and Arnold,
for bearing with my finicky eating habits
and for believing in me

KSB

Childhood Feeding Disorders

1 Introduction

Feeding from a
Biobehavioral Perspective

No human activity has greater biological and social significance than feeding. Because ingestive behavior is crucial to the survival of the species, eating and drinking—and the behaviors that support them—are imbued with emotional resonance for the individual, the family, and the community. An organism that does not consume energy effectively does not survive to reproduce; a species that does not feed its young effectively jeopardizes the transmission of its genes. The participants in a feeding relationship thus come well prepared by the selective contingencies of evolution to engage effectively in the give and take of feeding. A child's eating and drinking are sustained by immediate gustatory pleasures of taste and texture, the recurrent comforts of satiety, and the less direct but equally important pleasures of parent contact. For the parent, successful feeding is both inherently satisfying and a powerful affirmation of competence. It is no wonder that parent and child usually experience feeding as a synchrony of mutual satisfaction.

Childhood feeding also occurs in, and is supported by, broader social and cultural contexts. Feeding practices are transmitted from generation to generation, as are dietary customs and laws; and the community monitors and enforces—explicitly and implicitly—adherence to these practices. A parent learns to measure the success of feeding against a set of culture-specific standards, which includes the achievement of feeding milestones (e.g., beginning to eat solid foods, drinking from a cup), acquisition of appropriate social behavior ("table manners") during meals, and expectations for the child's physical growth. Feeding milestones help mark a child's progress through early developmental phases and are sources of pride for the parent. The maturation of a child's mealtime behavior facilitates participation in and sharing of family meals. A child's physical growth is monitored both by informal social comparisons and during health care visits. Optimal physical growth signifies the health and vitality of the child and affirms the skills and competence of the nurturing parent. By contrast, when feeding is technically or emotionally difficult, when feeding milestones are not met as anticipated, when mealtimes are charged with anger and distress, or when the child does not grow as expected, the experience usually elicits deep parental concern. Feeding problems can arouse powerful, atavistic, complicated feelings of personal rejection and inadequacy, fear of negative social evaluation, and both realistic and catastrophic appraisals of child health risks.

COMMON FEATURES OF CHILDHOOD FEEDING PROBLEMS

How does feeding, a process so integral to the child's health and well-being, go awry? Often there is no simple answer to this question. Rather, feeding problems commonly originate in, and are maintained by, an interaction of factors. Consider this case example of Joel, a "fussy" eater.

■ ■ ■

CASE 1.1. A "FUSSY" EATER
NAME: Joel
AGE AT INTERVENTION: 7 months

BACKGROUND

Joel, a 7-month-old boy, was referred by his pediatrician for behavioral assessment and treatment of what was described as "poor feeding." Joel's birth and early developmental history were unremarkable, and his growth and feeding were entirely satisfactory until 10 weeks of age, at which time he contracted a viral illness, running a high fever for 3 days. During this illness, his appetite was persistently poor, he often cried during feeding, and he frequently refused the bottle altogether. This pattern of "fussy" eating continued after the illness resolved, and by Joel's 4-month visit to his pediatrician, it was clear that his weight had been affected. Joel's weight-for-age, just above the 50th percentile at age 2 months, had fallen to just below the 25th percentile at age 4 months. His length continued to track at about the 50th percentile. He was subsequently referred to a number of medical specialists who were able to rule out any organic basis for Joel's poor weight gain. Joel also received two feeding evaluations, at different hospitals, that concluded that Joel was a completely healthy child with no evidence of oral-motor dysfunction or other developmental problem.

Joel was the first child of well-educated, professionally successful parents. They had become increasingly anxious, in part because, during one of many medical consultations, the term "failure to thrive" (FTT) had been applied to their son. This diagnostic label, though accurate, had elicited profound fears and a sense of parental inadequacy.

Since Joel became a "fussy eater," his parents had taken to feeding him his formula, by bottle, while he slept. They understood that this was a maladaptive practice and expressed frustration and embarrassment about their predicament. They were unable to discontinue sleep feeding, despite multiple professional recommendations to do so because they feared that Joel would "become malnourished." At 7 months of age, Joel was taking about 65% of his formula feeds during sleep. When he was offered the bottle during the day, he often refused it outright, despite increasing parental persistence, much cajoling, and desperate attempts to entertain and distract him during feeding. He had been introduced to cereal and to baby foods at about 4 months of age, and he would occasionally take 1–2 ounces of these. But he was just as likely to spit these out and to push away the spoon. According to his parents, Joel fed best when he was distracted by television or by play with a toy. Both parents were concerned, but Joel's mother was the primary feeder during the day and was especially anxious and overwhelmed.

FORMULATION

In considering the facts of this case, the following etiological sequence was hypothesized. During Joel's illness, he had diminished appetite, which led to decreased oral intake. Joel's appetite may have recovered more slowly than his parents had anticipated. They then became especially vigilant about monitoring daily formula intake; when the volume of Joel's feeds did not meet their expectations, their anxiety escalated, and they became more insistent in their attempts to feed. Eating became more aversive for Joel, and he consumed less, which resulted in even greater parental anxiety.

Joel's "fussy eating" began as a characteristic response to acute illness and would likely have recovered normally after the illness subsided. A chronic feeding problem, however, developed as a result of the parents' creative but maladaptive technique of feeding Joel while he was asleep. Sleep feeding, in turn, further reduced Joel's appetite for daytime feeding. It served to "disconnect" the act and the context of a behavior (sucking) from its biological consequence (satiation).

INTERVENTION

Intervention was provided, jointly by a psychologist and a pediatric nutritionist, in the form of weekly sessions with both parents, as well as through frequent telephone contact. The nutritionist reviewed the feeding diary, estimated Joel's daily nutritional needs, and monitored his weight and length. Considerable time was devoted to reassuring the parents about Joel's health, to providing education regarding normal variation in children's caloric intake, and to articulating the rationale for an intervention to "shift" Joel's appetite back to daytime feeding. A program to gradually and systematically reduce "sleep feeding," by reducing the volume of formula offered at night by a specific amount, was negotiated with the parents. An important therapeutic consideration was matching parent "readiness" and tolerance for change to each step of the sleep-feeding weaning program. The parents also were asked to feed Joel in a distraction-free environment and in a calm manner, reacting neutrally to fussiness and noncoercively to refusal. Similar feeding interaction guidelines had been offered before; but they had not been immediately effective because they were being applied to a child with diminished appetite and were prematurely abandoned by the parents. A careful coordination of all elements of the intervention (i.e., feeding interaction counseling, appetite promotion, growth monitoring, nutrition counseling), provided in a therapeutic context, was needed.

OUTCOME

Within 3 weeks, Joel was taking more than 85% of his formula during daytime feeds, was accepting more formula per feed, and was showing an increasing interest in solid foods. At this point, his parents were comfortable with discontinuing sleep feeding altogether. Joel maintained satisfactory weight gain throughout the intervention and was subsequently discharged to his pediatrician for follow-up.

■　■　■

Case 1.1 highlights some important features common to children with feeding problems. First, it illustrates that *multiple variables* often interact to maintain feeding difficulties. These variables include a number of biological (and medical) factors, such as the original acute illness, the accompanying loss of appetite, the dissociation of appetite as a result of sleep feeding, and the series of medical consultations, which failed to reduce parental concern and thereby contributed, indirectly, to persistence of the problem. These variables also include behavioral factors, such as the parents' night feedings; their use of distractions during meals; and their worried, insistent reactions when the child refused to eat. Additional child, caregiver, or systemic variables (which could include, for example, cognitive, emotional, or social aspects of the child and parents, as well as marital, work, or family pressures) may have played roles in the problem's persistence, as well.

Case 1.1 also demonstrates the *maladaptive learning* that often occurs in children and in parents as a result of the interaction of powerful biological and behavioral factors. Learning theory postulates that people learn to respond in characteristic ways to situations as a function of the immediate antecedents and consequences of their behavior (Skinner, 1953). These contingency relationships, together with the influence of previous experiences and organismic variables, shape individuals' behavioral repertoires (Kantor, 1959). Maladaptive learning occurs when behavior patterns that have an undesired or counterproductive effect emerge in response to environmental contingencies. In the case of children's health problems, patterns of parent and child responding often are established inadvertently in reaction to atypical or unexpected situations; yet these behavior patterns serve to maintain the problem even after the original precipitating factor (i.e., illness) has diminished (Russo & Budd, 1987).

Another point illustrated by Case 1.1 is the integral role of planned behavior change in feeding intervention. The case shows that feeding problems often are *responsive to behavioral intervention*, despite the fact that biological factors were involved in the problems' development and continuance. Subsequent chapters describe a wide range of feeding problems—many with a decidedly more biological basis—involving children with congenital or developmental delays, multiple impairments, and chronic illnesses. In these chapters, a biobehavioral conceptualization is applied to identify important components in the assessment process and to choose intervention procedures that have been useful in resolving the particular feeding problem. This book covers a diverse range of feeding interventions, emphasizing *empirically tested* treatments and *behavioral* intervention approaches, both of which are based on a tradition of laboratory research.

The remainder of this chapter provides a conceptual framework for discussing childhood feeding problems and introduces topics that are covered in greater detail later in the book. Topics include basic terminology; prevalence of children's feeding disorders; classification of children's feeding disorders, including etiological factors to be considered in assessment; an overview of potential intervention approaches; and feeding professionals' roles and interdisciplinary collaboration.

BASIC TERMINOLOGY

The term *feeding problem* is used to refer to variations in ingestive behavior that are sufficiently divergent from the norm to result in personal or familial distress, social or developmental risk, or negative health consequences. Feeding "problem" is used interchangeably with "disorder," granting that the latter term often suggests a greater degree of severity or departure from the norm. In some works, the term *disorder* suggests a problem that is symptomatic of a mental or emotional disturbance, whereas in other contexts "feeding disorder" has been used to refer to an exclusively organic problem. Neither of these meanings is implied in this book, unless so specified. The term *feeding* is chosen in preference to *eating* because, in infancy and early childhood, eating is most often a dyadic process. In addition, the term *eating disorder* commonly refers to anorexia nervosa and bulimia nervosa, problems usually emergent in adolescence and adulthood, and these are disorders specifically excluded from consideration in this book. The issue of a possible continuity between early childhood eating problems/disorders and later emerging eating disorders is considered briefly in the discussion of specific disorders throughout the book.

PREVALENCE OF CHILDREN'S FEEDING DISORDERS

Childhood feeding problems are apparently quite common, but precise prevalence figures are not available because there is a lack of consistent diagnostic criteria to identify feeding problems and an absence of large-scale studies using standard classification systems.

A classic, frequently cited source suggesting the frequent occurrence of feeding problems is Bentovim's (1970) review of several early studies, which reported rates of variable or finicky eating or feeding disturbances of 30%–45% in the general population. Bentovim also reviewed data from 10 years (1958–1967) of patient records at a London hospital, at which referrals were tracked for three types of feeding problems. One type was "feeding mismanagement" problems associated with initial establishment of feeding patterns, which showed a peak occurrence during the first 6 months of life. A second distribution of "feeding problems," presumably due to issues of children's developing autonomy, showed a peak occurrence during the second to fourth years of life. A third distribution—obesity problems—had a peak occurrence in children ages 8–12 years.

Studies in the 1980s and 1990s have reported eating or feeding problems at rates varying from 2% to 29% in children without other developmental or health problems (Beautrais, Fergusson, &

Shannon, 1982; Dahl, 1987; Dahl & Sundelin, 1986, 1992; Forsyth, Leventhal, & McCarthy, 1985; Marchi & Cohen, 1990). These studies employed different definitions of feeding problems, different age ranges, and different sources (e.g., parents versus professionals), and they may or may not include some consideration of the severity of the problems.

The prevalence of feeding disorders in certain "high-risk" populations, such as children with multiple impairments, children born prematurely, or children with traumatic brain injuries, may well be higher. Palmer and Horn (1978) reported that 33% of individuals referred to the nutrition division of an urban clinic for children with special needs had feeding problems (e.g., prolonged subsistence on puréed foods, difficulty chewing, mealtime tantrums, delays in self-feeding). The frequency of swallowing disorders following acquired brain injury (ABI) has been estimated to be 25%–50% (Logemann, 1989). This estimate is derived from studies of adults with ABI; studies of the prevalence of feeding and swallowing problems following pediatric ABI are not yet available.

Finally, the prevalence of at least some childhood feeding problems (e.g., pediatric obesity) has been increasing (Gortmaker, Dietz, Sobel, & Wehler, 1987), and the size of some child health populations (e.g., premature, low birth weight infants) in which feeding disorders are common also has been increasing. These estimates of the prevalence of some early childhood feeding problems, which are discussed more extensively in later chapters, suggest that feeding problems constitute a sizable and, in some child populations, a growing clinical concern.

CLASSIFICATION OF CHILDREN'S FEEDING DISORDERS

Although it is widely understood that a common nomenclature and taxonomy are prerequisites to meaningful research, accurate diagnosis, and selection of effective treatments or interventions (O'Brien, Repp, Williams, & Christophersen, 1991; Woolston, 1991), there is no universally accepted classification system for childhood feeding disorders. The absence of consensus on this issue is attributable to several factors, including the heterogeneity of feeding problems, the variety of professional disciplines involved in assessing and treating feeding difficulties, the presence of multiple theoretical perspectives, and the frequent overshadowing of feeding problems by other diagnostic, intervention, and treatment issues (Linscheid, 1992).

Children with feeding problems initially may present as being underweight or overweight, malnourished, noncompliant, colicky, depressed, or constipated; as having developmental delays; or as having a variety of other complaints directly or indirectly related to eating. When feeding problems occur in association with other urgent health care problems (e.g., malnutrition, cancer, gastrointestinal disease), feeding problems may be overlooked entirely, or their assessment and treatment may be viewed as secondary and, consequently, may be postponed.

There are various ways that a child can come to the attention of specific professionals. The child who is underweight or overweight first may come to the attention of a pediatrician; the child with delayed self-feeding skills may be seen by an occupational therapist; and the child with selective feeding may be identified by the psychologist treating oppositional disorder. Speech evaluations can uncover feeding problems, as can routine dental visits. Varying professional perspectives and nomenclatures may result in the "same problem" being characterized in different ways. As a result, diagnostic labels applied to children with feeding problems vary widely, depending on the professional context in which evaluation occurs and the predominant symptoms reported.

Nevertheless, the search continues for a common language to describe childhood feeding problems. Three basic approaches have been taken to classify childhood feeding problems: descriptive, causal, and multidimensional. Each approach is described briefly, and an integrated classification system is introduced.

Descriptive Classification

The most common approach to classifying early childhood feeding disorders is simply on the basis of some descriptive characteristic of the feeding problem. Table 1.1 lists several representative descriptive classification systems. These classification systems differ from each other appreciably because different aspects of feeding are being described and classified. Some descriptive systems classify on the basis of the amount and type of food ingested (e.g., eating too much, too little, or the wrong things [Ginsberg, 1988; Kessler, 1966; Woolston, 1988]), whereas others may include properties of the meal (e.g., excessive meal duration [Babbitt, Hoch, & Coe, 1994]). Other systems classify on the basis of specific descriptors of child behavior (e.g., food refusal [Luiselli, 1989; O'Brien et al., 1991]). Yet other systems classify on the basis of multiple aspects of the feeding occasion (e.g., child behavior, properties of the meal, amount consumed [Linscheid, 1992]). Some descriptive systems classify feeding disorders exclusively (e.g., Luiselli, 1989), whereas others are intended to incorporate disorders of both eating and growth (e.g., Lask

Table 1.1. Childhood feeding disorders: Descriptive classification

Authors	Descriptive categories
American Psychiatric Association (1994)	• Pica • Rumination disorder • Feeding disorder of infancy or early childhood
Babbitt, Hoch, & Coe (1994)	• Food refusal • Food selectivity • Tube dependence • Swallowing skill deficit • Self-feeding skill deficit • Mealtime tantrums and disruptive behavior • Excessive meal duration • Adipsia and polydipsia • Rumination and vomiting

Ginsberg (1988)	• Insufficient food consumption
	  Failure to thrive
	  Anorexia nervosa
	  Selective food refusal
	• Excessive food consumption
	  Obesity
	  Binging
	  Pica
	• Inappropriate interactions with consumed food
	  Rumination
	  Psychogenic vomiting
	  Purging

Kessler (1966)	• Eating too little • Eating too much • Eating the wrong things
Lask & Bryant-Waugh (1993)	• Anorexia nervosa • Food avoidance emotional disorder (FAED) • Food refusal • Pervasive refusal • Selective eating • Bulimia nervosa • Appetite loss secondary to depression
Linscheid (1992)	• Mealtime tantrums • Bizarre food habits • Multiple food dislikes • Prolonged subsistence on puréed foods • Delay or difficulty in chewing, sucking, or swallowing • Pica • Excessive overeating • Pronounced underintake of food • Rumination

(continued)

Table 1.1. *(continued)*

Authors	Descriptive categories
Luiselli (1989)	• Food refusal • Food selectivity • Limited food intake • Self-feeding deficits • Improper pacing • Mealtime behavior problems • Rumination and vomiting
Mayes & Volkmar (1993)	• Pica • Rumination disorder of infancy • Nonorganic failure to thrive • Psychosocial dwarfism
O'Brien, Repp, Williams, & Christophersen (1991)	• Food refusal • Grams or calories consumed low • Food-type selectivity • Food-texture selectivity • Liquid refusal or selectivity • Problems with sucking or swallowing • Problems with chewing • Delays in self-feeding • Delays in self-drinking • Lack of utensil use • Inappropriate utensil use • Problems with lunchbox or tray • Leaving table • Spitting • Throwing items • Aggression • Inappropriate verbalizations • Inappropriate noises • Amount of spillage • Rate of intake • Chewing with mouth open • Lack of napkin use

Woolston (1983, 1988)	• Disorders of insufficient weight gain and growth
	    Nonorganic failure to thrive
	    Psychosocial dwarfism
	    Rumination
	• Disorder of excessive weight gain: Obesity
	• Disorder of nonnutritive substances: Pica

Woolston (1991)	• Failure to thrive • Psychosocial dwarfism • Rumination • Pica • Obesity • Benign nutritional dwarfing • Prepubertal anorexia nervosa

& Bryant-Waugh, 1993; Mayes & Volkmar, 1993; Woolston, 1991). Some of these systems are purely descriptive, whereas others implicitly reference etiology (e.g., psychosocial dwarfism, nonorganic FTT). Although the diversity of these descriptive systems is especially salient, commonalities also are evident. For example, undereating, overeating, and eating the wrong things are important distinctions in several of these systems.

Causal Classification

The main alternative to descriptive classification has been the organization of feeding disorders by their suspected causes. Some representative causal classification systems are listed in Table 1.2. Feeding and growth disorders are frequently globally classified as having organic, nonorganic, or mixed etiologies (Budd et al., 1992; Homer & Ludwig, 1981). The binary classification of growth problems evolved naturally out of traditional medical practice for ruling out underlying illness or organ system dysfunction to account for growth failure (see Chapters 2 and 6). When the physical examination and medical tests used for differential diagnosis are "positive" for organic factors (e.g., due to endocrine disorder), the growth problem is classified as "organic." When these tests are "negative," growth

Table 1.2. Childhood feeding disorders: Examples of causal classifications

Authors	Classification of causal factors
Budd et al. (1992)	• Only organic • Primarily organic • Primarily nonorganic • Only nonorganic
Linscheid (1992)	• Neuromotor dysfunction • Mechanical obstruction • Medical/genetic abnormality • Behavioral mismanagement

Luiselli (1989)	• Organic influences
	    Neuromuscular
	    Anatomical
	    Physical disease/metabolic disorder
	• Nonorganic influences
	    Physical/emotional
	    Educational
	    Environmental
	    Behavioral mismanagement
	• Interaction of organic and nonorganic influences

failure is categorized as "nonorganic." Recognition that feeding and growth disorders rarely fit neatly into one category of a dichotomous system has led to categorizing many of these problems as having "mixed" etiologies. For example, Budd et al. (1992) found that children with feeding problems identified in a hospital-based outpatient clinic could be classified as follows: Only Organic, 26%; Primarily Organic, 40%; Primarily Nonorganic, 24%; and Only Nonorganic, 10%.

Even with the addition of a "mixed" category, the organic–nonorganic classification is overly general, begging the question of which specific environmental or organic factors induce individual feeding and/or growth problems. Linscheid's (1992) classification of feeding problems is somewhat more specific, including a causal classification dimension with four major etiological factors: neuromotor dysfunction, mechanical obstruction, medical/genetic abnormality, and behavioral mismanagement.

An even more detailed etiological classification—especially of nonorganic factors—has been suggested by Luiselli (1989). Physical/emotional factors (e.g., parental depression), educational factors (e.g., nutrition-specific knowledge), environmental factors (e.g., financial constraints), and behavioral mismanagement (e.g., social reinforcement of mealtime misbehavior) are identified as possible causal variables in the induction or maintenance of pediatric feeding problems.

Multidimensional Classification

Descriptive and causal categories can be combined to produce a multidimensional classification of feeding disorders. Multidimensional classification goes beyond the simple reduction of complex clinical phenomena into discrete, relatively homogeneous categories; relating descriptive categories to their presumed causes suggests strategies for assessment, intervention, and prevention. Linscheid's (1992) classification system (see section entitled Descriptive Classification) combined descriptive and causal dimensions into a matrix. Some feeding problems are presumed to be determined by a single factor, whereas others may be determined by multiple factors. For example, the model assumes that mealtime tantrums are largely determined by behavioral mismanagement, whereas prolonged subsistence on puréed foods is potentially determined by behavioral mismanagement, neuromotor dysfunction, mechanical obstruction, or some combination of these. The descriptive/causal matrix provides a framework for evaluating feeding problems and for guiding intervention planning.

Whereas Linscheid's (1992) model was intended to apply to the entire spectrum of feeding problems, some multidimensional conceptualizations focus on specific subcategories of feeding or growth disorders. For example, Chatoor and her colleagues (Chatoor, Dickson, Schaeffer, & Egan, 1985) proposed a developmentally based classification system for feeding problems seen in children with FTT. Based on the clinical and etiological characteristics of the problem, Chatoor et al. (1985) identified three subtypes of feeding disorders: homeostasis, attachment, and separation. They used this classification to delineate intervention options associated with specific subtypes of FTT.

A comprehensive, multidimensional classification, incorporating many of the descriptive and causal categories discussed in this section, has helped organize much of the material in this book and is described in the next section.

An Integrated Multidimensional Classification

The classification system used in this book is represented in Table 1.3. This classification of childhood feeding disorders incorporates and integrates descriptive and causal terminology from extant systems into a bidimensional classification system in an effort to provide a comprehensive framework for use with any child presenting with feeding problems. The challenge of proposing a new classification (in the absence of any new facts) is to incorporate most of what was believed to be important in previous systems, to add previously underappreciated material, to reconcile obvious discrepancies, and to offer an organizational schema with plausibly enhanced heuristic value.

The descriptive categories in this system are intended to be consistent with the definition of *feeding disorder* proposed previously: deviations of ingestive *behavior* with significant clinical *consequences*. Eating behavior and its outcome are the clinical data categorized in this system. Growth disorders plausibly related to eating behavior are therefore included, whereas those unrelated to eating are not. Superordinate descriptive categories are organized around three widely accepted global descriptive categories (eating too little, eating too much, eating the wrong things) as well as a fourth superordinate category of "feeding skill delays," which incorporates those disorders of feeding that are especially prevalent in children with developmental delays.

Each superordinate category classifies several specific feeding disorders. Mild selectivity (picky eating), extreme selectivity, FTT secondary to food refusal, benign nutritional dwarfism, and prepu-

Table 1.3. An integrated multidimensional classification of childhood feeding disorders

---

Descriptive categories

Children who eat too little

    Mild selectivity (picky eating)
    Extreme selectivity
    Failure to thrive secondary to undereating
    Nutritional dwarfism
    Prepubertal anorexia nervosa

Children who eat too much

    Obesity
    Hyperphagia

Children who eat the wrong things

    Pica (eating nonnutritive substances)
    Rumination (reconsumption of vomitus)

Children with feeding skill deficits

    Oral-motor delays
    Self-feeding delays
    Social feeding deficits
    Eating-rate extremes

Etiological constructs (with selected examples)

Diet

    Suboptimal caloric intake
    Micronutrient deficiency
    Developmentally inappropriate diet

Physical competence

    Cleft palate
    Dysphagia
    Hypotonia

Appetite

    Grazing/meal spacing
    Aversive conditioning
    Supplemental feeding

Illness (acute or chronic)

    Otitis media
    Celiac disease
    Cystic fibrosis

Interaction/management

    Misplaced social contingencies
    Cue insensitivity
    Distracting or unsupportive feeding environment

Child constitution

    Difficult temperament
    Attention-deficit/hyperactivity disorder
    Sensory deficit

(continued)

Table 1.3. *(continued)*

Caregiver competence
    Parent mental illness
    Maladaptive nutrition beliefs
    Nonnurturant parenting

Systemic
    Poverty
    Family stressors
    Multiple feeders

bertal anorexia nervosa are included as subcategories of "eating too little." Mild and extreme selectivity are self-restrictions on oral intake associated with varying degrees of social, developmental, and health consequences but generally are without significant implications for growth. FTT secondary to food refusal, benign nutritional dwarfism, and prepubertal anorexia nervosa are disorders of undereating resulting in growth deficiency. Some growth disorders (e.g., organic FTT, psychosocial dwarfism) are commonly included in the classification of early childhood eating disorders but are not included here because they do not originate in disorders of feeding. Obesity and hyperphagia are included under "eating too much." Pica (eating nonnutritive substances) and rumination (reconsumption of vomitus) are located under the more general category "eating the wrong things."

Feeding skill deficits—heavily emphasized in some classification systems and completely ignored in others—are included here because they represent disorders of consummatory behavior with significant social, developmental, and health consequences. Feeding skill deficits are partitioned into four subtypes: oral-motor delays, delays in self-feeding, social feeding deficits, and eating-rate extremes.

Any classification of causal variables should be both useful and comprehensive. On the one hand, the binary or tripartite etiological classification systems (organic/nonorganic/mixed) are logically comprehensive but have limited clinical utility because they provide insufficient direction to the assessment process. On the other hand, a complete listing of all causal variables potentially related to poor feeding would be comprehensive, but very long, very cumbersome, and, consequently, not very useful. The causal classification proposed here attempts the middle path between the overly global and the excessively specific. It organizes conceptually and clinically derived variables into eight causal constructs, beginning with the three logical requirements of effective ingestion. Eating requires 1) *something to eat* (i.e., diet), 2) the *ability to eat* (i.e., physical competence), and 3) *motivation to eat* (i.e., appetite). Five additional causal variables are constructed from a conceptual synthesis of many specific factors culled from research and practice in early childhood feeding disorders. These causal constructs—discussed after diet, physical competence, and appetite—are illness, interaction/management child constitution, caregiver competence, and systemic factors. Table 3.1 lists the eight major etiological constructs and three specific examples of each.

Diet An adequate diet has sufficient caloric content and balanced nutritional composition and is developmentally appropriate. All of these factors are necessary for adequate growth, and careful evaluations of children's diets are especially crucial in the assessment of children with poor growth (see Chapter 6). The quality of the diet is, of course, determined by a number of other variables (some are included in the discussion of Caregiver Competence and Systemic Factors), but the diet itself also should be examined as an important causal factor. Poor or inappropriate dietary content can have indirect effects on appetite, and a developmentally inappropriate diet can affect the child's ability to eat. For example, a deficiency of some micronutrients (e.g., zinc) may change taste perception and thereby contribute to feeding difficulty (Hambridge, 1981).

Physical Competence The ability to eat has significant anatomical and physiological dimensions, and both obvious and subtle problems of physical competence can contribute to childhood feeding disorders. Structural, anatomical, or neuromuscular dysfunction can complicate feeding in an otherwise healthy child (Morris & Klein, 1987). For example, cleft palate may make feeding by breast or normal bottle impossible. Dysphagia (physiological swallowing dysfunction) can be so severe that normal ingestion of solids or liquids is precluded or, in a milder form, it simply may make eating and drinking painful or unpleasant. A host of neurological conditions can complicate feeding by affecting muscle tone, coordination, skill acquisition, or the ability to communicate needs and wants. Children with severe developmental disabilities often require extensive training to learn self-feeding skills and also may exhibit behavior difficulties during meals.

Appetite The motivation to eat is a complex construct, which is determined by an exceedingly intricate interaction of many biological and environmental factors. Some are physiological and metabolic, some are related to the timing and size of meals, and some are related to the sensory properties of food. Children's appetites can seem capricious and highly variable, but most children demonstrate a robust ability to "self-regulate" energy intake (Birch, Johnson, Andresen, Peters, & Schulte, 1991). This apparently inherent capacity for energy regulation, however, depends on, and can be distorted by, many environmental factors.

Cultural/social factors affect the appeal of food, as do learning and conditioning (Birch & Fisher, 1995). For example, the association of negative events (e.g., acute gastroenteritis, accidental choking) with eating can result in a conditioned aversion, which may compromise appetite and feeding long after the pairing occurs. Associative conditioning also appears to play a role in the control of meal initiation and formation of children's food preferences. For example, children learn to prefer flavors paired with foods of high energy density, which produce pleasurable feelings of satiety (Birch & Fisher, 1995). Appetite is strongly affected by meal schedules, with diminished appetite resulting when children "graze" and snack indiscriminately throughout the day. Suboptimal appetite can, in turn, contribute to feeding interaction problems and disruptive mealtime behavior.

Appetite is also an especially critical factor to consider in oral feeding resistance associated with long-term gastrostomy feeding (Geertsma, Hyams, Pelletier, & Reiter, 1985). Children who are on long-term gastrostomy feeding programs may not be motivated to eat, both because they do not experience normative cycles of hunger and satiation and because ingestive behavior (e.g., sucking) has become dissociated from its normal consequence: hunger reduction. Finally, appetite may be impaired by severe psychosocial/interactional disturbance—a condition sometimes characterized as "infantile anorexia" (Chatoor, 1989).

Illness Feeding problems can be symptomatic of a wide variety of acute, recurrent, or chronic illnesses; and the possibility of underlying disease or organ dysfunction must always be considered when feeding problems are evaluated and treated. Acute and recurrent viral illnesses commonly reduce the child's appetite and intake. Medications used to treat these illnesses can further reduce appetite. At the same time, illness is often associated with increased caloric needs and, in combination with attenuated appetite, can result in rapid weight loss, which further compromises the child's health. Some chronic childhood health conditions (e.g., cystic fibrosis) are directly associated with altered nutritional status. Finally, the treatment of many chronic illnesses may have iatrogenic (i.e., induced inadvertently by medical treatment) effects on feeding, resulting from medications used to treat the illness, frequent hospitalization and surgeries, and the use of supplemental feeding.

Interaction/Management Parent–child interaction during infant feeding and mealtime management in early childhood can be significant factors in the etiology of feeding problems. Infant feeding problems can develop when the feeder fails to recognize, misinterprets, or ignores cues that represent the infant's efforts to communicate his or her needs during the feeding interaction (Barnard et al., 1989). As children take more responsibility for self-feeding, parents also may mismanage the feeding relationship by differentially attending to food refusal or fussiness rather than to oral intake and appropriate mealtime behaviors (Finney, 1986). Both child and parent variables may contribute to feeding interaction problems, and these are discussed in the description of the next two causal categories, child constitution and caregiver competence.

Child Constitution Just as diminished physical competence can place constraints on feeding, other, sometimes less obvious, child constitutional factors can influence feeding. The child who is persistently "fussy" or "difficult," the child with unusually passive temperament, the child with attention-deficit/hyperactivity disorder, the child with autism, and the child with sensory impairments all may present feeding challenges even when other conditions are optimal. Child constitution interacts with parent characteristics, and whether feeding becomes problematic may depend on the "goodness of fit" between parent and child (Chess & Thomas, 1986).

Caregiver Competence Parenting competence has many dimensions: Intellectual competence, child care and parenting skills, nutrition knowledge, and psychological status are among those most relevant to child feeding. Caregiver competence determines the availability and quality of the child's diet and contributes directly to the success of the feeding interaction. In some cases, significant preexisting emotional or personality problems may compromise the parents' ability to provide an appropriate diet and/or feeding environment.

Systemic Factors Finally, a host of more distal, contextual factors can contribute to the genesis or maintenance of feeding problems. Systemic factors are aspects of the broader "ecological" context that may affect feeding interactions. Family variables such as marital conflict and financial or health problems are sources of stress that can undermine parental competence in child care (Wahler & Hann, 1986). Systemic factors also may have an impact on feeding patterns outside the home environment; for example, when children are routinely fed by multiple feeders (e.g., on hospital or rehabilitation wards) or in multiple environments (e.g., mother's house, father's house, grandparents' house, child care center), inconsistencies, in feeding practices can create or exacerbate problems. Finally, a broad range of socioeconomic variables can affect all aspects of family functioning and child welfare.

The classification system discussed in this section represents one of many ways of organizing what is presently known about the causes of childhood feeding disorders. Some of the distinctions drawn by this classification system may seem arbitrary (e.g., the distinction between child physical competence and other child constitutional factors), whereas other constructs (e.g., systemic factors) may seem to be overly global or may obscure important distinctions. This classification of childhood feeding disorders, like its distinguished predecessors, awaits empirical validation.

It is also important to emphasize that the presence of one etiological factor does not necessarily rule out the influence of other factors. A single factor, some combination of factors, or all factors may play some role in a single case. When there are multiple factors, some factors may be more influential than others, and the presence and strength of individual factors can modify the expression of other factors. Figure 1.1 illustrates some ways that these factors can interact to affect feeding.

To see how this bidimensional classification system might work, consider again Joel, the young child who was fed in his sleep by his parents, described in Case 1.1. As displayed in Table 1.4, Joel's feeding problems would be classified under the superordinate descriptive category, "eating too little." Joel's undereating was an example of food refusal associated with suboptimal caloric intake and poor weight gain, and he would therefore be considered for a diagnosis of FTT, depending on the exact degree of growth deceleration (see Chapter 6). Several etiological factors were apparently responsible for Joel's feeding problem: 1) an acute *illness* (i.e., the original fever of unknown origin), 2) diminished *appetite* (i.e., resulting from the dissociation of sucking and satiety caused by sleep feeding), 3) feeding *interaction/management* problems (i.e., parental reliance on cajoling, distraction, and play during day feeds), and 4) *systemic* factors (i.e., multiple medical workups resulting in heightened parental anxiety).

The integrated classification system is offered primarily as a practical method for organizing the assessment of feeding problems. Table 1.5 provides some examples of diagnostic questions suggested by this organization of etiological factors. Methods for assessing potential etiological factors and their interaction are reviewed more thoroughly in Chapters 2 and 3, and methods of intervening to modify the impact of these factors are described in Chapters 4–10.

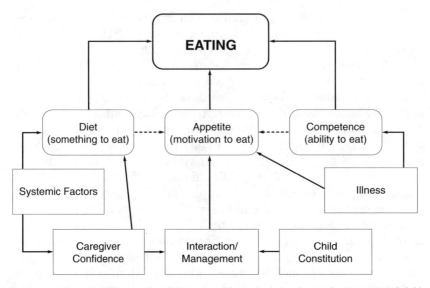

Figure 1.1. The potential interaction of major causal factors in the etiology and maintenance of childhood feeding disorders.

OVERVIEW OF INTERVENTION APPROACHES

An overview of treatment and intervention approaches that have been applied to feeding problems is offered next. *Biomedical* treatments focus on correcting physical defects or reducing the impact of organic anomalies; for example, surgery may be performed to repair malformations of the palate, esophagus, or intestine. Feeding tubes or intravenous lines are inserted to provide temporary nutritional support to children who cannot eat orally. Medications and special diets are among the biomedical techniques used to treat digestive problems or congenital growth abnormalities that cannot be medically resolved. Biomedical treatments are reviewed in Chapter 2.

Environmental interventions focus on changing the external and social conditions associated with feeding problems to decrease

Table 1.4. Multidimensional classification of Joel, the "fussy" eater

Descriptive	Etiological
Eating too little (failure to thrive secondary to undereating)	Appetite Illness (acute) Interaction/management Systemic

Table 1.5. Diagnostic questions suggested by causal classification

Causal factor	Some diagnostic questions
Diet	• Does the child get enough to eat? • Is the diet balanced? Are there adequate macronutrients and adequate micronutrients? • Is the child's diet developmentally appropriate?
Physical competence	• Does oral-motor dysfunction contribute to the problem? • Is neuromotor functioning adequate for independent feeding? • Does the child's neuromuscular status require adaptive utensils or seating?
Appetite	• Does the child graze (eat or drink continually throughout the day)? • Is there a history of traumatic events associated with eating? • How does supplemental feeding affect appetite?
Illness	• Is there a history of acute illness associated with the onset of feeding difficulty? • Does a current illness contribute to the problem? • Does the treatment of a current illness contribute to the problem?
Interaction/management	• Are parents sensitive to the child's hunger and satiety cues? • Are feeders overcontrolling? Are they undercontrolling? • Does social attention reinforce food refusal? • Does the feeding environment support effective feeding?
Child constitution	• Does the child have a "difficult" temperament? • Does the child have sensory impairments that influence feeding? • Does the child have a neurological impairment or developmental delay that affects learning and mealtime behavior?
Caregiver competence	• Do parents have maladaptive nutrition beliefs? • Does the parent have the intellectual ability to understand behavioral and nutritional recommendations? • Does the parent have a mental disorder that interferes with effective feeding or meal preparation?
Systemic	• Can the family afford an adequate diet? • Are recent family stressors (e.g., change of school, birth of sibling) correlated with the onset of feeding problems? • How many people feed the child, and do they use consistent feeding techniques?

or eliminate feeding difficulties. This book organizes environmental interventions into five topical areas: 1) *meal characteristics* (i.e., provision of a developmentally appropriate menu and repeated exposure to varied foods and textures), 2) *schedule of intake* (i.e., frequency and duration of meals), 3) *setting characteristics* (i.e., physical surroundings, feeding position and body support, and activities preceding and following eating), 4) *interactions* (i.e., reciprocity between feeder and child, and application of social contingencies using behavior management procedures), and 5) *other interventions* (e.g., nonnutritive sucking and adaptive feeding equipment).

In practice, feeding programs usually combine several intervention components in a clinical protocol. In some cases, interventions are directed at presumed deficits in the child's natural environment, such as behavioral mismanagement by the child's parents, inconsistent mealtime patterns, or nutritionally unbalanced diets. In other cases, environmental interventions are introduced to modify problems that result from the child's lack of exposure to typical eating practices because of developmental or health problems. Environmental interventions also may be used to facilitate a child's transition from reliance on biomedical procedures (e.g., feeding tubes, special diets) to normal eating conditions. Chapter 4 provides a more detailed description of environmental interventions.

PROFESSIONAL ROLES AND INTERDISCIPLINARY COLLABORATION

Because feeding is a biobehavioral process that involves the complex interaction of physiological and psychosocial systems, childhood feeding disorders commonly come to the attention of multiple professional disciplines during the course of assessment and intervention. Feeding problems are often first identified by the child's primary care physician; however, feeding assessment and intervention also may be initiated within special education or early intervention programs, acute care or rehabilitation settings, or therapeutic services and programs directed at other child issues (e.g., oppositional behavior, fine motor delays, communication problems). Professionals from different disciplines may see the child in sequence or in the context of a multidisciplinary process, such as a feeding team or pediatric specialty clinic, or concurrently manage different aspects of the problem in different settings. It is important, therefore, that the members of each discipline understand what other disciplines can contribute to the understanding of childhood feeding problems and to understand equally the extent and limits of their own expertise.

The professions most frequently involved—either by design or by accident—in the diagnosis and treatment of feeding problems are medicine, nutrition, nursing, occupational therapy, speech-language pathology/therapy, physical therapy, psychology, and social work. The following section provides a brief overview of areas of expertise commonly brought to childhood feeding disorders by different professionals. Chapter 3 describes alternative methods of collaboration across disciplines in feeding assessment.

Medicine

Early childhood feeding problems can come to the attention of a number of different medical specialties. The primary care physician, usually a pediatrician or family practitioner, may first uncover feeding problems during routine well-care visits or during the management of acute illness. Depending on the nature of the feeding problem, the primary care physician may address the problem directly (e.g., anticipatory guidance, brief developmental counseling, dietary guidelines). The physician also may order routine tests to rule out organic problems and/or may refer the child to a medical specialist or allied health professional for more specialized evaluation. A number of different medical subspecialists may be involved in more serious feeding problems, primarily on a consulting basis. A pediatric gastroenterologist may be consulted to diagnose gastrointestinal pathophysiology, a radiologist to help characterize swallowing problems, an endocrinologist to rule out specific hormonal dysfunction, a pediatric surgeon to place a gastrostomy tube, or a psychiatrist to evaluate for the presence of mental disorder in the child or parent. A related medical profession, dentistry, may be consulted to evaluate and possibly correct oral-structural impediments to feeding. It is not unusual for medical specialists to assume primary responsibility for treating or managing issues related to severe feeding problems. For example, a pediatric gastroenterologist may treat reflux and motility problems that have an impact on feeding, or a child psychiatrist may provide intervention for a dysfunctional parent–child relationship that is thought to be responsible for a child's suboptimal growth.

Nutrition

The clinical nutritionist or pediatric dietitian is frequently consulted to evaluate a child's nutritional status, the adequacy of a child's diet, the parent's knowledge of nutrition, and family dietary practices. The nutritionist effects changes in the child's diet by counseling parents directly, consulting with other professionals, or functioning within a feeding or medical team. The pediatric nutritionist plays a crucial role in the interventions for children with clinical disorders associated with altered nutrition (e.g., inborn errors of metabolism, pulmonary disease, pediatric burn patients) and who require highly specialized nutrition care plans.

Nursing

Hospitalized infants and young children often are fed by nurses, who then may be the first to be alerted to previously unappreciated feeding problems. Nurses generally document caloric intake and output, as well as changes in weight, and therefore play a critical role in monitoring the progress of feeding interventions. When feeding programs are conducted on an inpatient basis, nurses are often the primary agents of change. When intervention occurs on an outpatient basis, nurses may fulfill counseling and/or service coordination functions. Visiting nurses may provide intervention as well as guidance and support in the home. Nurses also may be responsible for obtaining the anthropometric data required to evaluate the progress of outpatient interventions.

Occupational Therapy

Traditionally, the pediatric occupational therapist is concerned with evaluation of and intervention for upper-extremity functioning, adaptive and self-help skills (e.g., dressing, grooming), and perceptual–motor interaction, especially as it involves self-help, play, or academic competence. In the evaluation and intervention for feeding problems, the occupational therapist may focus on a child's use of his or her upper extremities during feeding, on positioning, and on the teaching and facilitation of independent feeding skills. In some settings, the occupational therapist also evaluates and treats oral-motor problems. The occupational therapist may work individually with the child, help parents promote independent feeding, or function as a consultant or team member.

Speech-Language Pathology/Therapy

The speech-language pathologist/therapist (SLP) often is specifically trained to evaluate oral-motor dysfunction. The SLP frequently evaluates a child's oral-motor skills in the context of a feeding observation and may also collaborate with a radiologist in the assessment of swallowing dysfunction. The pediatric SLP may also be the primary intervention agent when feeding is, to some significant extent, due to oral-motor or swallowing problems. The SLP also evaluates and treats communication impairments that sometimes coincide with, and may contribute to, feeding problems.

Physical Therapy

The physical therapist has special expertise in gross motor development and functioning, with positioning of the child during feeding, and with adaptive equipment that can facilitate feeding. Children with cerebral palsy or other significant neuromuscular impairments who also have feeding problems are particularly likely to benefit from the consultation of a physical therapist. Physical therapists also may be responsible for carrying out interventions to foster adaptive and self-help skills.

Psychology

Pediatric psychologists are trained to evaluate and treat a wide spectrum of behavioral and developmental disorders of childhood and related parenting difficulties that present in pediatric settings. The pediatric psychologist with expertise in childhood feeding disorders may evaluate the quality of the parent–child interaction during feeding and nonfeeding activities, may assess for the presence of psychopathology or adjustment problems in individual participants in the feeding relationship, or conduct cognitive and developmental evaluations of children with feeding problems. The psychologist's role in intervention commonly involves the design of behavioral feeding protocols or involves working with parents and families to improve parent–child interactions and to reduce stress around feeding issues.

Social Work

The social worker may contribute to the assessment of feeding problems by evaluating family relationships and resources, gathering information on the home feeding environment, and surveying community resources. Social workers participate in interventions by providing therapeutic services (e.g., supportive counseling to individual parents, family therapy) or by securing and coordinating community services. Social workers sometimes serve as case managers on feeding teams.

Interdisciplinary Collaboration

As should be evident from this brief description of professional disciplines commonly involved with children with feeding problems, each profession offers special, sometimes unique, areas of expertise; but there also can be significant overlap in professional functioning. Sometimes overlapping functions occur as the result of commonalities in education and training; for example, psychologists, child psychiatrists, and social workers are all trained to provide psychotherapy. At other times, different professions have similar functions—not because of common training but because of prevailing clinical practices. This is exemplified when oral-motor problems may be treated by either a speech-language, occupational, or physical therapist, depending on the facility to which the child is referred. When professional resources are limited, many functions may be provided by a single professional (e.g., the occupational therapist may provide therapy for oral-motor problems, teach self-feeding skills, design adaptive equipment, and counsel parents regarding feeding interactions). When there is a relative abundance of professional resources (as is found on an interdisciplinary feeding team), professional roles may be defined more narrowly.

Interdisciplinary collaboration requires that each professional have enough understanding of the expertise brought by other disciplines to be able to problem-solve effectively to forge a coherent formulation of the feeding problem, as well as to generate a coordinated approach to treatment and intervention. Ongoing interchange and communication, as well as mutual respect and considerable professional tact, are essential to effective team functioning.

What may not be clear from the descriptions of professional roles and interdisciplinary collaboration is that professional membership may not ensure competence in the special issues relevant to childhood feeding problems. There is no certificate of "feeding expertise." Extensive clinical experience and keen interest still form the basis for much expertise in the area of feeding disorders.

Although there is a clear consensus that effective evaluation of and intervention for children with feeding disorders often requires the collaboration of professionals from multiple disciplines—and a growing appreciation that constructive collaboration is enhanced when children are seen by an interdisciplinary team—there are no clinical standards or guidelines for determining which child should be seen by which combination of professionals. For example, multidisciplinary feeding, growth, and nutrition teams are now the standard of care in many tertiary care centers, but recommendations for the staffing of these teams varies considerably (see Table 1.6), as does the actual staffing of existing teams and clinics.

Which professional disciplines actually become involved with a particular child and how they become involved depends on many

Table 1.6. Multidisciplinary teams concerned with feeding problems

Reference	Team members	Type of child
Bithoney et al. (1991)	• Pediatrician or pediatric gastroenterologist, M.D. • Nutritionist, R.D. • Developmental specialist, Ph.D. • Nurse practitioner, R.N., P.N.P. • Child psychiatrist, M.D. • Social worker, M.S.W.	Children with nonorganic failure to thrive
Cloud & Bergman (1991)	• Occupational therapist • Physical therapist • Speech pathologist • Nutritionist • Psychologist • Social worker • Dentist • Nurse	Children with developmental disabilities
Frank & Drotar (1994)	• Pediatric health care provider • Pediatric nutritionist • Social worker • Professionals with expertise in behavior, development, and family functioning	Children with failure to thrive
Morris & Klein (1987)	• Feeding therapist • Speech-language pathologist • Occupational therapist • Physical therapist • Physician • Nutritionist • Teacher • Dentist	Children with developmental disabilities
O'Brien, Repp, Williams, & Christophersen (1991)	• Physician • Nutritionist • Occupational therapist • Behavioral psychologist	Children with feeding disorders
Singer (1990)	• Pediatrician • Psychologist • Dietitians • Rehabilitation therapists	Children with chronic illness
Walter (1994)	Core team members • Developmental pediatrician • Gastroenterologist • Occupational therapist • Speech-language pathologist • Nutritionist • Nurse • Radiologist	Children with swallowing disorders

(continued)

Table 1.6. *(continued)*

Reference	Team members	Type of child
	Consulting members • Behavioral psychologist • Social worker • ENT surgeon/otolaryngologist • General surgeon • Dentist • Pulmonologist	
Wodarksi, Bundschuh, & Forbus (1988)	• Physician • Nutritionist • Psychologist or behavior specialist • Physical educator	Children with Prader-Willi syndrome
Wolf & Glass (1992)	• Occupational therapist • Physical therapist • Speech therapist • Nutritionist • Social worker • Nurse • Primary physician • Medical specialists	Infants with swallowing and feeding problems
Woolston (1991)	• Pediatrician • Nurse • Developmental psychologist • Child psychiatrist • Social worker • Nutritionist	Children with eating disorders

factors, including the nature and severity of the feeding problem, the clinical resources available, the organization of health care services within a facility or community, the policies of third-party payers, and somewhat less tangible factors such as the theoretical perspectives and referral practices of those managing a case. Much remains to be learned about how clinical resources should be organized to best serve children with feeding disorders and their families.

SUMMARY

Childhood feeding disorders consist of variations in ingestive behavior sufficiently divergent from the norm to result in personal or familial distress, social or developmental risk, or negative health consequences. Feeding problems are common in healthy children, but the prevalence of significant feeding disorders is greater in children with underlying medical conditions, developmental disabilities, or severe environmental deprivation. A biobehavioral perspective on childhood feeding disorders explicitly acknowledges that biological and environmental factors commonly interact in the etiology, maintenance, and treatment of feeding problems. Although there is no universally accepted classification of children's feeding problems, this chapter describes a multidimensional system of descriptive and etiological factors that incorporates many of the features of previous classification systems. General descriptive categories include eating too little, eating too much, eating the wrong things, and feeding skill delays, each of which is divided into subcategories representing more specific problems. Eight major etiological constructs are proposed: diet, physical competence, appetite, illness, interaction/management, child constitution, caregiver competence, and systemic variables. Potential interventions include both biological treatments and environmental approaches, and clinical interventions often combine several therapeutic components. Successful interventions for childhood feeding disorders often utilize the expertise of professionals from various disciplines, who work individually, in consultation with each other, or on interdisciplinary teams.

REFERENCES

American Psychiatric Association. (1994). *Diagnostic and statistical manual of mental disorders* (4th ed.). Washington, DC: Author.

Babbitt, R.L., Hoch, T.A., & Coe, D.A. (1994). Behavioral feeding disorders. In D.N. Tuchman & R.S. Walter (Eds.), *Disorders of feeding and swallowing in infants and children* (pp. 77–95). San Diego, CA: Singular.

Barnard, K.E., Hammond, M.A., Booth, C.L., Bee, H.L., Mitchell, S.K., & Spieker, S.J. (1989). Measurement and meaning of parent–child interaction. In F. Morrison, C. Lord, & D. Keating (Eds.), *Applied developmental psychology* (Vol. 3, pp. 40–76). New York: Academic Press.

Beautrais, A.L., Fergusson, D.M., & Shannon, F.T. (1982). Family life events and behavioral problems in preschool-aged children. *Pediatrics, 70,* 774–779.

Bentovim, A. (1970). The clinical approach to feeding disorders of childhood. *Journal of Psychosomatic Research, 14,* 267–276.

Birch, L.L., & Fisher, J.A. (1995). Appetite and eating behavior in children. *Pediatric Clinics of North America, 42,* 931–953.

Birch, L.L., Johnson, S.L., Andresen, G., Peters, J.C., & Schulte, M.C. (1991). The variability of young children's energy intake. *New England Journal of Medicine, 324,* 232–235.

Bithoney, W.G., McJunkin, J., Michalek, J., Snyder, J., Egan, H., & Epstein, D. (1991). The effect of a multidisciplinary team approach on weight gain in nonorganic failure-to-thrive children. *Journal of Developmental and Behavioral Pediatrics, 12,* 254–258.

Budd, K.S., McGraw, T.E., Farbisz, R., Murphy, T.B., Hawkins, D., Heilman, N., Werle, M., & Hochstadt, N.J. (1992). Psychosocial concomitants of children's feeding disorders. *Journal of Pediatric Psychology, 17,* 81–94.

Chatoor, I. (1989). Infantile anorexia nervosa: A developmental disorder of separation and individuation. *Journal of the American Academy of Psychoanalysis, 17,* 43–64.

Chatoor, I., Dickson, L. Schaeffer, S., & Egan, J. (1985). A developmental classification of feeding disorders associated with failure to thrive: Diagnosis and treatment. In D. Drotar (Ed.), *New directions in failure to thrive* (pp. 235–258). New York: Plenum.

Chess, S., & Thomas, A. (1986). *Temperament in clinical practice.* New York: Guilford Press.

Cloud, H.H., & Bergman, J. (1991). Eating/feeding problems of children: The team approach. *Nutrition Focus, 6,* 1–7.

Dahl, M. (1987). Early feeding problems in an affluent society: III. Follow-up at two years: Natural course, health, behaviour and development. *Acta Paediatrica Scandinavia, 76,* 872–880.

Dahl, M., & Sundelin, C. (1986). Early feeding problems in an affluent society: I. Categories and clinical signs. *Acta Paediatrica Scandinavia, 75,* 370–379.

Dahl, M., & Sundelin, C. (1992). Feeding problems in an affluent society. Follow-up at four years of age in children with early refusal to eat. *Acta Paediatrica, 81,* 575–579.

Finney, J.W. (1986). Preventing common feeding problems in infants and young children. *Pediatric Clinics of North America, 33,* 775–788.

Forsyth, B.W.C., Leventhal, J.M., & McCarthy, P.L. (1985). Mothers' perceptions of problems of feeding and crying behaviors: A prospective study. *American Journal of Diseases of Children, 139,* 269–272.

Frank, D.A., & Drotar, D. (1994). Failure to thrive. In R.M. Reece (Ed.), *Child abuse: Medical diagnosis and management* (pp. 298–325). Philadelphia: Lea & Febiger.

Geertsma, M.A., Hyams, J.S., Pelletier, J.M., & Reiter, S. (1985). Feeding resistance after parenteral hyperalimentation. *American Journal of Diseases of Children, 139,* 255–256.

Ginsberg, A.J. (1988). Feeding disorders in the developmentally disabled population. In D.C. Russo & J.H. Kedesdy (Eds.), *Behavioral medicine with the developmentally disabled* (pp. 21–41). New York: Plenum.

Gortmaker, S.L., Dietz, W.H., Sobel, A.M., & Wehler, C.A. (1987). Increasing pediatric obesity in the United States. *American Journal of Diseases of Children, 141,* 535–540.

Hambridge, K.M. (1981). Trace element deficiencies in childhood. In R.M. Suskind (Ed.), *Textbook of pediatric nutrition* (pp. 163–177). New York: Raven Press.

Homer, C., & Ludwig, S. (1981). Categorization of etiology of failure to thrive. *American Journal of Diseases of Children, 135,* 848–851.

Kantor, J.R. (1959). *Interbehavioral psychology.* Granville, OH: Principia.

Kessler, J.W. (1966). *Psychopathology of childhood.* Englewood Cliffs, NJ: Prentice Hall.

Lask, B., & Bryant-Waugh, R. (1993). *Childhood onset anorexia nervosa and related eating disorders.* Hillsdale, NJ: Lawrence Erlbaum Associates.

Linscheid, T.R. (1992). Eating problems in children. In C.E. Walker & M.C. Roberts (Eds.), *Handbook of clinical child psychology* (2nd ed., pp. 451–473). New York: John Wiley & Sons.

Logemann, J.A. (1989). Preface. Swallowing disorders and rehabilitation. *Journal of Head Trauma Rehabilitation, 4,* vii.

Luiselli, J.K. (1989). Behavioral assessment and treatment of pediatric feeding disorders in developmental disabilities. In M. Hersen, R.K. Eisler, & P.M. Miller (Eds.), *Progress in behavior modification* (Vol. 24, pp. 91–131). Beverly Hills, CA: Sage Publications.

Marchi, M., & Cohen, P. (1990). Early childhood eating behaviors and adolescent eating disorders. *Journal of the American Academy of Child and Adolescent Psychiatry, 29,* 112–117.

Mayes, L.C., & Volkmar, F.R. (1993). Nosology of eating and growth disorders in early childhood. *Child and Adolescent Psychiatric Clinics of North America, 2,* 15–35.

Morris, S.E., & Klein, M.D. (1987). *Pre-feeding skills: A comprehensive resource for feeding development.* Tucson, AZ: Therapy Skill Builders.

O'Brien, S., Repp, A.C., Williams, G.E., & Christophersen, E.R. (1991). Pediatric feeding disorders. *Behavior Modification, 15,* 394–418.

Palmer, S., & Horn, S. (1978). Feeding problems in children. In S. Palmer & S. Ekvall (Eds.), *Pediatric nutrition in developmental disorders* (pp. 107–129). Springfield, IL: Charles C Thomas.

Russo, D.C., & Budd, K.S. (1987). Limitations of operant practice in the study of disease. *Behavior Modification, 11,* 264–285.

Singer, L. (1990). When a sick child won't—or can't—eat. *Contemporary Pediatrics, 70,* 60–76.

Skinner, B.F. (1953). *Science and human behavior.* New York: Free Press.

Wahler, R.G., & Hann, D.M. (1986). A behavioral systems perspective in childhood psychopathology: Expanding the three-term operant contingency. In N.A. Krasnegor, J.D. Arasteh, & M.F. Cataldo (Eds.), *Child health behavior: A behavioral pediatrics perspective* (pp. 146–167). New York: John Wiley & Sons.

Walter, R.S. (1994). The multidisciplinary approach to management of swallowing disorders in the pediatric patient. In D.N. Tuchman & R.S. Walter (Eds.), *Disorders of feeding and swallowing in infants and children* (pp. 251–257). San Diego, CA: Singular.

Wodarski, L.A., Bundschuh, E., & Forbus, W.R. (1988). Inter-disciplinary case management: A model for intervention. *Journal of the American Dietetic Association, 88,* 332–335.

Wolf, L.S., & Glass, R.P. (1992). *Feeding and swallowing disorders in infancy.* Tucson, AZ: Therapy Skill Builders.

Woolston, J.L. (1983). Eating disorders in infancy and early childhood. *Journal of the American Academy of Child Psychiatry, 22,* 114–121.

Woolston, J.L. (1988). Eating disorders in infancy and early childhood. In B. Blinder, B.F. Chaitin, & R. Goldstein (Eds.), *The eating disorders* (pp. 275–283). New York: Spectrum Medical.

Woolston, J.L. (1991). *Eating and growth disorders in infants and children.* Beverly Hills, CA: Sage Publications.

2 Biological Factors in Feeding and Growth

Medical Approaches to Treatment

Robert Needlman, Robin H. Adair, and Karen Bresnahan

The foremost biological task of a young child is to grow. This chapter reviews the biological aspects of feeding, growth, and nutrition, and the medical approach to growth failure. A description of the gastrointestinal (GI) tract's anatomy, physiology, and regulation is followed by sections describing the fundamentals of nutrition and the mechanisms by which organ systems other than the GI tract influence growth. The final three sections of the chapter describe the clinical assessment of growth, the effects of various medications on nutrition, and the medical diagnostic approach to growth deficiency.

DIGESTION AS THE FOUNDATION OF GROWTH

The sequential process of taking in food, breaking it down into its constituent parts, and assimilating the parts into the bloodstream underlies all extrauterine growth. Arranged like work stations on an assembly line, the various components of the GI tract have specific tasks to perform as the body transforms food into nutrients and waste products. And, as in a well-designed factory, the operation of each component is tightly regulated for maximum efficiency. Dysfunction of the GI system is the most commonly identified "organic" contributor to failure to thrive (FTT) among both children who are hospitalized and children who are ambulatory and must always be considered in the differential diagnosis of growth failure (Berwick, Levey, & Kleinerman, 1982; Green, 1986). To understand the variety of GI problems that commonly affect growth, one requires a working knowledge of the physiology of the digestive

The authors wish to acknowledge the help of Jim Georgian, pharmacist, Franciscan Children's Hospital, Boston, Massachusetts, in the preparation of this chapter.

33

system and knowledge of the ways in which its components malfunction, and one should have an appreciation for the complexity of the regulatory mechanisms that keep the factory running smoothly.

Gastrointestinal Physiology: A Regional Atlas

The following section reviews the digestive system "from top to bottom," beginning with the mouth (see Figure 2.1). At each point, relevant aspects of typical functioning are discussed along with common malfunctions that regularly result in poor growth. Further details of GI anatomy and physiology can be found in Davenport (1978).

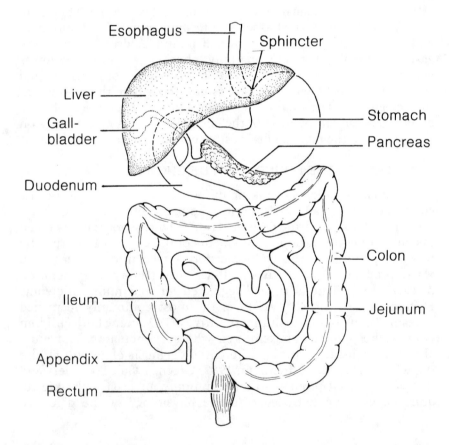

Figure 2.1. Atlas of the digestive tract. (From Eicher, P.S. [1997]. Feeding. In M.L. Batshaw [Ed.], *Children with disabilities* [4th ed., p. 627]. Baltimore: Paul H. Brookes Publishing Co.; reprinted by permission.)

The Mouth   During fetal life, the lower jaw develops more slowly than the upper part of the face, and—in keeping with the tongue's leading role in suckling—at birth the tongue is large relative to the oral cavity (Moore, 1977). Feeding proceeds through a series of reflexes: 1) rooting, in which the head turns toward the touched cheek; 2) latching on, with firm closure of the lips around the nipple; 3) rhythmic contractions of the tongue, first forcing the nipple up against the hard palate, then "stripping" it backward; 4) elevation of the soft palate to close off the back entrance to the nose; and 5) the initiation of a swallow (Carre, 1993). An infant breathes most comfortably through his or her nose and depends on this route during nursing; therefore, nasal obstruction commonly results in interrupted and uncomfortable feeding.

Saliva, stimulated by the presence of food or drink, contains a lubricant (mucin) and an enzyme that begins the process of breaking down starches. By acting as a solute for taste-bearing chemicals, saliva plays a role in enhancing the sensation of taste. Taste is sensed primarily by receptors on the tongue (taste buds) but also is sensed by the palate, pharynx, and other structures. Variations of flavor arise from different combinations of the four primary tastes (sweet, sour, salty, bitter) in conjunction with food textures and temperatures, odors sensed in the nose, and (particularly in toddlers) the colors of the food (Ganong, 1981).

With the introduction of solid foods, the tongue is called on first to move the food from side to side so that it can be chewed and then to separate off a small portion and push it back into the pharynx to be swallowed. The extent to which food is or is not chewed has little or nothing to do with how much nutrition is derived from it (Davenport, 1978). Dental abnormalities, however, can cause growth failure if the child is fed solids that are uncomfortable to swallow unchewed. Delayed tooth eruption (no tooth after 14–15 months of age) is sometimes a sign of endocrine or bone abnormalities. Severe dental caries (tooth decay) can cause pain with eating and are sources of ongoing infection, which can impair growth (Koch, Modeer, Puolsen, & Rasmussen, 1991).

Chewing and swallowing are mostly reflexive (although they can be performed voluntarily). Within the pharynx, another reflex is responsible for closing off the larynx and inhibiting breathing, preventing aspiration. Congenital abnormalities in oral-motor coordination can lead to loss of food across flaccid lips; slow, painstaking feeding; or frequent gagging. Abnormal tactile sensitivity—either too much or too little—can render eating aversive or unsatisfying. Such motor and sensory abnormalities may be subtle, yet potent enough to start a cycle of increasingly stressful and unproductive mealtimes (Mathisen, Skuse, Wolke, & Reilly, 1989).

Congenital facial malformations that commonly result in undernutrition include cleft lip, cleft palate, atypically large tongue (macroglossia), severe tongue-tie, or abnormally small jaw bones (micrognathia). In most cases, special feeding techniques can ameliorate the nutritional problem; for example, children with cleft palates often do well with cross-cut nipples, so that liquids flow into the mouth without having to be sucked in (Kaufman, 1991).

The Esophagus   The esophagus typifies the essential tube-like nature of the entire GI tract. The esophagus consists of several layers: a smooth inner layer similar to the lining of the mouth (the mucosa), a layer of connective tissue, and three layers of muscle—an inner layer (the muscularis mucosae), close to the mucosa; an intermediate layer whose fibers are arranged circularly; and an outer layer whose fibers are arranged longitudinally. The sole function of the esophagus is to transport ingested material from the pharynx to the stomach. Relaxation of the upper sphincter muscle allows food to enter the esophagus from the pharynx. The food is propelled by peristaltic waves of muscle contraction toward the lower esophageal sphincter, which relaxes momentarily to permit access to the stomach.

In rare cases, the lower sphincter fails to relax sufficiently, and the esophagus becomes distended with food and ceases to function (achalasia). More common, the sphincter is *too relaxed*, and acidic stomach contents flow up into the esophagus (gastroesophageal reflux, or GER). A certain amount of GER is normal, particularly in infants, and a few unconscious peristaltic waves quickly wash the acid back. When frequent and prolonged, however, GER results in inflammation of the mucosa (esophagitis) and in painful spasms of the esophageal muscles. Nerve fibers from both the esophagus and the heart travel together in the vagus nerve, and pain in the esophagus often is sensed as originating in the heart (hence heartburn). GER can result in poor weight gain, as well as respiratory symptoms (wheezing) and arching or unusual neck posturing in infants (Herbst, 1981; Orenstein, 1992). Medical treatment with drugs to strengthen the sphincter and to reduce stomach acidity is often helpful. With severe intractable GER, a surgical operation to create an artificial barrier between the stomach and the esophagus may be necessary. This operation, called a fundoplication, involves suturing the uppermost portion of the stomach (the fundus) around the lowermost stretch of esophagus (Hebra & Hoffman, 1993).

In the upper chest, the esophagus passes directly beneath the trachea and beneath the heart and great vessels in the midchest. These relationships are important because congenitally abnormal blood vessels can obstruct the esophagus, leading to pain on swallowing, as can food or other objects stuck in the trachea. Small openings connecting the trachea and esophagus (tracheo-esophageal fistulas, or TEFs) sometimes arise in embryonic development, leading to aspiration once the infant begins to nurse. These fistulas can be small and difficult to detect, requiring a skilled radiographer (Snyder & First, 1994).

The Stomach The mechanical grinding up of food occurs mostly in the stomach, not in the mouth. In the stomach, alternating bands of muscle contractions squeeze the contents first one way, then another, until the mass has been liquefied. Liquefaction is promoted by the secretion of large amounts of hydrochloric acid and of enzymes that break down proteins. Mucin also is secreted, lubricating the process. The stomach lining—made largely of protein—is protected from the acid and enzymes by special tight connections between adjacent cells, which prevent the acid from entering the tissues. When this barrier breaks down—as it does occasionally under the stress of infection, trauma (particularly burns), and certain drugs (e.g., caffeine, aspirin)—the stomach begins to digest itself, and gastric ulcers ensue. Since the late 1980s, the role of an unusual bacterium, *H. pylori*, has been recognized in the pathogenesis of gastric and duodenal ulcers (Marshall, 1990). Most, but not all, gastric ulcers are painful. They generally are diagnosed by a combination of occult blood in the stool and by abnormal barium swallow radiographs and are unusual causes of poor growth in children.

The stomach is funnel shaped, with a bulbus upper fundus and body and a narrow antrum at the bottom. At the end of the antrum, a circular mass of muscle called the pylorus functions as an outlet valve, intermittently relaxing to allow small portions of liquefied food to squirt through into the duodenum. A congenitally overgrown (hypertrophied) pylorus can obstruct this stomach outlet, resulting in stomach dilation, vomiting, dehydration, electrolyte disorders, and weight loss within the first 3–4 weeks of life. Hypertrophic pyloric stenosis (narrowing) arises for unknown reasons once in approximately 150 males and once in approximately 750 females (Behrman, Kliegman, & Nelson, 1992), and it is treated by a simple operation. Less common, the antrum is obstructed by masses in the stomach, such as tumors or bezoars (wadded up balls of nondigestible "stuff" that occur mostly in children with mental retardation or with emotional disturbance who habitually ingest hair). The principal symptom of obstruction of the stomach outlet is vomiting (Dodge, 1993).

The Small Intestine   Acidic stomach contents entering the small intestine are neutralized by bicarbonate and are further broken down by a barrage of enzymes secreted by the pancreas. Bile, secreted by the liver and stored in the gall bladder, emulsifies fats, allowing the fats to dissolve in the intestinal liquid. Most of the absorption of nutrients into the bloodstream occurs in the first part of the small intestine, the duodenum. The two more distal segments, the jejunum and the ileum, normally account for only 5%–10% of the absorption. These segments, however, provide a generous reserve capacity and play a critical role in the absorption of iron and vitamin B_{12}. To provide the maximum surface area for absorption, the inner surface of the small intestine is covered by leaf-like projections (villi, from the Latin for "shaggy hair"). The cells that make up the villi contain enzymes that break down complex carbohydrates, proteins, and fats into simple sugars, amino acids, and lipids. These components are taken up through the absorptive surface of the villi cells and are secreted across the lateral and basal membranes of the cells into nearby blood and lymph vessels.

There are numerous factors that can cause the complex processes of digestion and absorption to break down. The pancreatic secretions can be blocked by a tumor or by excessively sticky secretions as in cystic fibrosis, which is the most common cause of chronic malabsorption among North Americans. The flow of bile may be impeded anywhere on its path from the liver to the duodenum, either by gallstones or by malformations of the bile ducts. The cells covering the villi can be damaged by infection, by allergic reactions, or by some medical treatments, which result in impaired absorption of all or selected nutrients (Heitlinger & Lebenthal, 1988).

Whatever the cause of the malabsorption, the common effect is that substances that are not taken up from the intestines attract water by osmosis, resulting in diarrhea; unabsorbed nutrients also may predispose to the overgrowth of bacteria. If carbohydrates (i.e., sugars, starches) are unabsorbed, then they ferment, giving off hydrogen, which causes flatulence and which can be measured in the breath. Unabsorbed carbohydrates also raise the acidity of the stool, resulting in raw, painful diaper rashes.

The connection among intestinal dysfunction, malabsorption, and diarrhea is illustrated by lactase deficiency. Cow milk contains lactose, a two-part sugar that must be broken into its components by the enzyme lactase, which is contained in the cells of the villi. Few children are born lactase deficient, but many develop lactase deficiency as they mature; in addition, lactase is lost when the villi cells are damaged by infection, allergic reactions, or some medical treatments. Without lactase, lactose cannot be absorbed and remains in the intestine, where it attracts water and produces diarrhea. That is why continuing to give milk to a child with diarrhea sometimes makes the problem worse.

The small intestine is responsible for absorbing not only proteins, carbohydrates, and fats, but also most of the water taken in. A special "pump" in the villi cell takes up one molecule of glucose with one molecule of sodium; water follows, drawn by osmosis. The discovery of this one-for-one link between sodium and glucose transport has led to the development of oral rehydration solutions, which maximize the uptake of water from the small intestine, saving the lives of millions of children with diarrhea (Ghishan, 1988).

The small intestine takes its name from its diameter, not its length (about 10 feet in an adult). Blood vessels, lymphatic channels, and nerves reach the intestine along a thin sheet of tissue called the mesentery, which is anchored to the posterior abdominal wall. During embryonic development, an elegant sequence of growth and changes in position results in a precise arrangement of the mesentery within the abdominal cavity. If this sequence goes awry, then the mesentery can be prone to twisting on itself, resulting in bowel obstruction (Moore, 1977).

The intestine is in constant motion, mixing and propelling its contents along. If this stops for any time, then the contents build up, absorption fails, and vomiting ensues. This dreadful condition, called an ileus, sometimes accompanies serious infections, bowel obstruction, or abdominal surgery. Overly speedy passage of material through the small intestine also causes problems, as the large intestine finds itself overwhelmed by a mass of unabsorbed "stuff." This phenomenon, inelegantly termed "dumping," sometimes occurs after surgical removal of large segments of intestine, including the valve at the far end of the ileum. The most frequent reason for such massive surgery is necrotizing enterocolitis (NEC), a severe GI disease associated with extreme prematurity (Warner & Ziegler, 1993).

The Colon Under healthy conditions, material leaving the small intestine is nearly sterile and largely devoid of important nutrients. Much of what reaches the colon is indigestible fiber, which is necessary to give the stool bulk and a soft consistency. The colon, or large intestine, processes this residue by removing more of the water, salt, and minerals, and by adjusting the acidity. With the help of resident bacteria, the colon is responsible for producing and absorbing several necessary vitamins and packaging the waste in a compact (if not exactly neat) form.

It takes about 12 hours for residue to traverse the colon from the cecum at its beginning to the sigmoid (literally, "S-shaped") colon, just above the rectum. The sigmoid serves as a storage depot, and its strong contractions eventually provide the motive force behind defecation. When colonic transit proceeds too rapidly, excessive water escapes reabsorption, resulting in diarrhea.

When the transit is too slow, too much water is reabsorbed and the stool becomes hard and painful to pass. When this happens, children may struggle to retain stools in order to avoid the pain. The result is a cycle of ever-worsening constipation. Eventually, the colon becomes distended by hard, rock-like stool and ceases to move; liquid stool drips through the crevices between the "rocks" and passes out the anus, unnoticed by the child who has become habituated to the odor. Treatment includes laxatives to clean out the bowel, medicines to keep the stool soft, and regular toilet sitting. Chronic constipation is usually not a sign of mental illness, although it certainly can precipitate low self-esteem and depression (Levine, 1982).

Colonic bacteria, often termed "normal flora," produce vitamin K (necessary for clotting) and some B-complex vitamins. By competing for living space and resources, they also control the proliferation of other microorganisms such as fungi (or yeast). If the normal bacteria are killed off, then the fungus population explodes. Thus, children with ear infections frequently end up with irritating fungal diaper rashes as an unintended effect of the broad-spectrum antibiotics used to treat their ears.

Many distinctly unfriendly germs also favor the colon, causing colitis, with mucous and sometimes bloody diarrhea. Usually these infections are unpleasant but short lived. Noninfectious causes of ongoing inflammation of the colon include ulcerative colitis and Crohn disease, most often appearing in older school-age children and adolescents. The hallmark of these conditions is bloody diarrhea with cramping, but at the onset the only sign may be growth failure. Their cause is still largely unknown, although an abnormal response of the immune system appears to be the main engine of damage. Diagnosis is usually accomplished by a barium enema X-ray study (O'Gorman & Lake, 1993).

Control Mechanisms

So far, the individual components of the GI tract have been considered separately. Yet, for the system as a whole to function efficiently, these separate parts have to work together. This section surveys some of the hormonal and neurological mechanisms that control the processes of feeding, digestion, and elimination.

As foodstuff passes down the GI tract, its presence triggers activity of the appropriate muscles and secretion of the necessary substances. Thus, food in the mouth stimulates both chewing and the production of saliva. Protein in the stomach stimulates a hormone called gastrin, which in turn stimulates gastric contractions and triggers the secretion of acid and enzymes. Stomach contents entering the small intestine cause a hormone to be released into the bloodstream called cholecystokinin (CCK, literally "gall bladder activator"). CCK in turn stimulates the secretion of bile, bicarbonate, and pancreatic enzymes. Altogether, some 20 or more hormones have been recognized that exert effects on the functioning of the GI tract, such as stimulating or depressing secretion of particular enzymes or controlling the passage of various chemicals into or out of the cells lining the GI tract. The hormones have names such as somatostatin and motilin and acronyms such as VIP and GIP. Each has a role to play in fine-tuning the GI process, although for the most part the mechanisms remain poorly understood. It is interesting to note that many of these same substances are being found in the brain, in which they serve as messengers between adjacent neurons (Burke, 1993).

In conjuction with the hormones, a similarly intricate system of nerve signals also acts to regulate GI function. Nerves lying within the muscle layers of the esophagus, stomach, and intestine are responsible for establishing the underlying rhythm of contractions and peristalsis. This activity is further regulated by nerve impulses traveling back and forth to the brain in the vagus nerve. Impulses in the vagus nerve augment the gut musculature and glandular secretions. These vagal impulses constitute part of the parasympathetic nervous system, which is responsible for regulating many functions related to growth; the opposing sympathetic nervous system is activated in times of stress (the "fight-or-flight" response), and during these times GI activity is reduced to a minimum (Rubenstein, 1993).

There are also reflexes connecting one part of the GI tract with another. For example, the act of swallowing signals the stomach muscles to relax to accommodate the incoming meal. In a similar way, food in the stomach activates contractions in the sigmoid colon, clearing space below. This "gastrocolic" reflex is why infants often need their diapers changed right after eating. It may be that imbalances in these control systems contribute to problems such

as "functional abdominal pain" or "irritable bowel syndrome"—
entities that have long been suspected of having psychological
causes (Milla, 1988).

Perhaps the most complex and least well understood regulatory
mechanism concerns the control of hunger and satiety, the sine qua
non of digestion. How does the body signal that it needs more nourishment? In what ways does that mechanism malfunction to produce obesity, on the one hand, or anorexia on the other? Within a
small region at the base of the brain, the thalamus, lies one group of
cells, which, if stimulated, induces hunger, and another group that
induces satiety. The system appears to respond to a host of signals;
for example, the hormone CCK not only stimulates the gallbladder,
as described previously, but CCK also sends a satiety signal to the
brain. The hormone insulin, necessary for the uptake of fuel by the
cells of the body, also is sensed in the brain as a signal that sufficient nourishment has been taken in. Moreover, the body's degree
of fatness, or adiposity, appears to modulate the sensitivity of the
brain to insulin, such that people with high adiposity may be less
sensitive to the insulin signal. It is possible, but not proved, that
very lean people may be hypersensitive to the signal (Liebowitz,
Weiss, & Shor-Posner, 1988).

It is clear, too, that emotional factors impinge on this regulatory system in ways that are poorly understood. A loss of appetite
frequently accompanies depression, for example; but sometimes the
opposite effect occurs.

This degree of complexity is not surprising when one considers
the central role of digestion in survival and the necessity of coordination among the various parts of the system. In evolutionary
terms, the gut has roots in the deepest antiquity: Nearly all multi-
cellular organisms have a gut. By comparison, arms and legs are recent acquisitions. Embryologically, too, the gut is one of the first
structures to emerge, closely related in space, time, and cells of origin to the brain and spinal cord. The fact that many gut hormones
serve double duty in the brain is therefore not unexpected (Moore,
1977).

Clinically, a mechanistic view of the GI tract as an assembly
line is useful, assisting one to think of possible malfunctions at any
level—mouth, esophagus, stomach, small intestine, or colon. When
growth failure is related to GI dysfunction, the principal culprit is
usually malabsorption, and generally the symptoms of diarrhea,
flatulence, and cramps are all too apparent. The challenge then becomes localizing the area or areas of dysfunction and either "fixing"
the problem (e.g., by having the child ingest large quantities of a

missing enzyme) or eliminating from the diet those substances that the system cannot adequately process.

In most cases of growth failure, particularly among children who are not hospitalized, the main problem is not the GI tract at all but rather a failure to ingest adequate calories (Berwick, 1980; Frank & Zeisel, 1988). These cases call for an appreciation of the complexities of neural and hormonal regulation and the interaction of these systems with psychological and social influences. It is sad to note, however, that in the late 1990s the level of understanding of these regulatory mechanisms rarely suffices to indicate specific therapies, and effective treatments often require extensive psychological therapy and costly social supports (e.g., therapeutic child care) that are increasingly scarce (Peterson, Washington, & Rathbun, 1984). See Chapter 6 for a review of psychosocial interventions for children with poor growth.

NUTRITIONAL REQUIREMENTS

The previous section describes the GI tract as an assembly line or factory. This section looks at the raw materials for the factory, that is, the nutrients contained in the diet. Once absorbed into the bloodstream, these nutrients allow the body to grow, to exert itself, and to repair itself—processes that are collectively referred to as *metabolism*. What are these nutrients? How much of each is needed? How do these needs change with age, activity, and illness?

Nutrients can be grouped into four general categories: substances with caloric value, water, vitamins, and minerals. In addition to these four, the diet includes fiber that facilitates digestion despite having no intrinsic nutritional value.

Calories

Calories, simply stated, are units of energy. They can be used to fuel metabolism, much as a furnace burns fuel to heat a building, or to build up body tissue. Carbohydrates, protein, and fat all provide calories. Calories from these three sources are largely interchangeable, but each type of calorie source is required by the body. Ongoing caloric deficiency leads to weight loss, immune dysfunction, and developmental delay in children (Frank & Zeisel, 1988). Specific metabolic problems can arise from relative deficiency of any one source of calories.

The digestive system breaks down large carbohydrates, proteins, and fat into simple sugars, amino acids, and lipids, respectively. These components then are transported to tissue cells that either break them down further to release energy or use them to build new tissue. The body can manufacture most forms of sugars, amino acids, and lipids; those that cannot be made within the body must be consumed in the diet and are termed "essential."

Individuals need a balance among the various sources of calories for optimal health. As a general rule, younger children need more calories per unit of body weight than older children and adults because children have higher metabolic rates. Puberty is also a time of increased caloric need.

Carbohydrates, including sugars and starches, are built up of rings containing atoms of carbon, hydrogen, and oxygen. Carbohydrates provide a ready source of energy. In most developed countries, carbohydrates account for about 45% of caloric intake; in less-developed countries the percentage is higher, up to 90%. At a minimum, about 20% of calories must come from carbohydrates to prevent muscles and other tissues from being broken down for energy.

Proteins, the building blocks for most body tissues, are made of chains of amino acids. Of the 22 important amino acids, 8 are "essential" (as described previously). If even one essential amino acid is lacking, protein synthesis goes awry. Although both plants and animals provide protein, animal proteins contain more essential amino acids than do proteins derived from plants. It is difficult for strict vegan diets without any meat or dairy products to provide the needed variety of amino acids, although it is not impossible.

Lipids from vegetable and animal oils are critical for the functioning of many organs, particularly the nervous system. On a gram-for-gram basis, fats provide approximately two times as many calories as do carbohydrates or proteins. Calories from *any* source that are not needed immediately for fuel or for growth are stored in the body as fat. Excessive intake of fat can lead to heart and vascular disease in adult life, as well as obesity.

According to the American Academy of Pediatrics (1992), no more than 30% of daily calories should come from fats. Overzealous attempts to reduce dietary fat, however, can lead to impaired brain growth, particularly in infants under the age of 1 year.

Average requirements for calories and protein, according to age, appear in Table 2.1. The next section describes increased calorie and protein requirements in various illnesses.

Water

An adult's body is approximately 60% water by weight; a premature infant's is 80%. Of all the nutrients, water is the most critical to survival because of its role in many, diverse life-sustaining processes.

Table 2.1. Caloric requirements and growth

Age	Average caloric requirements (kcal/kg/day)[a]	Average protein requirements (grams/kg/day)[a]	Median daily weight gain (grams)	Median height gain (cm/month)
Birth to 3 months	108	2.2	24–30	3.4
3–6 months	108	2.2	20	2.2
6–9 months	98	1.6	14–15	1.5
9–12 months	98	1.6	11	1.3
1–3 years	102	1.2	6	.9
3–6 years	90	1.1	5	.5
6–10 years	70	1.0	7–8[b]	.5

Source: Frank et al. (1983).

[a] *Source:* Food and Nutrition Board, National Research Council (1989).

[b] Data elevated by inclusion of pubertal growth spurts in some children.

Water balance is primarily regulated by the kidneys and the digestive system.

The body's need for water is driven by metabolism, by loss through evaporation by the lungs and skin, and by excretion from the kidneys in the form of urine. A small amount of water is lost in the feces. With protracted or severe diarrhea or vomiting, or with decreased fluid intake, the loss of water can lead to dehydration—a potentially serious medical problem. Excessive water intake, common in infants fed overly diluted formula, can lead to brain swelling and seizures.

All beverages, such as juices and milk, contain water. In addition, many foods contain significant amounts of water, particularly fruits and vegetables. The staple diet of infants and toddlers contains a large amount of water, which is needed to maintain their higher metabolism and higher body water content.

Vitamins

Vitamins have no caloric value but are required by the body for a variety of metabolic processes. Vitamins must be taken in through the diet because the body cannot manufacture them. The fat-soluble vitamins—A, D, E, and K—can be stored in body fat if consumed in excess quantities. Water-soluble vitamins are the vitamin-B complexes (i.e., thiamine, riboflavin, niacin, folic acid, B_6, B_{12}, biotin) and vitamin C. Excessive amounts of the water-soluble vitamins are generally excreted in the urine. Children with ongoing malabsorption, as in cystic fibrosis or short-gut syndrome, may have difficulty absorbing vitamins and require large daily intakes. For most children, however, taking "megavitamin" supplements offers no known benefit. Vitamins from fresh vegetables have not been shown to be better than vitamins from a jar; although fresh vegetables also provide beneficial fiber. For children who find vegetables unpalatable, a daily multiple vitamin tablet can reduce tense struggles over food intake.

Minerals

Important minerals are calcium for the bones and teeth and iron and copper for the blood. Iodine is needed by the thyroid, which functions as a metabolic "thermostat." Zinc, chromium, and selenium are utilized in metabolic processes.

Other minerals also are found in the human body, some with known and others with unknown functions. Lead, for example, has no known benefit and is detrimental to children (Weitzman & Glotzer, 1992). Fluoride, although not absolutely required, helps prevent dental caries, particularly in young children (Latham, McGandy, McCann, & Stare, 1975).

NONGASTROINTESTINAL EFFECTS ON GROWTH

When a well-functioning GI tract delivers a healthy balance of nutrients to the bloodstream, the stage is set for growth. The true drama of growth, however, plays out on a million microscopic stages throughout the body as each cell burns or stores energy, synthesizes or breaks down complex molecules, dies off, or reproduces itself. For normal growth to occur, these processes all must operate in balance with each other. Just as the GI assembly line relies on an exquisite control system, so too are the nongastrointestinal aspects of growth controlled by an intricate network of neurological, hormonal, and physical signals. This section gives an overview of these regulatory factors and of other factors that can impair growth despite a healthy GI tract.

Hormonal Regulation

Nutrients are delivered to the bloodstream in bursts, interspersed with periods of time during which little or nothing is delivered. Despite this variation, the blood levels of various nutrients are relatively constant. The control of blood sugar (glucose) provides a good example. The rise in blood sugar after a meal triggers the release of insulin, a hormone that signals cells to take up and store sugar. As glucose levels fall, other hormones are released into the bloodstream causing cells to release sugar, which strikes a balance. A failure of insulin production or a failure of body cells to respond to the hormone causes diabetes: The blood sugar level rises even as cells are starving for the glucose that they cannot take up. The excess sugar (and vital calories) are wasted in the urine, and the child loses weight (Villee, Najjar, & Crigler, 1994).

Other hormones that affect growth include growth hormone, thyroid hormone, glucocorticoids secreted by the adrenal glands, and the hormones that control sexual development. Growth hormone has direct effects on the uptake and utilization of amino acids and glucose by growing tissues, as well as indirect effects mediated by substances called *somatomedins*. Measurement of growth hormone is difficult because it is secreted from the pituitary gland in a pulsating fashion. Endocrinologists use special techniques to stimulate secretion. The availability of potentially unlimited supplies of growth hormone, produced by genetic engineering, has raised practical and ethical questions about its use in children who are short in stature but may not be actually deficient in the hormone (Villee et al., 1994).

Thyroid hormone plays an important role in regulating the metabolic activity of the body—controlling how quickly cells burn glucose and other fuels. Classical symptoms of excessive thyroid hormone include heat intolerance, overactivity, inattention, heart palpitations, and weight loss. Symptoms are commonly more subtle and easily missed, however, and children may be mildly hyperthyroid for long periods of time before the diagnosis is suspected (Sills, 1994).

Glucocorticoids produced by the adrenal glands are hormones that play a role in the body's response to physiological stressors. Failure of the adrenal glands to produce sufficient glucocorticoids results in a serious, occasionally life-threatening condition called Addison disease. Pharmacological doses of glucocorticoids often are prescribed to combat inflammation in conditions such as severe asthma or arthritis. One side effect is that the body tends to shut off its own production of the hormone. If the medication is stopped too rapidly, then a critical insufficiency can result.

Cardiac and Respiratory Systems

The heart and the muscles of respiration influence growth in two ways: first, because their constant activity is necessary to supply the rest of the body with fuel and the oxygen to burn it and, second, because they have the potential to consume an inordinate amount of energy. These influences become apparent only when the systems malfunction.

A failure of fuel delivery, for example, occurs in certain forms of congenital heart disease in which poorly oxygenated blood returning from the body mixes with blood that has just passed through the lungs. As a result, the oxygen content of blood going to the body is low (hypoxia), giving the child a bluish (cyanotic) cast. Children with uncorrected cyanotic heart disease grow poorly. A similar effect occurs when lung function is so poor that the blood is never adequately oxygenated (Freed & Fyler, 1994).

Excessive fuel consumption occurs in a different class of congenital heart disease. In these cases, a percentage of the well-oxygenated blood may be diverted so that it passes back through the lungs a second time rather than flowing out to the body; for example, if 50% of the blood were "short-circuited" through the lungs, then the heart would have to pump twice as much volume to maintain the same net blood flow to the body. Children with this relatively common class of heart condition may require one and a half to two times the usual number of calories to sustain growth. Similarly, children with severe lung disease expend excess effort to move air in and out, and they may burn far more calories than children who can breathe easily. Bronchopulmonary dysplasia, a long-term complication of lung disease in very premature infants, can lead to growth failure because of excessive work of breathing as well as because of chronic hypoxia. Children with airway obstruction due to adenoid hypertrophy also may expend excessive calories in breathing and therefore grow poorly (Schiffman, Faber, & Eidelman, 1985).

Kidney and Liver Functions

As with the heart and the lungs, the effects of kidneys and liver on growth are apparent chiefly when the organs malfunction. Metabolic waste products normally excreted by these organs can lead to generally poor health and stunted growth. Although complete failure of either organ leads to rapid, severe illness, partial dysfunction can be insidious. The cause of the organ dysfunction may be an apparently mild infection, or it may not be apparent at all. Because of their crucial function, both systems have a great deal of excess capacity so that kidney or liver insufficiency generally does not become apparent until much greater than 50% of the organ is lost. This excess capacity allows kidney donors to sacrifice an entire kidney without any clinically noticeable loss of kidney function.

Prenatal Influences

Genetic endowment obviously affects growth potential. Children with chromosomal abnormalities are frequently—but not universally—short and have intellectual impairments. For example, children with Down syndrome (trisomy 21) or Turner syndrome are usually short; however, a few chromosomal abnormalities predispose to typical or tall stature (e.g., Klinefelter syndrome). Children with achondroplasia, or short-limbed dwarfism, have typical intelligence, as do children with Marfan syndrome, who tend to be tall and thin. In many genetic disorders, the number of chromosomes is normal, but one or more gene is defective.

A great number of nongenetic prenatal influences have an impact on growth. Common substances of abuse, including alcohol, cigarettes, marijuana, and cocaine, all are associated with impaired intrauterine growth. Other causes include prescription drugs, such as some anticonvulsants, and maternal infections, including Rubella, chickenpox, and cytomegalovirus among others. The degree to which such factors will affect any particular child is unpredictable. For example, only a small fraction of children whose mothers drink alcohol during pregnancy develop full-blown fetal alcohol syndrome (FAS), and some children born to heavy drinkers appear entirely unaffected (Jones, 1986).

Children who are born underweight for any reason are at greatly increased risk of *postnatal* growth failure. When growth failure occurs early in pregnancy, the typical result is low birth weight, length, and head circumference; the infant is a "perfect miniature." In contrast, when growth failure begins in the third trimester, the head size tends to be large relative to a smaller body. Infants with this "asymmetric" growth pattern have a better prognosis for normal growth and development than do infants with more pervasive or "symmetric" undergrowth (Frank, Silva, & Needlman, 1993).

Postnatal Infections

Ongoing or recurrent infections of any sort can lead to growth failure, as the immune system consumes large amounts of energy to fight infections. Food intake usually drops during an acute illness and increases above typical afterward. Poor growth is a common feature of acquired immunodeficiency syndrome and other immunocompromised conditions. Chronic undernutrition itself causes immune system dysfunction, contributing to a vicious cycle of infection and malnutrition. In developing countries, this downward spiral often leads to death. In developed countries, the side effects of multiple courses of antibiotics may contribute to poor growth among children with ongoing health conditions (Frank & Zeisel, 1988). The effects of other medications are described in the next section.

ASSESSING GROWTH

Physical well-being is a priority for all children and can be viewed as a function of growth, stamina, and resistance to disease. This section considers common means of assessing growth, including measurement of weight, height, head circumference, and skinfold thickness.

Growth Curves

Parents typically gauge growth by the rate at which clothes and shoes are outgrown; making pencil marks on a doorjamb is another tried and true method. Professionals plot anthropometric measurements on standard growth curves, based on population norms. The most commonly used norms for weight, height, and head circumference for age were derived by the National Center for Health Statistics and published in 1979 (Hamill et al., 1979).

There are separate growth curves for males and females; however, the same growth curves are used for all ethnic groups. Observed differences in average size among ethnic groups have more to do with different patterns of nutritional intake than with genetic potential. A classic study supporting this conclusion looked at the heights of Japanese living in Japan and of Japanese immigrants to the United States (Greulich, 1957). Second-generation immigrants ate a higher-protein diet than their parents and were considerably taller than both their parents and their contemporaries who had not emigrated, despite unchanged genetic make-up. Separate growth curves have been published for premature infants (Babson & Benda, 1976) and for children with Down syndrome (Cronk, Crocker, & Pueschel, 1988).

An example of a graph of standard growth curves for length and weight for girls birth to 36 months is shown in Figure 2.2. The curve is arranged with age plotted on the horizontal axis. The other measures—in this case, length and weight—are plotted on the vertical axis, usually in both metric and English units. Separate percentile curves for length and weight rise from the lower left corner and tend to diverge as they approach the upper right corner. Steep portions of the curves (e.g., from birth to 12 months) represent periods of relatively rapid growth.

As an illustration of how to interpret the percentile lines, consider a 15-month-old girl who is 80 centimeters tall. The intersection of the vertical line corresponding to 15 months and the horizontal line corresponding to 80 centimeters falls on the 75th percentile curve. Compared with girls her age in the standardization sample, this particular girl is taller than 75% of the girls and shorter than 25%.

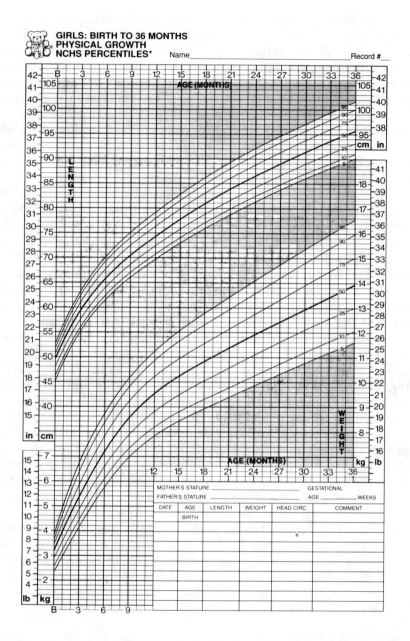

Figure 2.2. Standard growth curves for length and weight for girls birth to 36 months of age. (Adapted from Hamill, P.V.V., Drizd, T.A., Johnson, C.L., Reed, R.B., Roche, A.F., & Moore, W.M. [1979]. Physical growth: National Center for Health Statistics percentiles. *American Journal of Clinical Nutrition, 32,* 607–629; used with permission of Ross Products Division, Abbott Laboratories, Columbus, OH 43216; from NCHS Growth Charts, © 1982 Ross Products Division, Abbott Laboratories.)

The 50th percentile line represents the median measurement for each age (i.e., the weight or height at which half of the children fall below and half fall above). Depending on the edition of the charts, the lowest curve demarcates either the 3rd or the 5th percentile. By convention, this represents the lowest limits of "normal," although, of course, 3% or 5% of the children in the normative sample fell below this bottom curve. Statistically, as children fall farther below or above the limits of "normal," the likelihood increases that their size represents a pathological medical condition, rather than simply normal variation. Similar curves allow one to plot a child's head circumference.

In addition to the graphs of height, weight, and head circumference as a function of age, a fourth standard growth curve compares height on the x-axis against weight on the y-axis. An example of a graph of weight for height, for prepubescent boys, is shown in Figure 2.3. This weight-for-height curve indicates how heavy the child is compared with other children of the same height. The percentile curves are derived and interpreted in the same way as the other three growth curves. Weight-for-height provides a more accurate index of the degree of fatness, or adiposity, than does weight alone.

Percentiles should not be confused with percentages. When a child's weight falls outside the normal range, the percentile no longer conveys adequate information: A 12-month-old boy weighing 8 kilograms and a 12-month-old boy weighing 5 kilograms are both below the 5th percentile, but one is considerably more underweight than the other. In such cases, the weight is best expressed as a percentage of the median or "ideal" weight for age. At 12 months of age, the median weight for boys is 10 kilograms; thus, the first child is 80% of ideal weight (8 kilograms/10 kilograms), whereas the second is 50% (5 kilograms/10 kilograms) of ideal weight. Children with weights below 90% of ideal are classified as mildly (first degree) wasted; those with weights below 75% as moderately (second degree) wasted, and those with weights below 60% as severely (third degree) wasted (see Table 2.2). Percentages (rather than percentiles) for height-for-age and weight-for-height can be calculated in an analogous manner and compared with a standard grading system (see Table 2.2). These percentages provide a precise index of the degree of malnutrition and resultant growth impairment.

Patterns of Growth

A single point on a growth curve provides information about the child's size only in relation to a normative sample of children of the same age. Repeated measurements plotted over time allow the pe-

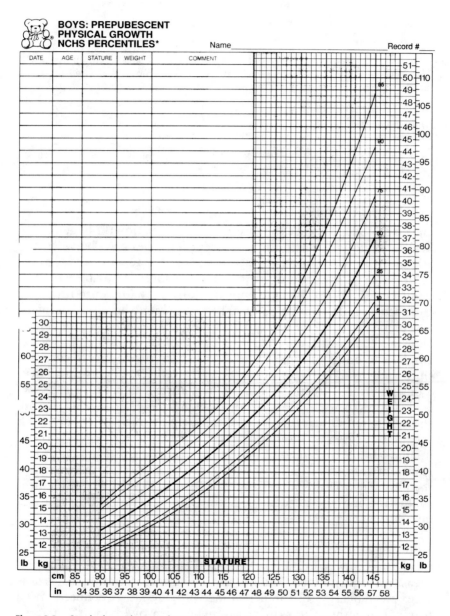

Figure 2.3. Standard growth curves for prepubescent boys. (Adapted from Hamill, P.V.V., Drizd, T.A., Johnson, C.L., Reed, R.B., Roche, A.F., & Moore, W.M. [1979]. Physical growth: National Center for Health Statistics percentiles. *American Journal of Clinical Nutrition, 32,* 607–629; used with permission of Ross Products Division, Abbott Laboratories, Columbus, OH 43216; from NCHS Growth Charts, © 1982 Ross Products Division, Abbott Laboratories.)

Table 2.2. Severity of malnutrition: Stunting and wasting

	Percent of median for age		
Grade of malnutrition	Weight for age (wasting)	Height for age (stunting)	Weight for height (wasting)
0	> 90	> 95	> 90
1 mild	75–90	90–95	81–90
2 moderate	60–74	85–89	70–80
3 severe	< 60	< 85	< 70

From Frank, D.A., Silva, M., & Needlman, R. (1993). Failure to thrive: Mystery, myth, and methods. *Contemporary Pediatrics, 10,* 114–133; reprinted by permission.

diatric provider to track the rate and pattern of growth. In general, a healthy child will settle into a percentile range—say, between the 5th and 10th percentiles—by age 2 years and stay within that range until puberty. Short-term, minor fluctuations are to be expected (Smith et al., 1976). Weight typically falls off with acute illnesses, and recovers afterward. Major shifts, in which the child's growth trajectory crosses 2 or more percentile groups, either up or down, alert the health care provider to possible medical problems. For example, the onset of hyperthyroidism might result in a downward shift of the weight curve, from the 75th to the 25th percentile over 3 or 4 months. Percentile shifts do not always signal disease, however. Children with constitutional growth delay, for example, are shorter than their contemporaries throughout grade school and high school, but catch up later and achieve typical adult height. Early in infancy and at the onset of puberty, percentile shifts are common. Apparent shifts may be caused by normal variation in the timing of the pubertal growth spurt (Tanner & Davies, 1985). Careful medical evaluation may be needed to distinguish between pathologic and normative short stature.

Other Measures

In addition to weight, height, and head circumference, several other measures and derived indices can be useful. Skinfold thickness gives an indication of the percentage of body fat. A caliper is used to pinch together the skin of the upper arm overlying the triceps muscle—a painless procedure that looks far worse than it feels! Normal values have been published (Frisancho, 1981). Derived indices include weight age, height age, and body mass index (Hammer, Kraemer, Wilson, Ritter, & Dornbusch, 1991). Definitions and uses of these indices are presented in Table 2.3.

Table 2.3. Definitions of common indices of growth

Index	Definition	Interpretation
Weight age	Age at which child's weight would be the median	Rough index of degree of wasting
Height age	Age at which child's height would be the median	Rough index of degree of stunting or short stature
Body mass index (BMI)	Weight/height^2 when weight is in kilograms and height in meters	Rough measure of obesity[a]

From Needlman, R. (1995). Assessment of growth. In R. Behrman & R. Kliegman (Eds.), *Nelson's textbook of pediatrics* (15th ed., pp. 63–67). Philadelphia: Saunders; reprinted by permission.

[a] Standards for BMI have been developed for Caucasian children, ages 1–19, based on the 1971–1974 National Health and Nutrition Examination Survey (NHANES). The BMI has a normal nadir between 4 and 8 years. Children whose BMI begins to rise before 5½ years may be at increased risk for adult obesity.

For infants and hospitalized children who are weighed relatively frequently, simple inspection of the growth curves may not be sensitive enough to reveal important variations in growth rate. In these cases, it is often helpful to calculate the average daily weight gain in grams. Median values for grams-per-day are listed in Table 2.1. The use of a chart that juxtaposes growth in grams-per-day with changes in medications, feeding regime, and events in the family or social environment can be of great value in identifying causes of inadequate growth.

EFFECTS OF MEDICATION ON THE GI SYSTEM AND NUTRITION

Medications can have an impact on the GI system and nutrition in several different ways. Some medications suppress the appetite (anorexia), others increase it. Others cause dysfunction of the digestive process with nausea (the urge to vomit), abdominal discomfort, vomiting, or diarrhea. These adverse GI effects can lead to loss of appetite. Nausea and vomiting may result from direct interactions between medications and specific areas in the brain. Medications occasionally will alter vitamin or mineral status; as a result, dietary supplements may be prescribed along with certain medications for some individuals.

The following section describes the benefits of many frequently prescribed medications and their common effects on the GI system and their interactions with nutrition. The medications are identified in the text and tables by their generic names; trade names also are provided in the text in parentheses. The *Handbook on Drug and Nutrient Interactions* (Roe, 1989) is the source for all drug information reported in this section.

The paragraphs and companion tables that follow are for general information only. The text and tables do not include all reported side effects (GI or other) and are not intended to substitute for medical advice. Readers with questions should consult with a health care provider.

Antibiotics

Antibiotics (see Table 2.4) are used to treat infections in different parts of the body, such as otitis media (middle-ear infection), cellulitis (deep skin infection), and pneumonia (lung infection).

Amoxicillin (e.g., Amoxil), an antibiotic used frequently in children, can cause diarrhea. This is particularly true for the amoxicillin-clavulanate combination (e.g., Augmentin). Infrequently, amoxicillin will lead to nausea or upset stomach. Erythromycin (e.g., EryPed, Ilotycin) often causes upset stomach, which may lead to vomiting; less often it can cause nausea and diarrhea. Amoxicillin and erythromycin do not usually depress appetite directly.

Sulfisoxazole (e.g., Gantrisin) is often used to treat urine infections and to prevent ear infections. It can cause nausea and, less commonly, other GI symptoms such as diarrhea or cramping.

The combination of trimethoprim-sulfamethoxazole (e.g., Bactrim, Septra) is used for ear infections and urine infections. It can cause nausea or upset stomach. Anorexia is less common.

Table 2.4. Antibiotics and their interactions with the GI system and nutrition

Antibiotic	Anorexia (loss of appetite)	Nausea	GI discomfort (vomiting)	Diarrhea
Amoxicillin	–	+	+	++
Erythromycin	–	+	++	+
Sulfisoxazole	+/–	++	+	+
Trimethoprim-sulfamethoxazole	+/–	+	+	+

Note: The data in this table are for general information only. They do not include all reported side effects (GI or other) and are not intended to substitute for medical advice. Readers with questions should consult with a health care provider.

Key: –, rarely reported side effect; +/–, occasionally reported side effect; +, commonly reported side effect; and ++, very commonly reported side effect.

Medications for the Gastrointestinal System

Most medications developed to treat disorders of the GI system understandably can have adverse effects on the GI system itself (see Table 2.5). The most frequent problem is alteration of vitamin status due to decreased absorption. Mineral oil, a nondigestible oil used to lubricate the colon to relieve constipation, can reduce absorption of fat-soluble vitamins, and it causes diarrhea if taken in excess. Glycopyrrolate (Robinul), which works to reduce stomach acidity, does not alter vitamin absorption but has been reported to cause nausea and vomiting.

Cimetidine (Tagamet) and ranitidine (Zantac) both control symptoms from ulcers and GER (see the section entitled The Esophagus) by reducing stomach acidity. Cimetidine sometimes causes diarrhea; ranitidine is more likely to cause nausea and stomach discomfort.

Dietary Supplements

Dietary supplements (see Table 2.6) are preparations of vitamins, minerals, and/or electrolytes (salts) taken when the diet is believed to be inadequate. Nearly all supplements can cause upset stomach or nausea.

Table 2.5.   GI medications and their interactions with the GI system and nutrition

Medication	Anorexia (loss of appetite)	Nausea	GI discomfort (vomiting)	Diarrhea	Other
Cimetidine	–	–	–	+/–	Altered vitamin status
Glycopyrrolate	–	+	+	–	
Mineral oil	–	–	–	+/–	Altered vitamin status
Ranitidine	–	+	+	–	Altered vitamin status

Note: The data in this table are for general information only. They do not include all reported side effects (GI or other) and are not intended to substitute for medical advice. Readers with questions should consult with a health care provider.

Key: –, rarely reported side effect; +/–, occasionally reported side effect; +, commonly reported side effect; ++, very commonly reported side effect.

Table 2.6. Dietary supplements and their interactions with the GI system and nutrition

Dietary supplement	Anorexia (loss of appetite)	Nausea	GI discomfort (vomiting)	Diarrhea	Other
Fluoride	−	−	−	−	
Iron (ferrous salt)	−	+	++	+	Constipation
Multivitamins	−	+	++	+	
Potassium chloride	−	+	+	+	

Note: The data in this table are for general information only. They do not include all reported side effects (GI or other) and are not intended to substitute for medical advice. Readers with questions should consult with a health care provider.

Key: −, rarely reported side effect; +/−, occasionally reported side effect; +, commonly reported side effect; ++, very commonly reported side effect.

Iron supplements (ferrous salts) (e.g., Fer-in-sol, Feosol), prescribed for prevention or treatment of some causes of anemia, may cause diarrhea or constipation. Multivitamins may cause diarrhea. Fluoride (e.g., Luride, Pediafluor), a prescription supplement used in communities with inadequate fluoridation of the drinking water, generally does not have GI side effects.

Potassium salts are prescribed for individuals taking certain medications that deplete the body's potassium supply or that make the body hypersensitive to potassium deficiency. Potassium chloride can cause diarrhea. Brand name potassium preparations often have the letter "K" in their names (e.g., K-Tab, Micro-K).

Cardiac and Blood Pressure Medications

Medications to treat heart conditions and elevated blood pressure commonly have GI side effects (see Table 2.7). Digoxin (e.g., Lanoxin) is used to increase the strength of the heart and stabilize the cardiac rhythm. GI effects include anorexia, nausea, upset stomach, vomiting, and diarrhea. Although digoxin does not cause electrolyte imbalance, it increases the body's sensitivity to electrolyte problems, requiring the use of potassium supplements.

Chlorothiazide (e.g., Diuril), furosemide (e.g., Lasix), and spironolactone (e.g., Aldactone) are prescribed to reduce blood pressure and reduce swelling of the body due to fluid buildup (edema). These medications work on the kidneys to increase water excretion and can alter electrolyte balance, necessitating potassium supplementation; and all are known to cause loss of appetite, nausea, gastric discomfort, vomiting, or diarrhea.

Table 2.7. Cardiac and blood pressure medications and their interactions with the GI system and nutrition

Medication	Anorexia (loss of appetite)	Nausea	GI discomfort (vomiting)	Diarrhea	Other
Digoxin	+	+	+	+	
Chlorothiazide	+	+	+	+	Electro-lyte imbal-ance
Furosemide	+	+	+	+	Electro-lyte imbal-ance
Spironolactone	+	+	+	+	Electro-lyte imbal-ance

Note: The data in this table are for general information only. They do not include all reported side effects (GI or other) and are not intended to substitute for medical advice. Readers with questions should consult with a health care provider.

Key: −, rarely reported side effect; +/−, occasionally reported side effect; +, commonly reported side effect; ++, very commonly reported side effect.

Respiratory Medications

Side effects of medications for pulmonary conditions frequently include GI upset (see Table 2.8). Wheezing is a common respiratory symptom usually caused by asthma. In addition to asthma, chronic lung damage due to prematurity (bronchopulmonary dysplasia) also can cause bronchospasm.

One of the mainstays of management of bronchospasm is albuterol (e.g., Proventil, Ventolin), which is taken orally or delivered by nebulizer or inhaler. Albuterol can cause loss of appetite, nausea, upset stomach, or vomiting.

Steroids reduce inflammation of the lungs related to bronchospasm. Prednisone (usually prescribed by its generic name), an oral steroid used extensively for both respiratory and nonrespiratory conditions, can cause nausea or vomiting. It also can cause increased appetite and weight gain. Beclamethasone, a related steroid administered by inhaler (e.g., Beclovent, Vancenase), also can cause nausea but rarely causes increased appetite or obesity.

Cromolyn (e.g., Intal) is delivered by inhaler or nebulizer and is used to prevent bronchospasm. Cromolyn is well known for causing nausea and also may cause vomiting or diarrhea.

Table 2.8. Respiratory medications and their interactions with the GI system and nutrition

Medication	Anorexia (loss of appetite)	Nausea	GI discomfort (vomiting)	Diarrhea	Other
Albuterol inhaler, nebulizer, oral	+	+	+	−	
Beclomethasone inhaler	−	+	−	−	
Cromolyn inhaler	−	++	+	+	
Prednisone[a]	−	+	+	−	Weight gain

Note: The data in this table are for general information only. They do not include all reported side effects (GI or other) and are not intended to substitute for medical advice. Readers with questions should consult with a health care provider.

[a] Effective treatment for other systems as well as respiratory.

Key: −, rarely reported side effect; +/−, occasionally reported side effect; +, commonly reported side effect; ++, very commonly reported side effect.

Antiseizure Medications

The antiseizure medications (see Table 2.9) have made significant contributions to the well-being of individuals with recurrent seizures (i.e., epilepsy). Ethosuximide (e.g., Zarontin), often the treatment of choice for petit mal (absence) seizures, can cause loss of appetite, nausea, vomiting, gastric discomfort, or diarrhea; other seizure medications have similar side effects. Carbamazepine (e.g., Tegretol) can cause altered taste, loss of appetite, nausea, vomiting, gastric discomfort, or diarrhea. Phenytoin (e.g., Dilantin) may alter an individual's vitamin status, reduce appetite, or cause nausea or gastric discomfort. Valproic acid (e.g., Depakene, Depakote) can cause deficiency of the vitamin carnitine, appetite loss, nausea, vomiting, or gastric discomfort. Phenobarbital (no brand name) is not reported to have frequent adverse effects on the digestive system.

Psychoactive Medications

Psychopharmacology is an increasingly important component of treatment for children and adolescents with emotional and behavior problems (Green, 1991). The side effects of psychoactive medications (see Table 2.10) commonly include changes in appetite and GI function. Psychoactive medications include several classes of medications that work on different symptoms; all are intended to normalize extreme forms of behavior, thinking, and emotions caused

Table 2.9. Antiseizure medications and their interactions with the GI system and nutrition

Medication	Anorexia (loss of appetite)	Nausea	GI discomfort (vomiting)	Diarrhea	Other
Carbamazepine	+	+	+	+	Altered taste
Ethosuximide	+	+	+	+	
Phenobarbital	−	−	−	−	
Phenytoin	+	+	+	−	Altered vitamin status
Valproic acid	+	+	+	−	Carnitine deficiency

Note: The data in this table are for general information only. They do not include all reported side effects (GI or other) and are not intended to substitute for medical advice. Readers with questions should consult with a health care provider.

Key: −, rarely reported side effect; +/−, occasionally reported side effect; +, commonly reported side effect; ++, very commonly reported side effect.

by basic biochemistry, detrimental experience, or complications of medical conditions.

The tricyclic antidepressants include imipramine (e.g., Tofranil), desipramine (e.g., Norpramin), nortriptyline (e.g., Pamelor), and amitriptyline (e.g., Elavil). "Tricyclic" refers to the antidepressants' characteristic three-ring molecular structure. In addition to their primary role treating depression, they also help in some cases of bedwetting, attention-deficit/hyperactivity disorder (ADHD), and chronic pain syndromes. These medications can cause nausea and stomach discomfort and occasionally will result in loss of appetite and diarrhea; liver function tests of the blood are obtained periodically to monitor for possible liver effects.

Stimulant medications have been shown to improve attention and concentration while reducing impulsivity and hyperactivity. They are used extensively in children and adolescents to treat ADHD; in adults, their most common application is as appetite suppressants in "diet pills." The most popular stimulants are methylphenidate (e.g., Ritalin), dextroamphetamine (e.g., Dexedrine), and pemoline (e.g., Cylert). They may cause a reduction in appetite for several hours following a dose; less often they cause nausea or stomach discomfort or, rarely, diarrhea. Reports of liver failure associated with pemoline have limited the usefulness of this medication.

Table 2.10. Psychoactive medications and their interactions with the GI system and nutrition

Medication	Anorexia (loss of appetite)	Nausea	GI discomfort (vomiting)	Diarrhea	Other
Antidepressants (tricyclic)	+/−	+	+	+/−	Liver effect
Antihistamines[a]	+/−	+/−	+/−	+/−	
Clonidine[a]	+/−	+	+	−	Increased appetite, dry mouth
Neuroleptics	−	−	+	−	Increased appetite, dry mouth
Stimulants	++	+	+	+/−	

Note: The data in this table are for general information only. They do not include all reported side effects (GI or other) and are not intended to substitute for medical advice. Readers with questions should consult with a health care provider.

[a] Effective treatment for other systems as well as psychoactive.

Key: −, rarely reported side effect; +/−, occasionally reported side effect; +, commonly reported side effect; ++, very commonly reported side effect.

Clonidine (Catapres) was first developed to reduce high blood pressure. Experience revealed that clonidine can be calming for agitated or anxious individuals. Clonidine can cause increased appetite or dry mouth, and less often, reduced appetite, stomach discomfort, or diarrhea.

The antihistamines, usually prescribed for allergic symptoms, are sometimes used for their mildly calming effect on agitated or anxious individuals. They are generally well tolerated by the GI tract; infrequently they will lead to loss of appetite, nausea, stomach discomfort, or diarrhea. Common examples are diphenhydramine (e.g., Benadryl, Benalyn) and hydroxyzine (e.g., Atarax, Vistaril).

Cyproheptadine (e.g., Periactin) is an antihistamine that may, as a desired side effect, stimulate the appetite, or more accurately, inhibit the sensation of satiety. Several published studies have documented a beneficial effect of cyproheptadine on growth in children who have ongoing health conditions (Kibel, 1969; Sanzgiri, Mohamad, & Raja, 1970; Silverstone & Schuyler, 1975); however, the medication is neither universally accepted for this use nor uniformly helpful.

Neuroleptic medications sometimes are referred to as major tranquilizers or antipsychotics because they are used to treat aggression and psychosis. This group of medications includes thioridazine (e.g., Mellaril) and haloperidol (e.g., Haldol). Increased appetite and related weight gain, as well as dry mouth, are the most frequent GI-related complaints. Neuroleptics occasionally cause GI discomfort.

Given the frequency with which commonly prescribed medications cause GI problems, a high level of suspicion is indicated whenever a child taking any medication shows signs of poor feeding or growth.

DIAGNOSTIC WORKUP OF FEEDING PROBLEMS AND GROWTH FAILURE

The medical diagnostic workup for feeding problems and growth failure always begins with a careful history and physical exam (Casey, 1992; Kempe, Silver, Obrein, & Fulginit, 1991). These, in turn, determine what, if any, laboratory testing may be needed. This section describes each of these three components—history, physical examination, and laboratory tests—and how they are integrated in the medical assessment of specific conditions associated with feeding problems and growth failure.

History

"Growth failure" brings to the pediatrician's mind a long list of possible causes and a host of factors that might interact to either exacerbate or lessen the problem. Virtually any serious medical, social, or psychological illness can lead to poor growth. For example, if a newborn returns to the doctor for a 2-week checkup with failure to gain weight, then the physician begins by asking questions that test a theory—perhaps that the poor weight gain is due to inadequate intake. The answers to the questions either support the theory or point toward an alternative hypothesis.

In addition to theory testing, the history provides a systematic database about the child and the family. A complete history includes 1) a history of the present illness, 2) a past medical history, 3) a review of systems, 4) a family medical history, 5) a social history, and 6) a developmental history. Each of these parts is described in the next sections.

History of the Present Illness   The history of the present illness includes questions about the onset of the feeding difficulty;

accompanying symptoms such as vomiting, diarrhea, and appetite; previous evaluations; and any interventions that were tried. On occasion, growth failure is first identified by the pediatrician; often, however, the parents have been concerned for some time and have tried various methods to get the child to eat. The child frequently arrives at the physician's office with a long list of failed interventions, including interventions devised by the parents, interventions recommended by friends or relatives, and interventions recommended by other professionals. Parents may be—secretly or openly—convinced that "nothing will work." The assessment of parental beliefs, motivation, and morale therefore constitutes an important goal of the history of the present illness.

One of the most revealing parts of the history is the pattern of growth itself. The growth charts reveal whether the child grew normally for a period before beginning to fail or whether there was poor growth from the start. The age of onset of growth problems provides important clues, as summarized in Table 2.11. When growth failure follows caloric deprivation, weight usually slows or stops increasing several weeks before height, and head circumference slows last of all. When height slows first, an endocrinological or other medical cause is more likely (Frank et al., 1993).

Of course, the history must include investigation of the child's diet. Few parents are able to report exactly what their child has eaten over the past weeks or month, but careful questioning sometimes can provide a reliable estimate. Often, this part of the history is taken by a pediatric nutritionist during a separate visit. A

Table 2.11.   Age of onset of growth problems: Diagnostic considerations

Age of onset	Diagnostic considerations
Prenatal (IUGR, prematurity)	"Symmetric" IUGR: prenatal infections, congenital syndromes, teratogenic exposures (associated with oral-motor dysfunction, attachment disorder)
Neonatal	Incorrect formula preparation; failed breast feeding; metabolic, chromosomal, anatomical abnormality; neglect
3–6 months	Inadequate monetary resources; improper formula preparation; milk protein intolerance; oral-motor dysfunction
7–12 months	Autonomy struggles; overly fastidious parent
After 12 months	Acquired illness; new psychosocial stressor (e.g., divorce, job loss, new sibling)

history of low caloric intake, late introduction of solid foods, or food intolerance may suggest a diagnosis and treatment direction.

Past Medical History   The past medical history includes questions about the prenatal course, any significant postnatal illnesses, hospitalizations, operations, allergies to medications, and immunizations. The prenatal history is particularly important because low birth weight is so commonly associated with later feeding and growth problems (Brandt, 1979). Critical, and difficult, questions assess the possibility of exposure to toxins (e.g., alcohol, tobacco, other licit and illicit drugs) or infectious agents (e.g., toxoplasmosis, cytomegalovirus) known to depress intrauterine growth. Other questions focus on the general health of the mother, the length of the pregnancy, labor and delivery, and whether the doctors were ever concerned about the health of the infant. The past medical history also includes the newborn nursery course, any neonatal concerns (e.g., high bilirubin, frequent vomiting), and the early feeding history.

A history of frequent or complicated medical illness (e.g., recurrent ear infections, congenital heart disease, respiratory illness) may suggest a cause for the growth failure. In many cases, however, the situation is more complex. An identified medical problem may result in a feeding problem indirectly, either through inordinately heightened parental concern resulting in overly intrusive feeding or through parental disengagement and understimulation. Parents of children who have ongoing health conditions may be so stressed—emotionally and financially—that they lack the resources necessary to provide adequate feeding. For some children who are seriously ill or for children with major disabilities, the requirements for feeding may be so great as to over-stress even the most competent and committed of parents (Berwick, 1980).

The history of immunizations is important in that it can suggest a pattern of neglect. A lack of immunizations does not, however, establish neglect nor does a completed immunization series rule it out.

Review of Systems   This part of the history—the review of systems—comprises a loosely standardized set of questions intended to detect problems in any body system that may have been overlooked in the preceding parts. The review may lead to associations that might not be obvious to the reporter but are nonetheless important. For instance, a parent may report that a child urinates unusually frequently. The physician might follow up with questions about eating and drinking habits, pain on urination, and bowel habits that then may lead to a diagnosis of urinary tract infection, diabetes, or chronic constipation. Systems reviewed during this part of the history include the central nervous system, the skin, the cardiovascular and respiratory systems, the muscles and joints, and, of course, the GI system. Questions about mouth breathing, snoring, and irregular breathing during sleep are particularly important because a common cause of poor appetite is oversized adenoids with consequent blockage of the airway during eating (Schiffman et al., 1985).

Family History The family medical history is important in identifying disorders such as cystic fibrosis, inflammatory bowel disease, and sickle-cell disease. It also can provide information about the family's experience with illness. The history that "everyone in the family was small as a child" is sometimes advanced by parents to explain a child's growth pattern. In cases in which both parents are short in stature, there is indeed an increased likelihood of the child having "short genes"; it is also possible that multiple generations have been affected by undernutrition, particularly in cases in which poverty is a factor.

Social History Across the globe, the most common cause of deficient growth is simply a lack of access to nutritious food. Even in wealthy, developed nations, hunger is a major factor. Food stamps, temporary assistance for needy families, and other government supports are often unavailable; or if present, they are inadequate (Frank et al., 1993). Food may be available, but high-protein, high-calorie foods such as red meat may be unavailable or available intermittently.

Parents may be reluctant to admit that they cannot provide food for their children. It may be necessary to ask about the presence in the home of certain foods *at the end of the month*, before the next paychecks or assistance checks arrive. A home visit by an experienced social worker or nutritionist may be required to establish a lack of food resources as the cause of growth failure. One study that documented an increase in children in Boston who were underweight during the winter months suggested that parents may be forced to choose between eating and heating (Frank et al., 1993).

The social history also includes the family constellation and an assessment of the family supports and stressors. Growth failure in a child may appear when the balance between social stresses and social supports tilts too far in the direction of stress. Family violence may be associated with growth failure, perhaps because of the severe and ongoing anxiety engendered in children who witness violence. Growth failure associated with physical abuse, although uncommon, carries an inordinately high mortality.

Developmental History The developmental and behavioral history includes questions that examine a child's ability to meet major motor and language milestones. Early neurological insults may result in poor ability to suck, swallow, and self-feed. Such early feeding disabilities then may set up a vicious cycle of tense feeding interactions, parental pressure to eat, resistance on the part of the child, and so forth. By the time the child comes to medical attention because of poor growth, the original oral-motor dysfunction may be discernible only to a specialist (Mathisen et al., 1989).

Another important area of investigation involves the contribution of temperament and goodness of fit in the maternal–child interaction (Chess & Thomas, 1986; Zuckerman & Frank, 1992). On the one hand, children who by temperament respond negatively to new experiences may do well with parents who are temperamentally persistent and "low key." On the other hand, with parents who are easily discouraged or overly assertive, the feeding interaction may quickly deteriorate to one of mutual distaste. Highly distractible children may do well with parents who are energetic and imaginative but do poorly with parents who are easily distracted themselves. In the latter case, the history may reveal meals that last only a few minutes before the parent decides that the child "wasn't hungry."

Developmental delays may be either a cause or a consequence of undernutrition, or both. The first 2 years of life is a time of rapid brain growth and the development of connections among neurons. Caloric deprivation during this period is associated with lasting learning impairments, particularly in the areas of fine motor function and attention (Drotar & Sturm, 1992; Galler & Ramsey, 1989).

Physical Examination

The physical examination provides a systematic assessment of a child's condition, starting with the general appearance of the child. Is the child well-developed and healthy-appearing, or is the child small, thin, and wasted appearing? Is he or she happy and interactive or irritable, fussy, and difficult to console? The general appearance may provide some clue as to what the child brings to the interaction that may have an impact on feeding and growth. For instance, irritable children who are easily overstimulated may have difficulty with feeding because of the amount of stimulation during feeding time. This sort of observation also can be used in intervening with the parents. With easily overstimulated children, for example, it may be possible to demonstrate an improved ability to interact and eat when the television is turned off, the kitchen is cleared of extraneous people, and the adult doing the feeding speaks quietly and slowly.

The child's body as a whole is evaluated for proportionality and minor or major anomalies or malformations that may provide diagnostic hints. Examples include the characteristic facial configuration of FAS, the transverse palmar creases of Down syndrome, and the disproportionately long trunk characteristic in certain skeletal disorders (Rimoin & Horton, 1978).

Each body system is examined. Assessment of the skin and the hair is important as an indication of nutritional status and of general health. Certain rashes and nail and hair changes may signal specific nutritional deficiencies or diseases. The head, eyes, ears, nose, and throat are examined for signs of acute or ongoing health conditions such as ear or sinus infections, dental caries, or gum disease. The lungs and heart are evaluated, as disease in either system may lead to increased caloric demand. The abdominal exam, including a rectal exam, may reveal bloating, tenderness, constipation, or a mass that was overlooked in the history. The genitourinary tract is inspected, as hormonal disorders may alter the appearance of the external genitalia. Abnormalities of the musculoskeletal and neurological systems may point to inherited or acquired metabolic disorders associated with arrested growth or difficulty with feeding.

The physical exam is also a good time to observe the parent–child interaction. Young children, in particular, often find being examined by a stranger stressful. The way in which the parent responds to the child's distress, and the way in which the child uses the parent as a source of comfort provides valuable information about their relationship (Lyons-Ruth & Zeanah, 1993). It is important to remember that neither the history nor the physical is done in isolation. Although the history may point to certain areas for especially close physical assessment, the physical examination may indicate further lines of questioning to be pursued.

Laboratory Tests

The fact that virtually any serious medical condition can lead to growth failure might suggest that the diagnostic battery should include an extensive menu of tests intended to rule out every possible cause. This is not so: In almost every case, a careful history and physical examination suggest the diagnosis, which then may be confirmed by testing. Poorly targeted test batteries ("fishing expeditions") may actually delay the diagnosis while exacting a high cost in pain and laboratory fees (Sills, 1978). A limited number of simple tests are defensible as routine because they can detect relatively common conditions that can result in growth failure without any other clues to their existence. With this caveat, however, the diagnostic workup is dictated by the findings on history and physical exam, and there is no standard laboratory workup of growth failure.

Some of the routine laboratory and radiological tests described in the following paragraphs include blood electrolytes, the complete blood count (CBC), and urinalysis. Further discussion of specific tests can be found in general pediatrics texts (Avery & First, 1994; Wallach, 1978).

Blood Cell Counts   A CBC enumerates each of the three classes of blood cells: red cells, white cells, and platelets. Red blood cells may be deficient in number and/or abnormally small because of iron deficiency. Lead poisoning may result in a similar picture. Both low iron and high lead are common contributors to growth problems, particularly among children from lower-income families (Weitzman & Glotzer, 1992). Ongoing or acute health conditions also may lower red cell production. Abnormally shaped red cells are found in sickle-cell anemia and in other inherited anemias that are associated with stunted growth. Lymphocytes, a subset of white cells, may be depressed in states of malnutrition. In rare cases, extremely high white cells, or very low platelets, point to a diagnosis of malignancy.

Blood Chemistry and Toxicology   A typical chemistry profile includes measurements of the electrolytes (i.e., sodium, potassium, chloride, bicarbonate), glucose, total protein and albumin (a particular protein), substances excreted by the kidney, and substances made and broken down by the liver. Electrolyte balance is important to maintain efficient body functioning at the cellular level; imbalance can be either the cause or the result of illness. Abnormally high glucose (blood sugar) signals possible diabetes (see the section on Hormonal Regulation).

Children with protein–calorie malnutrition may have low levels of blood protein in general and of albumin in particular. Low albumin results in fluid shifts and inefficient functioning at the cellular level. Both the liver and the kidneys remove waste materials from the blood and also produce numerous enzymes, hormones, and other substances. Elevated blood levels of certain "liver enzymes" can signal liver damage. Kidney dysfunction may result in altered levels of blood electrolytes or other chemicals.

Iron deficiency or lead toxicity may be reflected in abnormal red blood cells (see Blood Cell Counts). Blood concentration of both iron and lead also can be measured directly, and there are other tests that may reflect the chronicity or severity of a problem. With the exception of iron, vitamins and minerals are rarely measured directly because of a lack of reliable assays. The best indicator remains the diet history.

Urine Analysis   Analysis of urine can aid in the diagnosis of kidney disease, metabolic disease, and infections. Bladder and kidney infections may be surprisingly difficult to detect, by history or physical exam, in children because symptoms often mimic trivial viral illnesses. Ongoing or recurrent infections sometimes lead to growth failure and may first be detected by urine analysis or culture.

Stool Analyses   Stool analyses may provide evidence of malabsorption, GI tract inflammation, or infection. Significant GI dysfunction rarely exists without at least intermittent abdominal discomfort, bloating, diarrhea, or other unpleasant symptoms. Young children, however, may not localize discomfort or may not be able to communicate the nature of their symptoms clearly. Intestinal parasites occasionally will blunt the appetite without causing other obvious symptoms. Tests that look for evidence of parasites are therefore prudent when there is a history of travel to areas in which disease is endemic (including anywhere in the developing world as well as parts of the western United States), of exposure to immigrants from developing countries, or of living in shelters, in barracks or in other group situations.

Tests of Immunological Function   Growth failure may be the earliest symptom of human immunodeficiency virus (HIV) infection in children. Unless HIV can reliably be excluded by a recent negative test result for the mother, HIV testing is indicated in any infant with unexplained growth failure. More mundane, but no less important, is the Mantoux, or "PPD," test for tuberculosis. This test involves injecting into the skin a small quantity of material made from killed tuberculosis bacteria. A raised lump at the site of injection indicates a past exposure to tuberculosis, and further diagnostic work is needed to rule out active disease. The absence of a response to the test may mean either that the child has not been exposed or that the child's immune system is not able to mount a response to the test material. To exclude the latter possibility, another injection is made with a substance to which most children should respond. A negative (nonreacting) response to this "control" test is evidence of an immunological impairment. One possible cause of such an impairment is ongoing undernutrition.

Radiographic Studies   Commonly encountered radiographic studies include X rays of the chest, abdomen, and bones; studies using radiographic contrast materials; fluoroscopy; nuclear medicine scans; ultrasound; computed tomography (CT); and magnetic resonance imaging (MRI). Radiographic studies are never part of the routine evaluation because they often involve considerable discomfort, expense, and the risk of radiation exposure. When indicated by the history and the physical exam, however, they can prove invaluable.

A chest X ray may show evidence of heart or lung disease as well as abnormalities of bone. Abdominal films may show abnormal accumulations of stool or gas in the intestines or show radiographically opaque materials that have been swallowed, such as paint chips containing lead. X rays of the hands and knees are used to gauge bone maturity, an important factor in assessing short stature (Tanner et al., 1983).

Detailed information about GI tract structure and function is provided by X rays using radiographic contrast materials, that is, materials that appear a characteristic white color on X-ray film. Commonly used contrast materials include a suspension of barium in a clear liquid and a water-soluble material called Gastrografin. Contrast materials are not absorbed into the bloodstream; swallowed from above, they outline the shape of the oral cavity, pharynx, and esophagus, and they reveal any obstruction. The upper GI imaging study (e.g., "barium swallow") is done under fluoroscopy—essentially an X-ray movie—allowing assessment of the muscular coordination of swallowing and the propulsion of the barium down into the stomach. Reflux of contrast material back into the esophagus also is visualized (Riddlesberger, 1988). The contrast can be tracked from the stomach down through the small intestines, called the "small bowel follow-through" study. This study provides information about the rate of stomach emptying and the anatomy of the small intestine. Rare causes of recurrent vomiting, such as obstruction or malpositioning of the small intestine, can be seen with a barium swallow.

Barium, or other contrast material, also is instilled from below as a lower GI imaging study (e.g., "barium enema") to define the anatomy of the rectum and large intestine. Inflammatory changes in the bowel wall, found in ulcerative colitis and Crohn disease, sometimes show up on the barium enema; when there is retained fecal material, the test may not be helpful. Perforation of the intestine, with contamination of the abdominal cavity by contrast materials and feces is a dreaded but, thankfully, rare complication of the test. As a rule, contrast studies are not painful, but they do involve an amount of prodding and positioning, which is upsetting to many young children, and there is often considerable radiation exposure.

The urinary system also is studied radiographically. Water-soluble contrast materials are instilled via catheter to outline the bladder and ureters (e.g., the "voiding cystourethrogram," or VCUG test) or are given intravenously to reveal the anatomy and functioning of the kidney (the "intravenous pyelogram," or IVP test).

In many cases, nuclear medicine studies provide equivalent or greater information with less radiation exposure than with radiographic studies. Nuclear medicine studies involve the injection into the bloodstream or instillation into the bladder of tiny amounts of radioactive chemicals, bound to other chemicals that define specific functions. The child then is placed next to a special "camera" that registers the radioactivity as black dots on film. For example, a radioactive "label" may be bound to a chemical that is taken up selectively by white blood cells actively fighting infection. Areas of infection that might be inapparent on physical examination show up as black smudges on this nuclear medicine scan.

Nuclear medicine scans also are used to assess GI function. In the "milk scan," an infant is given radioactively labeled milk to drink. Any radioactivity later detected within the lung fields is evidence of aspiration of the milk. Another study looks at the time it takes for a meal of radioactively labeled food to pass from the stomach into the small intestine. Prolonged presence of radioactivity in the stomach may be evidence of abnormal stomach function (Riddlesberger, 1988).

Ultrasound, CT, and MRI scans are useful primarily when the clinical examination or blood tests suggest a tumor or degenerative condition of the central nervous system. As the technology improves, more and more conditions will be diagnosable with these tests; their role in the evaluation of feeding disorders, however, remains limited.

Other Tests   In addition to blood tests and radiography, tests that often are helpful in the diagnosis of feeding and growth failure include endoscopy and biopsy, the pH probe, and the sweat chloride test. Endoscopy allows the gastroenterologist to see the working surface of virtually any part of the GI tract. With modern flexible fiber optics, no child is too small to be "scoped." Inflammation and ulcers that might have been subtle or invisible by X-ray are seen plainly. Biopsies can be taken, allowing much more accurate diagnoses. In the diagnosis of giardia infection of the small intestine, for example, the biopsy is able to detect the parasite much more sensitively than the available stool tests.

The pH probe commonly is used to diagnose GER. The test involves having the child swallow a tiny electronic sensor attached to a thin wire that sits within the esophagus, just above the entrance to the stomach. As acidic stomach contents reflux up into the esophagus, the probe registers the changes in pH over a 24-hour period. Prolonged episodes of low pH indicate excessive reflux and make the diagnosis. Despite its conceptual simplicity, the test is technically difficult, requiring precise placement of the probe, careful monitoring of the child's diet and activity, and the cooperation of the child. Few toddlers will tolerate a wire coming out of their nose for a full day without trying to pull it out! Although a positive pH probe establishes the presence of reflux, an endoscopic study often is required to detect whether there is actual inflammation or ulceration of the esophagus (esophagitis) (Orenstein, 1992).

In the sweat chloride test, the sweat glands are stimulated by a small electric current, and the sweat is analyzed for chloride. Elevated chloride concentrations are diagnostic of cystic fibrosis. In experienced hands, the test is highly accurate, with very few false positive results. Inadequate sweat collection occasionally may result in a falsely reassuring result, and the test may need to be repeated.

It is tempting to view the causes of poor feeding and growth as either medical ("organic") or psychosocial ("nonorganic"), and this distinction is well ensconced within the medical literature (Frank et al., 1993). In most instances, however, medical and nonmedical causes coexist; often, they reinforce one another. For example, many children with congenital heart disease require meticulous, intensive feeding. If a family is unable to provide this extraordinary level of intervention, then growth failure may ensue. Because of the interplay between medical and nonmedical factors, the medical assessment must always be viewed within the wider psychosocial context.

SUMMARY

Behavior disorders of feeding originate in the interaction among the biological and the interpersonal, intrapsychic, and social domains. This chapter has reviewed the fundamental biological mechanisms underlying feeding and growth. The GI tract functions like an assembly line, systematically converting food into the building blocks of growth. Each station along the line has defined functions, all tightly coordinated by the parasympathetic nervous system and an intricate system of hormones. Dietary nutrients provide the raw materials that link feeding with growth, activity, and health. In addition, the chapter reviewed medications that commonly affect GI function and feeding and explored medical approaches to the diagnosis of feeding and growth problems.

74 ■ ■ ■ Childhood Feeding Disorders

REFERENCES

American Academy of Pediatrics, Committee on Nutrition. (1992). Statement on cholesterol. *Pediatrics, 90,* 469–473.

Avery, M.E., & First, L.R. (Eds.). (1994). *Pediatric medicine* (2nd ed.). Baltimore: Williams & Wilkins.

Babson, S.G., & Benda, G.I. (1976). Growth graphs for the clinical assessment of infants of varying gestational age. *Journal of Pediatrics, 89*(5), 814–820.

Behrman, R.E., Kliegman, R.M., & Nelson, W.E. (Eds.). (1992). *Nelson textbook of pediatrics.* Philadelphia: W.B. Saunders.

Berwick, D.M. (1980). Nonorganic failure to thrive. *Pediatrics in Review, 1*(9), 265–270.

Berwick, D.M., Levey, J.C., & Kleinerman, R. (1982). Failure to thrive: Diagnostic yield of hospitalization. *Archives of Diseases of Children, 57,* 347–351.

Brandt, L. (1979). Growth dynamics of low birthweight infants with emphasis on the perinatal period. In F. Falkner & J. Tanner (Eds.), *Human growth, neurobiology and nutrition.* New York: Plenum.

Burke, V. (1993). Gut hormones. In M. Gracey & V. Burke (Eds.), *Pediatric gastroenterology and hepatology* (pp. 211–223). Boston: Blackwell Scientific.

Carre, I.J. (1993). Some physiologic mechanisms of the upper gastrointestinal tract. In M. Gracey & V. Burke (Eds.), *Pediatric gastroenterology and hepatology* (pp. 22–23). Boston: Blackwell Scientific.

Casey, P.H. (1992). Failure to thrive. In W.B. Levine, W. Carey, & A.C. Crocker (Eds.), *Developmental-behavioral pediatrics* (pp. 375–383). Philadelphia: W.B. Saunders.

Chess, S., & Thomas, A. (1986). *Temperament in clinical practice.* New York: Guilford Press.

Cronk, C., Crocker, A.C., & Pueschel, S.M. (1988). Growth charts for children with Down syndrome: 1 month to 18 years of age. *Pediatrics, 81,* 102–110.

Davenport, H.W. (1978). *A digest of digestion* (2nd ed.). Chicago: Yearbook Medical Publishers.

Dodge, J.A. (1993). The stomach. In M. Gracey & V. Burke (Eds.), *Pediatric gastroenterology and hepatology* (p. 107). Boston: Blackwell Scientific.

Drotar, D., & Sturm, L. (1992). Personality development, problem solving, and behavior problems among preschool children with early histories of non-organic failure to thrive: A controlled study. *Journal of Developmental and Behavioral Pediatrics, 13,* 266–273.

Eicher, P.S. (1997). Feeding. In M.L. Batshaw (Ed.), *Children with disabilities* (4th ed., pp. 621–642). Baltimore: Paul H. Brookes Publishing Co.

Food and Nutrition Board, National Research Council. (1989). *Recommended daily allowances* (10th ed.). Washington, DC: National Academy Press.

Frank, D.A., Silva, M., & Needlman, R. (1993). Failure to thrive: Mystery, myth, and method. *Contemporary Pediatrics, 10,* 114–133.

Frank, D.A., & Zeisel, S.H. (1988). Failure to thrive. *Pediatric Clinics of North America, 35*(6), 1187–1206.

Freed, M., & Fyler, D.S. (1994). Cardiology. In M.E. Avery & L.R. First (Eds.), *Pediatric medicine* (p. 376). Baltimore: Williams & Wilkins.

Frisancho, A. (1981). New norms of upper limb fat and muscle areas for assessment of nutritional status. *American Journal of Clinical Nutrition, 34*, 2540–2545.

Galler, J.R., & Ramsey, F. (1989). A follow-up study of the influence of early malnutrition on development: Behavior at home and at school. *Journal of the American Academy of Child and Adolescent Psychiatry, 30*(1), 254–261.

Ganong, W.F. (1981). *Review of medical physiology.* Los Altos, CA: Lange Medical Publications.

Ghishan, F. (1988). The transport of electrolytes in the gut and the use of oral rehydration solutions. *Pediatric Clinics of North America, 35*(1), 35–51.

Green, M. (1986). *Pediatric diagnosis* (4th ed.). Philadelphia: W.B. Saunders.

Green, W. (1991). *Child and adolescent clinical psychopharmacology.* Baltimore: Williams & Wilkins.

Greulich, W.W. (1957). A comparison of the physical growth and development of American born and native Japanese children. *American Journal of Physical Anthropology, 14*, 489.

Hamill, P.V., Drizd, T.A., Johnson, C.L., Reed, R.B., Roche, A.F., & Moore, W.M. (1979). Physical growth: National Center for Health Statistics percentiles. *American Journal of Clinical Nutrition, 32*, 607–629.

Hammer, L.D., Kraemer, H.C., Wilson, D.M., Ritter, P.L., & Dornbusch, S.M. (1991). Standardized percentile curves of body-mass index for children and adolescents. *American Journal of Diseases of Children, 145*, 259–263.

Hebra, A., & Hoffman, M.A. (1993). Gastroesophageal reflux in children. *Pediatric Clinics of North America, 40*(6), 1233–1251.

Heitlinger, L.A., & Lebenthal, E. (1988). Disorders of carbohydrate digestion and absorption. *Pediatric Clinics of North America, 35*(2), 239–253.

Herbst, J.J. (1981). Medical progress: Gastroesophageal reflux. *Journal of Pediatrics, 98*, 859–870.

Jones, K. (1986). Fetal alcohol syndrome. *Pediatrics in Review, 8*(4), 122–126.

Kaufman, F.L. (1991). Managing the cleft lip and palate patient. *Pediatric Clinics of North America, 38*(5), 1127–1147.

Kempe, C.H., Silver, H.K., Obrein, D., & Fulginit, V.A. (1991). *Current pediatric diagnosis and treatment* (10th ed.). Norwalk, CT: Appleton & Lange.

Kibel, M. (1969). Appetite and weight gain in children: A double-blind trial using cyproheptadine and methandrostenolone. *Central African Journal of Medicine, 15*, 229–232.

Koch, G., Modeer, T., Puolsen, S., & Rasmussen, P. (1991). *Pedodontics—A clinical approach.* Copenhagen, Denmark: Munksgaard.

Latham, M.C., McGandy, R.B., McCann, M.B., & Stare, F.J. (1975). *Scope manual on nutrition.* Kalamazoo, MI: The Upjohn Company.

Levine, M.D. (1982). Encopresis: Its potentiation, evaluation, and alleviation. *Pediatric Clinics of North America, 29*(2), 315–330.

Liebowitz, S., Weiss, G., & Shor-Posner, G. (1988). Hypothalamic serotonin: Pharmacological, biochemical, and behavioral analyses of its feeding–suppressive action. *Clinical Neuropharmacology, 11*(Suppl.), S51–S71.

Lyons-Ruth, K., & Zeanah, C.H. (1993). The family context of infant mental health: I. Affective development in the primary caregiving relationship. In C.H. Zeanah (Ed.), *Handbook of infant mental health* (pp. 14–37). New York: Guilford Press.

Marshall, B.J. (1990). Campylobacter pylori: Its link to gastritis and peptic ulcer disease. *Review of Infectious Disease, 12*(Suppl. 1), S87–S93.

Mathisen, B., Skuse, D., Wolke, D., & Reilly, S. (1989). Oral-motor dysfunction and failure to thrive among inner-city infants. *Developmental Medicine and Child Neurology, 31,* 293–302.

Milla, P.J. (1988). Gastrointestinal motility disorders in children. *Pediatric Clinics of North America, 35*(2), 311–330.

Moore, K.L. (1977). *Before we are born: Basic embryology and birth defects* (2nd ed.). Philadelphia: W.B. Saunders.

O'Gorman, M., & Lake, A.M. (1993). Chronic inflammatory bowel disease in childhood. *Pediatric Clinics of North America, 14*(12), 475–480.

Orenstein, S. (1992). Gastroesophageal reflux. *Pediatrics in Review, 13*(5), 174–182.

Peterson, K.E., Washington, J., & Rathbun, J. (1984, July). Team management of failure to thrive. *Perspectives in Practice, 84,* 810–815.

Riddlesberger, M.M. (1988). Evaluation of the gastrointestinal tract in the child: CT, MRI, and isotopic studies. *Pediatric Clinics of North America, 35*(2), 281–310.

Rimoin, D.L., & Horton, W.A. (1978). Short stature, Part I. *Journal of Pediatrics, 92,* 523–528.

Roe, D.A. (1989). *Handbook on drugs and nutrient interactions: A problem oriented reference guide.* Chicago: American Dietetic Association.

Rubenstein, J.S. (1993). The autonomic nervous system and adrenergic receptors in pediatric practice. *Pediatric Clinics of North America, 14*(12), 489–492.

Sanzgiri, R., Mohamad, H., & Raja, Z. (1970). Appetite stimulation and weight gain with cyproheptadine: A double-blind trial in underweight children. *Journal of Postgraduate Medicine, 16,* 12–17.

Schiffman, R., Faber, J., & Eidelman, A.I. (1985). Obstructive hypertrophic adenoids and tonsils as a cause of infantile failure to thrive: Reversed by tonsillectomy and adenoidectomy. *International Journal of Pediatric Otorhinolaryngology, 9,* 183–187.

Sills, I.N. (1994). Hyperthyroidism. *Pediatrics in Review, 15*(11), 417–421.

Sills, R.H. (1978). Failure to thrive: The role of clinical and laboratory evaluation. *American Journal of Diseases of Children, 139,* 967–969.

Silverstone, T., & Schuyler, D. (1975). The effect of cyproheptadine on hunger, caloric intake, and body weight in man. *Psychopharmacologia, 40,* 335–340.

Smith, D.W., Truog, W., Rogers, J.E., Greitzer, L.J., Skinner, A.L., McCann, J.J., & Harvey, M.A.S. (1976). Shifting linear growth during infancy: Illustration of genetic factors in growth from fetal life through infancy. *Journal of Pediatrics, 89*(2), 225–230.

Snyder, J., & First, L.R. (1994). Gastroenterology. In M.E. Avery & L.R. First (Eds.), *Pediatric medicine* (pp. 472–473). Baltimore: Williams & Wilkins.

Tanner, J.M., & Davies, P.S.W. (1985). Clinical longitudinal standards for height and height velocity for North American children. *Journal of Pediatrics, 107*(3), 317–329.

Tanner, J.M., Whitehouse, R.H., Cameron, N., Marshall, W.A., Healy, M.J.R., & Goldstein, H. (1983). *Assessment of skeletal maturity and prediction of adult height (TW2 Method).* New York: Academic Press.

Villee, D., Najjar, S., & Crigler, J. (1994). Endocrinology. In M.E. Avery & L.R. First (Eds.), *Pediatric medicine* (p. 909). Baltimore: Williams & Wilkins.

Wallach, J. (1978). *Interpretation of diagnostic tests.* Boston: Little, Brown.

Warner, B.W., & Ziegler, M.M. (1993). Management of the short bowel syndrome in the pediatric population. *Pediatric Clinics of North America,* 40(6), 1335–1358.

Weitzman, M., & Glotzer, D. (1992). Lead poisoning. *Pediatrics in Review,* 13(12), 461–468.

Zuckerman, B.S., & Frank, D.A. (1992). Infancy and toddler years. In M.D. Levine, W.B. Carey, & A.C. Crocker (Eds.), *Developmental-behavioral pediatrics* (pp. 27–38). Philadelphia: W.B. Saunders.

ABOUT THE AUTHORS

Robert Needlman, M.D., Division of Developmental and Behavioral Pediatrics, Department of Pediatrics, Case Western Reserve University School of Medicine, 11100 Euclid Avenue, Cleveland, Ohio 44106. Dr. Needlman is Assistant Professor of Pediatrics at Rainbow Babies and Children's Hospital, and Director of Resident Training in Continuity Care. Dr. Needlman is Co-founder of Reach Out and Read, a national model pediatric literacy program, and author of the Growth and Development section of *Nelson's Textbook of Pediatrics.*

Robin H. Adair, M.D., M.M.H.S., Master of Management Program, Heller Graduate School, MS035, Brandeis University, Waltham, Massachusetts 02254. As the Associate Director of the Master of Management Program, Dr. Adair is responsible for the development, writing, implementation, and quality management of student and academic policies. She is also a project director for the Institute of Health Policy at the Heller Graduate School and is a pediatrics consultant to the Healthy Steps Initiative, a national program that integrates developmental/behavioral and family services with general pediatric care. She was Medical Director of the Cognitive-Behavior Program and Coordinator of the Division of Developmental and Behavioral Pediatrics at Franciscan Children's Hospital and Rehabilitation Center in Boston.

Karen Bresnahan, M.D., Center for Children with Special Needs, 750 Washington Street, NEMC #334, Boston, Massachusetts 02111. Dr. Bresnahan is Assistant Professor of Pediatrics, Staff Developmental/Behavioral Pediatrician at the Center for Children with Special Needs, Division of Pediatric Neurology, Department of Pediatrics, Tufts University School of Medicine, The Floating Hospital for Children at New England Medical Center. She evaluates and treats children and adolescents with a variety of developmental, learning, and behavioral disorders. She completed training in child and adolescent psychiatry and has an interest in psychiatric and behavioral difficulties and their impact on school, community, and family functioning.

3 Assessment of Environmental Factors in Feeding

An Overview

Understanding and treating a feeding disorder begins with a thorough assessment of the problem and related factors. In conjunction with the consideration of biological factors, as described in Chapter 2, a host of behavioral and environmental factors needs to be considered. Behavioral assessment is fundamentally a problem-solving expedition to identify behavior–environment relationships in feeding problems and to suggest relationships amenable to change via intervention (Babbitt et al., 1994; Iwata, Riordan, Wohl, & Finney, 1982; Linscheid, Budd, & Rasnake, 1995). Behavioral assessment serves four major functions: 1) to clarify target behaviors, adaptive skills, historical factors, and current environmental variables related to the presenting problems; 2) to establish realistic intervention goals given available resources and obstacles; 3) to identify appropriate intervention strategies; and 4) to provide a baseline from which to evaluate progress (Hersen & Bellack, in press; Mash & Terdal, 1997).

This chapter considers referral problems that justify a feeding evaluation and presents possible frameworks for assessment. The chapter outlines relevant information to be gathered (including developmental and medical functioning, feeding history and habits, current dietary intake, feeding interactions, and family stressors), and it discusses the integration of assessment findings for development of an intervention plan.

REFERRAL CRITERIA FOR FEEDING EVALUATION

Children's food preferences and eating habits are highly variable over short periods of time, particularly among toddlers and preschoolers. Thus, an initial consideration for assessment is whether a child's growth and eating patterns fit within "normal" variation or suggest problematic patterns meriting more focused attention. A related consideration is recognizing feeding problems in children with chronic illnesses or developmental disabilities. Linscheid (1992), for example, described a child with a hearing impairment who initially was referred by her speech-language pathologist for behavior management because of minor behavior problems (e.g., resistance to wearing hearing aids). Only after behavioral intervention was well under way did her mother mention casually to the behavior therapist that she had to feed the child in the bathtub to get her to eat (T.R. Linscheid, personal communication, October 1992). Once the therapist became aware of the feeding problem, he counseled the mother to apply behavioral strategies that she had been learning for managing other problems to modify the child's eating behavior.

Table 3.1 lists 13 criteria to consider in referring a child for a feeding evaluation. These criteria are organized into nutritional and growth factors (e.g., diet, anthropometric measures), developmental patterns (e.g., oral-motor skills, utensil use), and behavior characteristics (e.g., mealtime tantrums, rumination) that are potentially indicative of feeding disorders (Linscheid & Rasnake, 1985; Palmer, 1978; Queen, 1984). It should be emphasized that no single item or set of items identifies a child as having a feeding disorder; the list represents broad screening criteria rather than diagnostic elements. The presence of one or more items, however, identifies a child as a possible candidate for feeding assessment.

In some cases, referral information is too vague to determine whether feeding evaluation is warranted; for example, the authors have received referrals for behavioral feeding assessment of children hospitalized for medical treatment who continued to display restricted appetite 2–3 days after medical procedures were completed. These children were referred with the question, "Is the child anorectic?" In such cases, the items in Table 3.1 could serve as a guide for questioning the referring professional about feeding-related concerns to determine whether feeding evaluation is appropriate.

FRAMEWORKS FOR BEHAVIORAL FEEDING ASSESSMENTS

Feeding evaluations vary with regard to the professionals, locales, and specific assessment protocols involved. These variations depend on the agency (or team) performing the evaluation and the individuals being served. Evaluations also are influenced by concerns of the individual being treated and by professional expertise. Ideally, evaluations should be family centered (i.e., tailored to the individual child's and family's needs and interests). Two basic components

Table 3.1.   Referral criteria for potential feeding evaluation

NUTRITIONAL AND GROWTH INDICES

- Child is notably below or above normal levels on standard growth charts (i.e., weight or length/stature is below 5th percentile, weight is above 95th percentile).
- Child's rate of growth has increased or decreased dramatically without sufficient medical explanation.
- Child has a restricted dietary range, rejects textures, or has insufficient or excessive total food intake.
- Health professional has recommended that the child take high-calorie supplements (e.g., Polycose, nutritional milkshakes) for catch-up growth.
- Nutritional deficiency is suggested by physical signs (e.g., anemia, unusual body odor).

DEVELOPMENTAL INDICES

- Oral-motor problems exist in sucking, swallowing, or chewing.
- Child's feeding skills are below the level anticipated by developmental age (e.g., resists self-feeding or utensil use despite having sufficient motor coordination).

BEHAVIORAL INDICES

- Child has bizarre food habits (e.g., pica, steals food) or maladaptive mealtime habits (e.g., eats only in front of television).
- Mealtimes routinely last less than 10 minutes or more than 30 minutes.
- Child (excluding infant) eats more than three meals and three snacks per day, or child of any age eats less than three times per day.
- Child is disruptive or has tantrums at mealtimes.
- Child gags, vomits, or ruminates on food during or after meals.
- Inappropriate affect is indicated around feeding (e.g., persistent lack of interest in feeding, strong fears related to food).

of the evaluation are clinical interview of one or more caregivers (e.g., parent, nurse) and direct observation of the child and caregiver during feeding. The next section reviews common assessment formats and their advantages and disadvantages.

Team versus Individual Approach

Feeding evaluation teams exist in many pediatric hospitals and clinics (e.g., Berkowitz, 1985; Bithoney et al., 1991; Walter, 1994). Feeding teams usually consist of four to eight professionals from various disciplines (see Chapter 1 for more detail). The strength of the team approach lies in its broad coverage and comprehensiveness, which usually is beneficial for the individual as well as for the professionals. As Holm and McCartin (1978) commented, team members have the opportunity to associate with people having similar interests but with different tools of the trade, and thus they can learn from each other.

Feeding teams typically operate by sharing professional responsibilities in a *multidisciplinary* or an *interdisciplinary* manner. In a multidisciplinary model, team members work parallel to one another, often in a sequential fashion. For example, a nutritionist evaluates the adequacy of a child's diet, an occupational therapist assesses oral-motor skills, a psychologist examines intellectual and psychosocial competence, and so forth. Team members then share their findings with each other. If areas of responsibility are delineated clearly and are agreed on by different disciplines, then the multidisciplinary team can operate efficiently (Holm & McCartin, 1978); this mode of interaction, however, does not take full advantage of the range of skills each professional offers nor does it promote development of new skills.

Interdisciplinary teams work by seeing children concurrently or by sharing roles and by encouraging members to substitute for each other (Holm & McCartin, 1978). Decisions about who fulfills which role are made around each child and family. In one case, the nurse may interview a caregiver about feeding patterns; in another case, the social worker may complete the interview; in a third case, the nutritionist and physical therapist together may interview a parent to elaborate on information from a previous medical workup. The speech-language pathologist may feed the child to assess tongue lateralization and swallowing patterns and afterward may try alternative feeding strategies suggested by other team members. Interdisciplinary teams thus capitalize on the expertise of individual team members as well as on collective observations and impressions obtained from the shared evaluation process.

The conditions that constitute the strengths of the interdisciplinary evaluation team also potentially limit the team's effectiveness. Professionals who lack a shared philosophy of child development and treatment goals will have difficulty interacting as a team. Also, a team approach typically reduces the time any one specialist interacts directly with a child and family. A team is particularly useful for initial screening and periodic follow-up, whereas other approaches may be more efficient for detailed evaluation regarding specific aspects of feeding.

The effect of a team approach on feeding assessment and treatment is difficult to evaluate empirically. Walter (1994) noted that, although the team approach has many "anecdotal champions," objective data are sparse on actual utilization of the approach for pediatric feeding disorders. Given that teams may operate in a variety of formats (e.g., multidisciplinary, interdisciplinary, consultant-referral), it is important to assess what team members actually do when one evaluates each member's impact on feeding interventions. In one of the few evaluations of a team approach to feeding treatment, Bithoney and colleagues (1991) compared a multidisciplinary team with a pediatric primary care model for children with nonorganic failure to thrive (NFTT). These authors found that the multidisciplinary team resulted in significantly greater catch-up growth in children older than a mean of 6 months, suggesting that a coordinated team approach has tangible advantages for the individuals being treated. Bithoney and colleagues (1991) attributed the success of the multidisciplinary team to its provision of comprehensive services (e.g., high-calorie diets, behavioral intervention, social/family services) targeted specifically at problems often associated with NFTT.

As an alternative to a team approach, an individual feeding specialist consults or serves as the primary therapist for a child with feeding difficulties. Ideally, referrals are based on features of the case that appear relevant to the professional's area of expertise. In comparison to a team approach, an individual approach typically is more cost-efficient, which is a significant factor influencing the design of health care services. Because the full range of knowledge and skills regarding feeding cannot be offered by a single practitioner—however skilled—it is important that consultation and support be available from other disciplines and critical that the individual specialist know how to use them appropriately.

Evaluation Setting

A second major source of variation in behavioral feeding assessment is the physical setting, which has implications for how the evaluation proceeds. A child may be hospitalized because of severe feeding problems, or feeding difficulties may be diagnosed during a course of hospitalization initiated for other reasons. In these cases, feeding evaluation occurs on an *inpatient* basis, usually in the child's room or in a central pediatric feeding area. For well children, feeding evaluation typically occurs in an *outpatient* (ambulatory care) setting in a clinic room equipped with a high chair or with a table and chairs. Less often, assessment occurs in a *natural* setting, such as the child's home, school, or chronic care facility, as discussed later in this section. Each of these locales has strengths and weaknesses for gathering relevant information regarding feeding problems (Linscheid et al., 1995).

Inpatient and outpatient feeding assessments differ to some extent in the people involved and types of information that are accessible. During inpatient evaluations, a representative of the ward staff, such as the primary nurse, usually participates along with a parent to provide information about the child's behavior in the hospital. Medical records are easily accessible to inpatient feeding evaluators. By contrast, during outpatient evaluations, the parent or primary caregiver often is the sole informant, and only selected medical records may be available. Inpatient status provides an opportunity to observe feeding behavior over several meals rather than on a single occasion, as is common in outpatient evaluations. Multiple observations enhance the reliability of information about a child's behavior, given day-to-day variability in children's eating patterns. Depending on the child's health status, however, inpatient evaluation may or may not reflect the child's intake patterns outside the hospital.

Some differences exist in the types of presenting problems at inpatient and outpatient feeding evaluations. Children are hospitalized because of severe feeding difficulties, extensive medical involvement, or highly unstable home environments. Thus, the feeding problems seen in inpatient evaluations are likely to require more extensive or complicated interventions than those seen in outpatient evaluations. One question relevant to inpatient feeding evaluation is whether services should be conducted on an inpatient or outpatient basis. Decisions about the appropriate locus for treatment are influenced by the child's medical stability; the caregiver's willingness and ability to carry out recommended treatment procedures; availability of inpatient professional staff to carry out procedures; and, increasingly, by fiscal concerns (Linscheid, Oliver, Blyler, & Palmer, 1978). These issues are discussed further in Chapter 4.

Space is almost always at a premium in clinical facilities, whether inpatient or outpatient. As a result, the physical setting for feeding assessment may be busy, cramped, or otherwise distracting; and it is likely to bear little similarity to the child's typical feeding environment. These differences, unfortunately, may reduce the validity of mealtime observations made as part of the evaluation. To increase the representativeness of feeding observations, it is important to simulate the child's usual feeding context as much as possible. Variables to consider are the length of time since the child's last feeding, the child's usual seating position for meals, the person serving as feeder, the types and preparation of foods and liquids offered, the distractions present, and the objects available to the child during the meal. Recommended procedures for conducting mealtime observations are discussed later in this chapter in the section entitled Feeding Interactions.

Whereas most feeding evaluations occur in inpatient or outpatient settings, it occasionally may be feasible to conduct the feeding assessment in the child's natural environment (e.g., home, school, child care, residential care facility). Home visits provide a rich source of information about feeder–child interactions, environmental features, and mealtime routines (Budd, Chugh, & Berry, 1998; Drotar & Crawford, 1987). For example, Mathisen, Skuse, Wolke, and Reilly (1989) compared feeding patterns of inner-city failure to thrive (FTT) infants with demographically matched comparison children during home observations and found several group differences. The infants with FTT were fed in the main living room in the midst of high ambient noise and movement, whereas comparison infants were fed in the kitchen or dining room. Meals for infants with FTT were much shorter than for comparison cases (8.5 minutes versus 21 minutes on average, respectively), and mothers of infants with FTT perceived their children as providing less clear cues during feeding interactions.

Although observation in the natural environment is relatively uncommon in clinical practice, the approach merits consideration, especially when clinic-based procedures provide limited information or with families that are not easily engaged in the clinic. The major disadvantages are the logistical and financial arrangements implicit in professional field visits and with the reduced number of disciplinary professionals who can be present. Some feeding therapists recommend conducting an occasional visit in the child's natural feeding environment as a complement to other assessment procedures to gather initial information or problem-solve persistent feeding difficulties (Bernal, 1972; Budd et al., 1998; Drotar & Crawford, 1987). Luiselli (1994) incorporated direct observation and staff interviews in a residential habilitation setting to identify potential reinforcers prior to beginning feeding intervention with children who had multiple developmental disorders. A few research-oriented feeding programs have used home observations to evaluate intervention outcome (e.g., Stark, Bowen, Tyc, Evans, & Passero, 1990; Werle, Murphy, & Budd, 1993). When observing a child's natural feeding setting is not an option, asking caregivers to audiotape or videotape a typical meal is another means of gaining valuable information about the everyday feeding environment (Madison & Adubato, 1984).

Family-Centered Assessment Protocol

Presenting problems, informants, and prior records vary considerably across cases. Professional roles vary as well, particularly on interdisciplinary feeding teams. For these reasons, professionals often determine the specific protocol to be followed in a feeding evaluation on a case-by-case basis. General guidelines, however, have been developed by various feeding specialists (e.g., Babbitt et al., 1994; Linscheid, 1992; Pipes, Bumbalow, & Glass, 1993; Queen, 1984) that can be adapted to individual cases, as discussed in the next section.

In addition to focusing the content of assessment on patient concerns, family-centered assessment includes the child's parents or caregivers as collaborators in the evaluation process. They are uniquely qualified to describe the everyday nature of the child's feeding problems, report on methods they have tried for dealing with the problems, identify potential resources and obstacles to modifying feeding difficulties, and respond to professional suggestions regarding intervention strategies (Drotar, 1995). Because carrying out assessment recommendations usually is left in parents' hands, it is essential that their perspective be heard and understood by feeding specialists. Techniques for engaging parents in the assessment process are described in the next section and in Chapter 4.

INFORMATION TO BE COLLECTED

Several basic content areas are integral to a comprehensive behavioral feeding assessment: general medical and developmental functioning, feeding history and habits, current dietary intake, feeding interactions, and family stressors. These areas, and information relevant to each topic, are outlined in Table 3.2. The following sections discuss these areas in detail and illustrate how they contribute to comprehensive behavioral assessment of feeding.

General Medical and Developmental Functioning

Behavioral feeding assessment includes a review of the child's medical history and screening of several health and developmental parameters, such as growth, oral-motor, cognitive, and behavioral functioning.

Medical History Whereas formal evaluation of biomedical factors is outside the scope of a behavioral feeding assessment, *review* of the child's medical history and current medical status *is* a crucial part of the behavioral feeding assessment. In particular, it is important to be aware of biological conditions that can affect diet, interfere with intake or digestion, or increase or decrease growth rate. Medical abnormalities affecting the nervous system also must be identified because these conditions affect neuromuscular functioning and, in turn, may interfere with eating responses. Potentially

Table 3.2. Components of a comprehensive feeding assessment

Areas	Relevant information
General medical and developmental functioning	Health records and screening: • congenital, perinatal, and acquired conditions • illnesses and accidents • medications and hospitalizations • growth parameters • oral-motor development • cognitive and behavioral development
Feeding history and habits	Caregiver interview: • onset and nature of feeding problems • feeding milestones • mealtime routines • current feeding concerns • feeding techniques tried
Current dietary intake	Food/liquid intake records: • total caloric intake • nutrient content • food groups and textures • developmentally appropriate diet • access to food
Feeding interactions	Observation of mealtimes: • foods/liquids accepted, refused, and expelled • disruptive or atypical behaviors • self-feeding skills • feeder prompts and reactions • adaptive and maladaptive feeding techniques
Family stressors	Health records and screening: • parent emotional distress • marital conflict • financial problems • abuse/neglect • lack of parent knowledge • major social transitions • other health problems

important biological factors include congenital anomalies, inherited conditions, chronic illnesses, constitutional factors, and medications. Chapter 2 describes biological factors affecting feeding and their clinical implications for treatment of feeding disorders.

Previous illnesses, hospitalizations, and accidents (e.g., choking, swallowing poisonous substances) also should be identified. These conditions may affect current feeding problems by providing an aversive conditioning history even though the biological effects are no longer contributory. They also may have prevented the child from progressing through the normal feeding stages (see Oral-Motor Development). Linscheid (1992) noted that often it is not the medical complication itself that prevented the succession of typical stages but the fact that development of proper eating in the child was considered of much less importance in light of the medical condition.

Growth Parameters Anthropometric records (particularly weight, height, and head circumference) provide another vital source of information relevant to behavioral feeding assessment. Reviewing growth percentiles for an individual child as plotted graphically on standardized National Center for Health Statistics charts indicates where the child ranks relative to all contemporary U.S. children of the same age and sex (Hamill et al., 1979). Interpretation of growth status in children with developmental disabilities can be complicated, however, because of difficulties obtaining reliable weight and height measurement or because of the inapplicability of standards based on normally active children (Stevenson, 1995). Useful growth indices for monitoring feeding problems and guidelines for clinical interpretation are provided in the section on Assessing Growth in Chapter 2 and also in Chapter 6.

Oral-Motor Development Children with feeding problems may show delays in oral-motor skills involved in adaptive mealtime behaviors (Gisel & Alphonce, 1995; Lewis, 1982; Reilly, Skuse, Mathisen, & Wolke, 1995). Review of the child's oral-motor development and current skills is thus integral to the behavioral feeding assessment. Figure 3.1 presents an outline of the normal progression of mealtime skills and texture acceptance from birth to beyond the second year of life.

Initially, the infant's feeding responses consist of reflexive reactions to the breast, bottle, or another stimulus to the oral area. These primitive reflexes typically begin to disappear between 3 and 5 months of age, except for the gag reflex, which continues throughout life. Persistence of primitive reflexes past this time frame can delay or prevent the development of adaptive feeding behaviors (Lewis, 1982; Morris & Klein, 1987).

Chewing and swallowing skills develop progressively through a hierarchy of functional eating behaviors (Lewis, 1982; O'Brien, Repp, Williams, & Christophersen, 1991; Stevenson & Allaire, 1991). As Figure 3.1 shows, the child typically begins to munch on foods at around 5 months of age, develops tongue lateralization and begins biting at about 7 months of age, and refines tongue and jaw movements into mature chewing skills between 8 and 36 months of

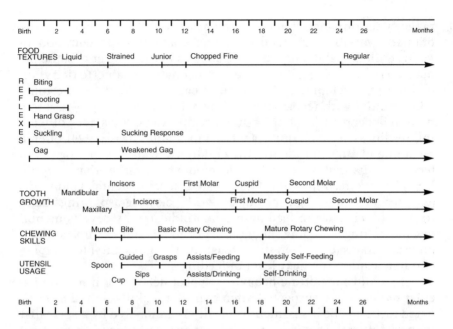

Figure 3.1. The child's acquisition of mealtime skills and food textures. (From O'Brien, S., Repp, A.C., Williams, G.E., & Christophersen, E.R. [1991]. Pediatric feeding disorders. *Behavioral Modification, 15,* 394–418; reprinted by permission.)

age. As the child progresses from suckling to chewing, the textures of foods that the child can handle also change. Infant diets consist mainly of liquid formulas or breast milk until 4–6 months of age. Strained or puréed foods then can be introduced, followed by junior foods (i.e., ground textures; small, soft lumps) at around 10 months, finely chopped textures at 10–12 months, and regular textures by 24 months of age.

A similar developmental progression occurs in the use of feeding utensils (see Figure 3.1). A child begins to self-feed by finger feeding at about 7 months of age, grasps the spoon at 10–12 months, assists in self-feeding at 12–18 months of age, and engages in messy self-feeding by 18–24 months. Weaning from the breast or bottle usually occurs between 6 and 18 months. Cup drinking begins at 8–10 months of age, drinking with assistance begins at 12–14 months, and independent drinking begins at 18–20 months.

Whereas the developmental feeding guidelines outlined in Figure 3.1 describe the typical feeding progression in young children, identifying that a specific child is functioning outside the normal range of oral-motor feeding skills can be quite difficult (Linscheid, 1988; Pipes & Glass, 1993). This difficulty is due in part to the wide range of performance characterizing healthy child development, the dramatic variations in food preferences and appetite common in young children, and individual differences in the impact of some pediatric conditions (e.g., prematurity, neonatal cocaine toxicity) on oral-motor development. Likewise, it can be difficult to determine when a child with recognized feeding delays is able to progress to a more independent level of feeding because the child's cues of feeding readiness may be quite subtle. Pipes and Glass (1993) offered recommendations for identifying children's readiness to progress in feeding skills that are based on developmental rather than chronological markers. Pipes and Glass listed developmental landmarks (e.g., reaches for and grasps objects with scissor grasp, brings hand to mouth), changes in feeding method indicated by developmental level (e.g., finger-feeding large pieces of food), and examples of appropriate foods (e.g., oven-dried toast, teething biscuits) for helping children acquire the next level of feeding skills.

If a child's mealtime behaviors appear delayed or if neuromuscular problems are suspected, then oral-motor skills should be evaluated further. The assessment typically is conducted by a specialist in occupational therapy, speech-language pathology, or physical therapy. Evaluation areas include facial symmetry, muscle tone, mandible deviations, oral hygiene, tactile sensitivity, and oral reflexes (Lewis, 1982; Morris & Klein, 1987; Palmer & Horn, 1978). Functional movements involved in eating, drinking, swallowing, and utensil use are examined in detail (Reilly et al., 1995). When severe oral-motor impairment exists, the time involved in chewing different textures also may be a relevant assessment dimension (Gisel & Patrick, 1988).

Morris and Klein (1987) provided a comprehensive checklist of prefeeding skills that lists the typical sequence of oral-motor skills from birth to 2 years of age, organized by specific skill areas (e.g., feeding positions, oral reflexes, swallowing liquids, jaw movements in biting, lip movements in chewing). This checklist serves as a standard reference for oral-motor assessment of children with significant oral-motor delays. Pipes et al. (1993) provided a screening tool for assessing oral-motor feeding abilities as part of a comprehensive feeding team evaluation. Other researchers (e.g., Gisel, Appelgate-Ferrante, Benson, & Bosma, 1996) described oral-motor assessment protocols for use with specialized populations, such as children with cerebral palsy.

One measure, the Schedule for Oral Motor Assessment (SOMA) (Reilly et al., 1995), broadens the assessment tools available by providing a standardized measure of oral-motor skills in infancy and early childhood. The SOMA is designed to detect oral-motor dysfunction in children with an intact neurological system as well as those with a range of neurological impairments. Oral-motor behaviors are rated on a variety of food textures, and normative levels allow for clinical identification of children with atypical skills. An abbreviated version of the SOMA also has been developed and appears to be useful for screening purposes (Skuse, Stevenson, Reilly, & Mathisen, 1995).

Cognitive and Behavioral Development   Mealtime problems have been estimated to occur in roughly one third of children with developmental disabilities (Palmer, Thompson, & Linscheid, 1975). It is important to determine whether a child's feeding-related behaviors are reflective of overall developmental delays or whether the problems are specific to feeding. Developmental performance estimates are diagnostically useful in assessing for mental retardation, central nervous system dysfunction, and other conditions that affect global functioning. Also, because cognitive and communication skills are integral to feeding interactions, it is important to screen the child's abilities in these areas.

Several methods are available for assessing developmental status in infants and children. A standardized parent-report inventory is an option when the primary caregiver is available. Examples include the Kent Infant Development Scale (Reuter & Bickett, 1985) and the Minnesota Child Development Inventory (Ireton & Thwing, 1972). Another option is a developmental screening inventory, such as the Denver II (Frankenburg et al., 1992) or the Vineland Adaptive Behavior Scales (Sparrow, Balla, & Cicchetti, 1984). The latter scales are administered by a psychologist, nurse, or other trained practitioner. For in-depth cognitive evaluation, standardized psychological tests such as the Bayley Scales of Infant Development–II (Bayley, 1993), the Stanford Binet Intelligence Scale (Thorndike, Hagen, & Sattler, 1986), the McCarthy Scales of Children's Abilities (McCarthy, 1972), or the Wechsler Intelligence Scale for Children (Wechsler, 1991) are used with measures of adaptive functioning.

A related area of inquiry is the child's behavioral and emotional adjustment. How does the child compare with similar-age children in following instructions, interacting with others, waiting for a turn, sleeping through the night, finishing chores, and the like? An index of global psychosocial functioning is useful for determining the appropriate scope of intervention. When feeding is one of several areas in which the child displays behavior difficulties, intervention may need to occur across several aspects of child behavior. In contrast, if the child's behavior is generally adaptive and cooperative except for feeding interactions, then a more focused intervention is indicated.

Methods of assessing behavioral and emotional adjustment include standardized parent-report inventories such as the Eyberg Child Behavior Inventory (Eyberg & Ross, 1978) and the Child Behavior Checklist (Achenbach, 1991, 1992). Temperament scales (Carey & McDevitt, 1978) based on parental report can be used to assess infants' and young children's responses to a variety of common events, social situations, and caregiving routines. For school-age children, self-report measures such as the Child Depression Inventory (Kovacs, 1981) or the Piers-Harris Children's Self-Concept Scale (Piers, 1984) may be appropriate, depending on the referral concerns. Clinicians also informally observe the child's activity level, response to instructions, social interactions, and impulse control to assess behavioral adjustment. Interested readers are referred to more comprehensive sources on developmental and behavioral assessment in children (e.g., Mash & Terdal, 1997; Schroeder & Gordon, 1991; Walker & Roberts, 1992). Considering that the primary referral concern is feeding, however, any additional measures should be selected to amplify understanding of factors related to the feeding disorder.

Feeding History and Habits

Obtaining a thorough picture of the child's past and current feeding patterns by interviewing the caregivers is an essential ingredient of behavioral assessment. The interview provides the caregivers' perspective of how feeding problems developed and specifies present behavioral concerns. It also may suggest child–feeder interactions that relate to feeding problems. Relevant topics of inquiry are displayed in the Parent Interview form (Budd, 1992) in Figure 3.2. This form includes sections specifically relating to the child's feeding patterns (i.e., feeding history, mealtime habits, current feeding problems, feeding techniques), as well as to other general topics (i.e., demographics, general developmental background, treatment plans) to be covered as part of the behavioral feeding assessment. The Parent Interview is adapted and expanded from a questionnaire developed by Linscheid and Rasnake (1985) for assessing behavioral feeding problems in children with NFTT, as well as drawing on other sources (Iwata et al., 1982). Several clinical feeding references (e.g., Macht, 1990; Pipes et al., 1993; Queen, 1984) provide useful

BEHAVIORAL FEEDING ASSESSMENT
PARENT INTERVIEW

Date_____ Location _____ Interviewer _____

Demographics

Child _____ B.D. _____ Age _____
Parent/Guardian(s) _____
Address _____ Phone _____
_____ _____

Mother:

Relationship to child:

____ Natural parent   ____ Other relative (describe) _____
____ Adoptive parent   ____ Other (describe) _____
____ Foster parent (how long?) _____
Age ____ Ethnicity_____
Total years of formal education (beginning with grade 1) _____
Occupation_____
Number of hours worked per week _____

Father:

Relationship to child:

____ Natural parent   ____ Other relative (describe) _____
____ Adoptive parent   ____ Other (describe) _____
____ Foster parent (how long?) _____
Age ____ Ethnicity_____
Total years of formal education (beginning with grade 1) _____
Occupation_____
Number of hours worked per week _____

Family:

Marital status:

____ Single   ____ Divorced
____ Married   ____ Widowed
____ Separated   ____ Other_____

Household composition:

____ Married couple   ____ Extended family
____ Unmarried,   ____ Single parent
      stable couple

Persons living in home other than parent(s) and child: _____

(continued)

Figure 3.2. Behavioral Feeding Assessment Parent Interview form. (This project was supported in part by a grant from the National Institute of Mental Health [No. MH 47539].) (© 1992 by K.S. Budd, *Behavioral Feeding Assessment Parent Interview form.*)

General Developmental Background

Pregnancy/birth history: _____

_____

Health conditions/problems (inherited conditions, chronic diseases, medications, neuromuscular conditions, etc.):

_____

_____

_____

Illnesses, accidents, traumatic events, or hospitalizations (i.e., aversive conditioning history):

_____

_____

_____

Overall development (gross and fine motor, language, social, etc.):

_____

_____

_____

Variations or stresses in day-to-day living conditions (moves, job changes, sibling births, serious illnesses in family, etc.):

_____

_____

_____

Feeding History

Onset of feeding problems (e.g., when and how began):

_____

_____

_____

Changes in feeding problems over time:

_____

_____

_____

Feeding milestones achieved (in months):   Note help
                                                   needed:

____ Strained foods (4–6)   ____ Finger feed   _____
____ Junior foods (6–10)   ____ Cup   _____
____ Chopped fine (10–12)   ____ Spoon   _____
____ Regular foods (18–24)   ____ Fork   _____
                               ____ Knife   _____
                               ____ Straw   _____
                               ____ Pours drink   _____
                               ____ Gets food   _____

Medical restrictions on certain foods or liquids:

_____

_____

Mealtime Habits

Foods and liquids child currently and regularly accepts:

_____

_____

Check types child accepts:

_____ fruits	_____ meats	_____ breads/cereals
_____ vegetables	_____ dairy products	_____ sweets/snacks

Check textures child accepts:

_____ strained/puréed	_____ chopped	_____ crunchy
_____ blenderized	_____ crisp	_____ regular
_____ mashed	_____ chewy	_____ liquid

Foods and liquids child accepted at one time but no longer accepts:

_____

_____

_____

Foods and liquids child regularly rejects:

_____

_____

_____

Person who regularly feeds child (e.g., mother, father, varies):

_____

_____

Extent to which child feeds self (e.g., uses fingers, fork) for preferred/ nonpreferred foods:

_____

_____

Typical meal schedule (example in parentheses):

Meal	Time of Day	Length of Meal	Location	Where Seated	Other Eaters
(Lunch)	(9:00)	(30 mins)	(Kitchen)	(on lap)	(sister)

(continued)

Typical sequence in which food is offered (e.g., liquids last, preferred foods first):

_____

Best description of child's appetite (e.g., poor, variable, strong):

_____

Proportion of daily intake outside meals (i.e., snacks, breast feeds):

_____

Current Feeding Problems

____ Eats too fast	____ Eats too little
____ Eats too slow	____ Eats too much
____ Fails to chew food	____ Pushes food away
____ Vomits or gags	____ Fails to suck
____ Spits food out	____ Refuses to open mouth
____ Throws or drops food	____ Takes food from others
____ Drools	____ Cries or tantrums
____ Turns away from spoon	____ Messy eater
____ Plays with food	____ Refuses to swallow food
____ Leaves table	____ Finicky eater
____ Eats non-food items	____ Ruminates
____ Sneaks or steals food	____ Other _____

Feeding Techniques

Techniques currently used during meals:

____ Coax	____ Forced feeding	____ Ignore
____ Threaten	____ Change foods offered	____ Model
____ Offer reward	____ Distract with play/toys	____ Spank
____ Send in room/ time-out	____ Change meal schedule	____ Praise
____ Limit foods	____ Mini-meals	____ Use t.v.

Other/explain _____

_____

Feeding environment used most often for meals:

____ lap	____ booster seat	____ floor
____ infant seat	____ table/chair	____ couch
____ high chair	____ stand/roam	____ other ____

Impressions of most effective techniques:

_____

_____

Professional recommendations received (e.g., vitamins, food supplements, feeding techniques) and results:

_____

_____

Major sources of feeding information (e.g., parent, friend, spouse) and agreement/disagreement with suggestions received:

_____

_____

Treatment Plans

Parents' priorities regarding feeding:

_____

_____

Obstacles to environmental treatment (child's health, parents' availability, etc.):

_____

_____

Parents' availability to participate in treatment (times, location, etc.):

_____

_____

Plan for next contact and instructions given to parent:

_____

_____

ideas for interview questions and strategies, depending on the nature of the child's feeding disorder.

Linscheid and Rasnake (1985) described how caregiver responses during the feeding history can provide indications of behaviorally based feeding problems. Long mealtimes (e.g., longer than 20–25 minutes for children without oral-motor impairments) suggest that parents are switching strategies during meals, coaxing the child to eat, or in other ways reinforcing the child's noneating behavior. If the caregiver reports that the child has strong food preferences or has narrowed the range of accepted foods, then the parents may have responded by changing the types of foods offered and thus in effect supported the child's selectivity. The lack of set mealtimes, a practice of feeding the child in locations other than at the table or high chair, and making food available for the child to "graze" freely across the day are additional signs that parent management strategies play a role in feeding problems.

Although the preceding examples pertain to children with insufficient intake or selective eating patterns, parenting practices also are likely to influence eating in children who are overweight. Observations in the homes of families with children who are obese and non-obese indicate that parents encourage their offspring who are obese to eat more frequently and give them more food prompts than they do their children who are non-obese (Klesges et al., 1983). Because food serves social as well as dietary functions, the evaluator should examine the extent to which food is used as a reward or a punishment for the child's behavior and for social activities that involve food.

In addition to inquiring about feeding patterns, it is also relevant for the interviewer to ask about parents' sources of information regarding their feeding practices. For example, do caregivers agree on how to feed the child, have they received pressure to use particular techniques from extended family members, or are they following recommendations of a professional? These questions may elucidate parental conflicts in management strategies, idiosyncratic or culturally derived beliefs about feeding, or negative experiences with professionals that are likely to affect the caregiver's receptivity to intervention recommendations.

To supplement the interview, it may be helpful to gather information about caregivers' perceptions of the child's feeding patterns from a written questionnaire. The Children's Eating Behavior Inventory (CEBI) is one such measure, which was designed to screen for feeding/mealtime problems in children ages 2–12 years (Archer, Rosenbaum, & Streiner, 1991). The CEBI has been shown to differentiate clinical from nonclinical populations, but to date little research has examined its usefulness in assessing clinical feeding problems. Another example of a parent inventory is the Child Feeding Questionnaire, which assesses attitudes and experiences around parents' and children's adiposity and eating styles (Johnson & Birch, 1994). This measure explores parents' beliefs about eating in relation to overweight status.

Questionnaires are useful sources of clinically relevant information, but they are subject to methodological problems due to use of retrospective reports, global ratings, and terms that may be interpreted differently across reporters (Jensen & Haynes, 1986). The psychometric adequacy of caregiver reports can be strengthened by focusing the reports on specific behavior instances and by collecting samples across repeated occasions. Sanders, Patel, Le Grice, and

Shepherd (1993) used this approach as one means of comparing children with persistent feeding difficulties with matched nonproblem feeders. Parents were asked to keep a mealtime diary for a 2-week period, detailing the occurrence or nonoccurrence of five disruptive behaviors (e.g., playing with food, leaving the table) during each meal and rating the child's difficulty during the meal on a 7-point scale. The group with feeding difficulties differed significantly from the nonproblem feeders in the percentage of meals in which parents reported that disruptive behaviors occurred and the average difficulty rating of meals. In an intervention outcome study using the same measure, Turner, Sanders, and Wall (1994) found significant reductions in parents' reports of disruptive behavior and mealtime difficulty following both behavioral parent training and standard dietary education. The work of Sanders and his colleagues points to the clinical usefulness of structured caregiver reports, both for assessing feeding problems at the outset of intervention and for evaluating treatment.

Current Dietary Intake

The caregiver interview regarding feeding history and habits, as described in the preceding section, provides some information about a child's intake patterns and food preferences; however, it focuses mainly on behavior patterns involved in feeding problems rather than on the precise content of intake. More specific information about the child's food and fluid intake is needed to assess the nutritional adequacy of the child's diet.

Nutrient intake can be examined by first interviewing the caregiver about a child's diet for a typical day using focused questions, such as "When does the child first have something to eat?" (Pipes et al., 1993). This sample will provide an indication of whether the child is receiving appropriate nutrients and whether the parents have knowledge of appropriate nutrition and food preparation procedures. Nutritionists look for signs that the child is at nutritional risk, such as inappropriate preparation of infant formula, too little or too much milk intake, excessive use of vitamin supplements, refusal of an entire group of foods, or developmentally inappropriate food textures (Krug-Wispe, 1993; Pipes et al., 1993; Queen, 1984). If the child appears to be at nutritional risk, then more precise information should be obtained through recordings of actual food intake.

Food diaries kept for a 3- or 7-day period are the most common method of quantitatively assessing intake. The caregiver is instructed to measure and record everything that the child consumes.

Typical forms include a place to record when the food or drink was consumed, the type of food, the method of preparation, and household measures (fractions of measuring cups, level teaspoons, or tablespoons) of food consumed. Recipes for mixed dishes should accompany the food records. Vitamin and mineral supplements also should be recorded.

Food intake then is evaluated with regard to total caloric intake, protein, vitamins, and minerals for the child's weight or age, using standard Recommended Daily Allowances established by the U.S. Food and Drug Administration. Computer software programs (e.g., Food and Nutrition Information Center, 1992) are available for calculating the nutritional adequacy of diets. Nutritional excesses or deficiencies may call for intervention under the supervision of a nutritional specialist.

As a general guide, it can be helpful to compare a child's diet to recommended daily servings of each food group for typically developing children of different ages. Figure 3.3 shows a sample chart from a pamphlet entitled *A Food Guide for the First Five Years*, published by the National Live Stock and Meat Board (1992). As stated in the guide, the pamphlet material has been reviewed favorably by the American Academy of Family Physicians Foundation and the American Academy of Pediatrics. Minimum serving sizes for children are defined in the guide as 1 measuring tablespoon of cooked food for each year of a child's age. Expected intake obviously would vary from the norm for children on hyper- or hypocaloric diets.

One limitation of food diaries is that there is a likelihood of substantial inaccuracy in reporting: Even motivated parents forget to document information, miscalculate amounts, or simply do not notice some aspects of a child's food consumption. More precise records can be obtained for actual intake during the feeding evaluation by weighing food before and after the meal or by counting actual bites eaten (Linscheid, 1992; Riordan, Iwata, Finney, Wohl, & Stanley, 1984). These methods also can be used by feeding professionals during ongoing monitoring of a child's progress in feeding sessions. In addition, parents may be taught to provide more accurate reports of food consumption using food scales or plastic food models, which provide standardized reference points for estimating the size of servings (Stark et al., 1990; Turner et al., 1994).

Feeding Interactions

A child's immediate feeding environment consists of physical attributes (e.g., location, furnishings, seating arrangement, people pres-

FOOD GROUPS CHART

	FOODS INCLUDED IN THIS GROUP ARE:	SERVING SIZES 1 Year	2-3 Years	4-5 Years	DAILY RECOMMENDED SERVINGS	KEY NUTRIENTS SUPPLIED
MILK AND DAIRY PRODUCTS	**3 servings daily in the amounts recommended from a variety of foods listed in this group**					
	milk, yogurt and milk base soups	1/2 c.	1/2 c.	1/2 c.-3/4 c.	3 servings daily	Calcium, Riboflavin, Protein
	cottage cheese	2-4 T.	4-6 T.	6 T.	For children around 1 year, additional calories and nutrients may come from breast milk, infant formula and cow's milk.	
	custard, milk pudding and ice cream (served only after a meal)					
	cheese (1 oz. = 1 slice or a 1" cube)	1/3 oz.-2/3 oz.	2/3 oz.-1 oz.	1 oz.		
MEAT AND MEAT ALTERNATES	**2 servings daily in the amounts recommended from a variety of foods listed in this group**					
	beef, pork, lamb, fish and poultry liver (every few weeks)	2 T. or 1 oz.	2-3 T. or 1½ oz.	4 T. or 2 oz.	2 servings daily	Protein, Niacin, Iron, Thiamin
	eggs	1	1	1		
	cooked legumes, dried beans or peas	1/4 c.	1/3 c.	1/2 c.		
	nuts	Nuts and chunks of unspread peanut butter are not recommended for children under 4 because they can cause choking.				
FRUITS AND VEGETABLES	**5 servings daily in the amounts recommended from a variety of foods listed in this group**					
	VITAMIN C SOURCE FRUITS, VEGETABLES AND JUICES citrus fruits, berries, melons, tomatoes, peppers, cabbage, cauliflower, broccoli, chilies and potatoes	1/3 c.	1/2 c.	1/2 c.	1 Vitamin C source daily	Vitamin C, Carbohydrates including fiber
	VITAMIN A SOURCE FRUITS AND VEGETABLES (DEEP GREEN AND YELLOW) melons, peaches, apricots, carrots, spinach, broccoli, squash, pumpkin, sweet potatoes, tomatoes, brussels sprouts	1-2 T.	3-4 T.	4-5 T.	1 Vitamin A source 3-4 times per week	Vitamin A, Carbohydrates including fiber
	FRUITS	1/4 c.	1/4 c.	1/2 c.	3 servings of other fruits and vegetables daily	Carbohydrates including fiber
	VEGETABLES	1-2 T.	3-4 T.	4-5 T.		
BREADS AND CEREALS	**6 servings daily in the amounts recommended from a variety of foods listed in this group**					
	whole-grain, enriched or restored breads	1/2 slice	3/4 slice	3/4-1 slice	6 servings daily	Thiamin, Iron, Niacin, Carbohydrates including fiber
	cooked cereals, rice and pasta	1/4 c.	1/3 c.	1/2 c.		
	whole-grain or fortified ready-to-eat cereals	1/2 oz.	3/4 oz.	1 oz.		
FATS/OILS	margarine, butter, oils, mayonnaise and salad dressings (1 Tablespoon = 100 calories)	1 tsp.	1 tsp.	1 tsp.	3 servings daily in the amounts recommended	This group is a significant source of fats for which there is no U.S. RDA.
OTHER FOODS	jams, jellies, sweet desserts, gravies, and catsup	USE IN MODERATION			NO AMOUNT RECOMMENDED 3 servings daily is maximum	This group is a significant source of carbohydrates and fats for which there is no U.S. RDA.

Figure 3.3. Children's recommended daily servings by food group. (From National Live Stock and Meat Board. [1992]. *A food guide for the first five years*. Chicago: Educational Department, Author, pp. 2-3; reprinted by permission courtesy of National Cattlemen's Beef Association.)

ent, objects available), temporal characteristics (e.g., time since the child's last feeding, type of activity immediately preceding meal), foods and liquids offered, and behavior of the feeder who interacts with the child during meals. Any of these environmental variables may be functionally related to the child's behavior during mealtimes such that changes in the environmental variables will result in systematic changes in the child's behavior. Observing feeding interactions provides a direct context for studying possible relationships between child behaviors and environmental variables. Thus, examining feeder–child interactions is a fundamental part of the behavioral feeding assessment (Babbitt et al., 1994; Linscheid et al., 1995; Linscheid & Rasnake, 1985).

To make the observation most informative, it is important to prepare the caregiver by stating that the goal of observation is to allow feeding clinicians to see the child's typical feeding behavior and the usual feeding routine as much as possible. This includes how the child is positioned during the meal, the foods offered, food containers and utensils used, and feeding techniques that the caregiver uses during the meal. It is helpful to provide both preferred and nonpreferred foods in order to see how the child responds to both types of foods at the meal. To increase the likelihood of hunger, the child should not be fed for 2 hours prior to the evaluation. (If a typical feeder is not available, then the evaluator can feed the child to try various feeding techniques.) Some evaluators interact with the feeder and child throughout the observation by asking questions, by making suggestions, or by trying out feeding techniques. As an alternative, the professional can take a passive, observer role during the feeding session to approximate a more natural sample of feeder–child interactions.

The feeding observation permits examination of how the caregiver structures the feeding situation, the child's responses to specific caregiver behaviors, and the caregiver's reactions to particular child behaviors. The professional attends closely to the sequence of interactions and looks for recurring patterns. Consider the following examples: How does the child react when preferred as opposed to nonpreferred foods are presented? How does the feeder respond when the child refuses or spits out food? Does the child attempt to self-feed, and is this allowed or encouraged? Which child behavior immediately precedes instances of the feeder's positive attention to the child? Is the pace of intake too fast or too slow, and who determines the rate? How do interactions change as the mealtime proceeds? Is the child positioned to provide adequate physical support to facilitate eating?

There are many possible ways of organizing information from feeding interactions. Clinicians often take informal notes or tally occurrences of specific child and feeder behaviors of interest. Some formal observational coding systems have been developed for applied research purposes, and aspects of these systems can be modified for clinical use. Table 3.3 lists features of 11 observational systems that were designed variously for children with FTT, ongoing food refusal, dysphagia, obesity, and delayed feeding skills.

Inspection of Table 3.3 shows that most of the observation systems provide information on the occurrence of pertinent behaviors in short time intervals (e.g., 20-second or 1-minute periods) or on consecutive offers of food and liquid across a feeding session. Sample child behaviors commonly recorded in the systems include food acceptances, refusals, swallows, spitting out food, leaving the table, playing with food, and crying. Some coding systems (e.g., Luiselli, 1993) document the child's performance of specific components of feeding (e.g., grasping spoon, moving it to mouth, touching lips with spoon), whereas others (e.g., Mathisen et al., 1989; Sparling & Rogers, 1985) focus on oral-motor skills exhibited by the child. Categories for recording the texture or dietary content of foods offered, eaten, and refused are provided within some coding systems (e.g., Mathisen et al., 1989; Munk & Repp, 1994; Werle et al., 1993).

Whereas all of the observational methods displayed in Table 3.3 document child behaviors, only some (e.g., Klesges et al., 1983; Sanders et al., 1993; Werle et al., 1993) also include feeder behaviors. Sample feeder responses coded are presenting food, modeling eating, verbally encouraging the child to eat, and providing positive or negative attention. Environmental variables, such as the location at which feeding occurs, salient objects present (e.g., television on, toys within child's reach), and other people present, are denoted in a few of the observation systems (e.g., Klesges et al., 1983; Mathisen et al., 1989).

Another approach to organizing information about feeding interactions involves rating feeder and child characteristics on specific dimensions for the entire session by means of standardized feeding scales. The first two entries in Table 3.3 represent this approach. Barnard and her colleagues developed the Nursing Child Assessment Feeding Scale (NCAFS) for assessing parents and their infants from birth to 1 year of age (Barnard et al., 1989). The NCAFS includes four parent subscales measuring parent's sensitivity to cues, response to the child's distress, social-emotional growth-

Table 3.3. Summary of selected feeding observation systems

Reference and instrument	Purpose	Description
Barnard et al. (1989)—Nursing Child Assessment Feeding Scale (NCAFS)	Assess dyadic interactions and emotional responsivity between parents and infants	Score presence of 50 parent and 26 infant characteristics on binary scale across feeding session
Chatoor (1986)—Mother–Infant/Toddler Feeding Scale	Evaluate quality of parent–child interactions and diagnose type of feeding disorder	Rate 26 parent and 20 child characteristics on 4-point scale across feeding session
Klesges et al. (1983)—Bob and Tom's Method of Assessing Nutrition (BATMAN)	Assess child, parent, and social-environmental variables related to obesity	Score 9 child, 7 parent, and 6 environmental codes in 10-second intervals during family meal
Lamm & Greer (1988)	Evaluate behavioral treatment to induce swallowing in infants with dysphagia	Record occurrence of swallows to each prompt with specific feeding implements and quantity eaten
Luiselli (1993, Study 1)	Assess self-feeding skills in children with multiple disabilities	Code independent performance of 6 component steps on 10 feeding trials
Mathisen, Skuse, Wolke, & Reilly (1989)—Feeding Assessment Scale (FAS)	Assess oral-motor functioning, ecological aspects, and feeding behavior in children at risk for FTT	Score oral-motor skills on standard presentations of textures, code ecological context, and interview feeder in home
Munk & Repp (1994)	Evaluate selectivity to food types and textures in individuals with severe disabilities	Score acceptance, rejection, expulsion, and negative behavior to different types and textures of foods
Riordan, Iwata, Finney, Wohl, & Stanley (1984)	Evaluate behavioral treatment to reduce food refusal in children with disabilities	Record occurrence of acceptances, expulsions, disruptive behaviors for each bite, and quantity eaten
Sanders, Patel, Le Grice, & Shepherd (1993)—Mealtime Observation Schedule	Compare mealtime interactions of problem and nonproblem feeders	Score 17 child behaviors and 14 parent behaviors in 10-second intervals during clinic meals

(continued)

Table 3.3. *(continued)*

Reference and instrument	Purpose	Description
Sparling & Rogers (1985)—Feeding Interaction Report Scale and Treatment (FIRST)	Assess oral-motor skills and parent–child interactions in children at risk for developmental disabilities in conjunction with oral-motor treatment	Record 4 oral-motor and 8 interactional items in 20-second intervals from videotapes of home visits
Werle, Murphy, & Budd (1993)—Feeding Observations Code	Evaluate behavioral treatment to increase food acceptance in children with chronic food refusal	Record 7 child and 12 parent behaviors, and code food group and texture for each bite offered in 1-minute intervals from videotapes of home visits

fostering, and cognitive growth-fostering. It also contains two child subscales measuring clarity of cues and responsiveness to parent. Scores on the NCAFS have been shown to differentiate infants whose FTT is attributable to interactional problems from infants whose FTT is due to organic etiology. Preterm infants score lower on the feeding scale than do term infants, and maternal education level correlates positively with total parent scores (Barnard et al., 1989). The NCAFS has been used extensively in research and clinical practice, and it offers valuable normative information on feeding patterns with infants.

Chatoor (1986) also developed a qualitative observational feeding scale, which is designed for children from birth to 3 years of age and their mothers. Scores on the scale are used to classify children's feeding disorders into one of three developmental categories: homeostasis, attachment, and separation. Although research on this instrument has yet to be published, its diagnostic focus offers a potentially valuable contribution to feeding assessment.

Family Stressors

In addition to child, parent, and immediate environmental influences on the feeding situation, more global family variables may affect feeding problems. Feeding occurs within the ecological context of the family, which includes siblings, marital and extended family relationships, friendships, financial and health status, and parental mental health status. These variables are sources of support or stress, which serve to promote or undermine parental competence in moment-to-moment interactions with the child (Belsky, Robins, & Gamble, 1984; Galler, Ricciuti, Crawford, & Kucharski, 1984). It is likely that these conditions interact with feeding problems and can interfere with the success of intervention. Thus, it is important to identify significant family stressors as part of behavioral feeding assessment.

Family variables such as poverty, single parenthood, and marital conflict have been cited in correlational studies as risk factors for some feeding problems, particularly NFTT and growth deficiency. (More explicit definitions of these terms are provided in Chapter 6.) For example, Casey, Bradley, and Wortham (1984) conducted a prospective study of families of NFTT infants and a demographically matched control group of healthy infants. Compared with controls, mothers of NFTT children were significantly less responsive and accepting of the children, and their home environments were more disorganized, suggesting that poor parenting patterns may have contributed to the development of NFTT. Other studies (e.g., Drotar, Eckerle, Satola, Pallotta, & Wyatt, 1990), however, showed fewer and more isolated differences between NFTT and non-NFTT infants and their families than were suggested by earlier studies. Even when significant group differences are found, there appears to be considerable heterogeneity in the NFTT population. Black, Hutcheson, Dubowitz, and Berenson-Howard (1994) found significantly more neglectful, undercontrolling mothers of NFTT children than mothers of comparison children; but they also found subgroups of authoritarian, overcontrolling mothers and nurturant mothers within the NFTT group. Other findings (Bithoney, Van Sciver, Foster, Corso, & Tentindo, 1995) implicate decreased child adaptability as a contributory factor to growth deficiency. The overall findings lend credence to Woolston's (1985) hypothesis that nonorganic feeding disorders are influenced by psychosocial stress but are not necessarily caused by it.

Budd and her colleagues measured parent emotional distress in families of children with differing etiologies of feeding disorders (Budd et al., 1992). High levels of parent emotional distress in their sample were associated with low levels of child feeding skills, older children, parents who used less positive disciplinary practices, and parents with higher educational and occupational status. The high emotional distress scores for some parents indicate that, rather than focus mainly on the child's functioning, clinical services also need to consider and promote parents' emotional adjustment.

With respect to the feeding evaluation, clinical interviews and case records provide the main sources of information about family stressors. The topic can be raised during the interview by asking how the family is getting along in areas other than the child's feeding. It is useful to inquire about recent or upcoming social transitions (e.g., birth of sibling, unemployment, recent move) likely to exacerbate family pressures. The Parent Interview form (displayed in Figure 3.2 and discussed in the Feeding History and Habits section) includes some questions regarding potential family stresses.

Standardized self-report instruments are another source of information about family stressors. Examples include the Symptom Checklist 90–R (Derogatis, 1983) for assessing emotional distress; the Dyadic Adjustment Scale (Spanier, 1989) for measuring quality of the marital relationship; the Daily Hassles Scale (Lazarus & Folkman, 1989) for measuring perceived stressful events in daily living; and the Parenting Stress Index (available in both long and short forms) (Abidin, 1995) for screening global parent, child, and interactional stressors. When specific concerns arise about maladaptive parenting practices, it may be appropriate to administer the Child Abuse Potential Inventory (Milner, 1986), which assesses child-rearing attitudes and parent symptoms associated with physical child abuse. These scales are rarely used in routine clinical assessment of children with feeding problems but rather are more likely to be applied within a research context.

In considering the use of formal measures regarding family functioning or stressors as part of behavioral feeding assessment, a cautionary statement is in order. Many family-related measures exist, but few have adequate specificity, reliability, or predictive validity for making inferences to an individual case (Jensen & Haynes, 1986). As when determining which assessment measures to include regarding the child's developmental, behavioral, and emotional functioning, the choice of which, if any, family-related measures to employ should be guided by the referral concerns. Parents are understandably sensitive about being asked to reveal confidential information about themselves and their family relationships during an evaluation of their child's feeding problems. The information gained from such measures may not be worth the expense in terms of family comfort and trust in the evaluation process.

CASE FORMULATION AND INTERVENTION PLANNING

After the evaluator collects information from various sources, his or her task is to integrate assessment findings into a behavior analysis that provides a blueprint for intervention. The behavior analysis specifies 1) problem conditions to be changed, 2) fixed states not available to change, 3) environmental variables that potentially function to maintain current problems, 4) skills and resources that may be utilized in intervention, and 5) potential obstacles to the change process (Kanfer & Schefft, 1988). A behavior analysis takes into account medical, developmental, and social factors relevant to feeding problems; and it considers the consequences of therapeutic intervention on child and family adjustment. Discrepancies in findings should be examined to determine whether more information is needed to complete the analysis.

Organizing information from disparate disciplines, sources, and areas of functioning into a coherent whole is perhaps the most challenging part of the behavioral feeding assessment. First, it is useful to reconsider the child's feeding problems in light of evaluation data, using the descriptive categories of the multidimensional classification system offered in Chapter 1. Salient features of feeding problems can be organized according to subcategories of four major areas: eats too little, eats too much, eats the wrong things, and feeding skill delays. Second, it is helpful to review assessment findings relating each of the potential etiological variables impinging on feeding problems to determine which aspects are relevant in the present case. The eight areas, as outlined in Chapter 1, are as follows: diet, physical competence, appetite, illness, interaction/management, child constitution, caregiver competence, and systemic factors. The five key issues for the behavior analysis, cited at the beginning of this section, then need to be articulated. Third, the results of behavior analysis are used to make tentative decisions about case disposition, such as whether immediate intervention is required, whether additional evaluations are needed, whether to recommend intervention, and, if so, appropriate intervention strategies.

SUMMARY

Behavioral assessment of feeding disorders, an important first step in the intervention process, serves four major functions: 1) to clarify target behaviors, adaptive skills, historical factors, and current environmental variables related to feeding problems; 2) to establish realistic intervention goals; 3) to identify appropriate intervention strategies; and 4) to provide a baseline from which to evaluate progress. Behavioral feeding assessment can take the form of a team or individual approach; occur in inpatient, outpatient, or natural settings; and include various disciplinary professionals. Ideally, it is family centered, which implies that assessment content and structure are tailored to referral, child, and family concerns. Core components include review or screening of medical and developmental status, interview with the primary caregiver(s), and direct observation of feeder–child interactions during a meal. Major content areas for the feeding evaluation are general medical and developmental functioning, feeding history and habits, current dietary intake, feeding interactions, and family stressors. Once information is obtained, the evaluator integrates assessment findings into a behavior analysis that provides a blueprint for intervention. The following chapters describe and illustrate the process of case formulation, intervention planning, and ongoing evaluation with various types of feeding disorders.

REFERENCES

Abidin, R.R. (1995). *Parenting Stress Index: Professional manual* (3rd ed.). Odessa, FL: Psychological Assessment Resources.

Achenbach, T.M. (1991). *Manual for the Child Behavior Checklist/4–18 and 1991 profile.* Burlington: University of Vermont, Department of Psychiatry.

Achenbach, T.M. (1992). *Manual for the Child Behavior Checklist/2–3 and 1992 profile.* Burlington: University of Vermont, Department of Psychiatry.

Archer, L.A., Rosenbaum, P.L., & Streiner, D.L. (1991). The Children's Eating Behavior Inventory: Reliability and validity results. *Journal of Pediatric Psychology, 16,* 629–642.

Babbitt, R.L., Hoch, T.A., Coe, D.A., Cataldo, M.F., Kelly, K.J., Stackhouse, C., & Perman, J.A. (1994). Behavioral assessment and treatment of pediatric feeding disorders. *Journal of Developmental and Behavioral Pediatrics, 15,* 278–291.

Barnard, K.E., Hammond, M.A., Booth, C.L., Bee, H.L., Mitchell, S.K., & Spieker, S.J. (1989). Measurement and meaning of parent–child interaction. In F. Morrison, C. Lord, & D. Keating (Eds.), *Applied developmental psychology* (Vol. III, pp. 40–76). New York: Academic Press.

Bayley, N. (1993). *Bayley Scales of Infant Development* (2nd ed.). San Antonio, TX: The Psychological Corporation.

Belsky, J., Robins, E., & Gamble, W. (1984). The determinants of parental competence: Toward a contextual theory. In M. Lewis (Ed.), *Beyond the dyad* (pp. 251–279). New York: Plenum.

Berkowitz, C. (1985). Comprehensive pediatric management of failure to thrive: An interdisciplinary approach. In D. Drotar (Ed.), *New directions in failure to thrive: Implications for research and practice* (pp. 193–210). New York: Plenum.

Bernal, M.E. (1972). Behavioral treatment of a child's eating problem. *Journal of Behavior Therapy and Experimental Psychiatry, 3,* 43–50.

Bithoney, W.G., McJunkin, J., Michalek, J., Snyder, J., Egan, H., & Epstein, D. (1991). The effect of a multidisciplinary team approach on weight gain in nonorganic failure-to-thrive children. *Journal of Developmental and Behavioral Pediatrics, 12,* 254–258.

Bithoney, W.G., Van Sciver, M.M., Foster, S., Corso, S., & Tentindo, C. (1995). Parental stress and growth outcome in growth-deficient children. *Pediatrics, 96,* 707–711.

Black, M.M., Hutcheson, J.J., Dubowitz, H., & Berenson-Howard, J. (1994). Parenting style and developmental status among children with nonorganic failure to thrive. *Journal of Pediatric Psychology, 19,* 689–707.

Budd, K.S. (1992). *Behavioral Feeding Assessment Parent Interview form.* Unpublished manuscript, DePaul University, Chicago.

Budd, K.S., Chugh, C., & Berry, S.L. (1998). Parents as therapists for children's food refusal problems. In J.M. Briesmeister & C.E. Schaefer (Eds.), *Handbook of parent training: Parents as co-therapists for children's behavior problems* (2nd ed., pp. 418–440). New York: John Wiley & Sons.

Budd, K.S., McGraw, T.E., Farbisz, R., Murphy, T.B., Hawkins, D., Heilman, N., Werle, M., & Hochstadt, N.J. (1992). Psychosocial concomitants of children's feeding disorders. *Journal of Pediatric Psychology, 17,* 81–94.

Carey, W.B., & McDevitt, S.C. (1978). Revision of the Infant Temperament Questionnaire. *Pediatrics, 61,* 735–739.

Casey, P.H., Bradley, R., & Wortham, B. (1984). Social and nonsocial home environments of infants with nonorganic failure-to-thrive. *Pediatrics, 73,* 348–353.

Chatoor, I. (1986). *Mother–Infant/Toddler Feeding Scale.* Unpublished manuscript, Children's Hospital National Medical Center, Washington, DC.

Derogatis, L.R. (1983). *SCL-90–R: Administration, scoring, and clinical procedures manual–II.* Towson, MD: Clinical Psychometric Research.

Drotar, D. (1995). Failure to thrive (growth deficiency). In M. Roberts (Ed.), *Handbook of pediatric psychology* (2nd ed., pp. 516–536). New York: Guilford Press.

Drotar, D., & Crawford, P. (1987). Using home observation in the clinical assessment of children. *Journal of Clinical Child Psychology, 16,* 342–349.

Drotar, D., Eckerle, D., Satola, J., Pallotta, J., & Wyatt, B. (1990). Maternal interactional behavior with nonorganic failure-to-thrive infants: A case comparison study. *Child Abuse and Neglect, 14,* 41–51.

Endres, J., & Rockwell, R. (1980). *Food, nutrition, and the young child.* St. Louis: C.V. Mosby.

Eyberg, S.M., & Ross, A.W. (1978). Assessment of child behavior problems: The validation of a new inventory. *Journal of Clinical Child Psychology, 7,* 113–116.

Food and Nutrition Information Center. (1992). *Microcomputer software collection.* Beltsville, MD: U.S. Department of Agriculture.

Frankenburg, W.K., Dodds, J., Archer, P., Bresnick, B., Maschka, P., Edelman, N., & Shapiro, H. (1992). *Denver II: Training manual* (2nd ed.). Denver, CO: Denver Developmental Materials.

Galler, J.R., Ricciuti, H.N., Crawford, M.A., & Kucharski, L.T. (1984). The role of the mother–infant interaction in nutritional disorders. In J.R. Galler (Ed.), *Nutrition and behavior* (pp. 269–304). New York: Plenum.

Gisel, E.G., & Alphonce, E. (1995). Classification of eating impairments based on eating efficiency in children with cerebral palsy. *Dysphagia, 10,* 268–274.

Gisel, E.G., Appelgate-Ferrante, T., Benson, J., & Bosma, J.F. (1996). Oral-motor skills following sensorimotor therapy in two groups of moderately dysphagic children with cerebral palsy: Aspiration vs. nonaspiration. *Dysphagia, 11*, 59–71.

Gisel, E.G., & Patrick, J. (1988, February 6). Identification of children with cerebral palsy unable to maintain a normal nutritional state. *Lancet*, 283–286.

Hamill, P.V.V., Drizd, T.A., Johnson, C.L., Reed, R.B., Roche, A.F., & Moore, W.M. (1979). Physical growth: National Center for Health Statistics percentiles. *American Journal of Clinical Nutrition, 32*, 607–629.

Hersen, M., & Bellack, A.S. (in press). *Behavioral assessment: A practical handbook* (4th ed.). Needham Heights, MA: Allyn & Bacon.

Holm, V.A., & McCartin, R.E. (1978). Interdisciplinary child development team: Team issues and training in interdisciplinariness. In K.E. Allen, V.A. Holm, & R.L. Schiefelbusch (Eds.), *Early intervention: A team approach* (pp. 97–122). Baltimore: University Park Press.

Ireton, H.R., & Thwing, E.J. (1972). *Minnesota Child Development Inventory*. Minneapolis, MN: Behavior Science Systems.

Iwata, B.A., Riordan, M.M., Wohl, M.K., & Finney, J.W. (1982). Pediatric feeding disorders: Behavioral analysis and treatment. In P.J. Accardo (Ed.), *Failure to thrive in infancy and early childhood: A multidisciplinary team approach* (pp. 297–329). Baltimore: University Park Press.

Jensen, B.J., & Haynes, S.N. (1986). Self-report questionnaires and inventories. In A.R. Ciminero, K.S. Calhoun, & H.E. Adams (Eds.), *Handbook of behavioral assessment* (pp. 150–175). New York: John Wiley & Sons.

Johnson, S.L., & Birch, L.L. (1994). Parents' and children's adiposity and eating style. *Pediatrics, 94*, 653–661.

Kanfer, F.H., & Schefft, B.K. (1988). *Guiding the process of therapeutic change*. Champaign, IL: Research Press.

Klesges, R.C., Coates, T.J., Brown, G., Sturgeon-Tillisch, J., Moldenhauer-Klesges, L.M., Holzer, B., Woolfrey, J., & Vollimer, J. (1983). Parental influences on children's eating behavior and relative weight. *Journal of Applied Behavior Analysis, 16*, 371–378.

Kovacs, M. (1981). Rating scales to assess depression in school-aged children. *Acta Paedopsychiatrica, 46*, 305–315.

Krug-Wispe, S. (1993). Nutritional assessment. In P.A. Queen & C.E. Lang (Eds.), *Handbook of pediatric nutrition* (pp. 26–82). Rockville, MD: Aspen Publishers, Inc.

Lamm, N., & Greer, R.D. (1988). Induction and maintenance of swallowing responses in infants with dysphagia. *Journal of Applied Behavior Analysis, 21*, 143–156.

Lazarus, R.S., & Folkman, S. (1989). *The Daily Hassles Scale*. Palo Alto, CA: Consulting Psychologists Press.

Lewis, J.A. (1982). Oral motor assessment and treatment of feeding difficulties. In P.J. Accardo (Ed.), *Failure to thrive in infancy and early childhood: A multidisciplinary team approach* (pp. 265–295). Baltimore: University Park Press.

Linscheid, T.R. (1988). The role of development and learning in feeding disorders. In D.E. Russo & J.H. Kedesdy (Eds.), *Behavioral medicine with the developmentally disabled* (pp. 43–48). New York: Plenum.

Linscheid, T.R. (1992). Eating problems in children. In C.E. Walker & M.C. Roberts (Eds.), *Handbook of clinical child psychology* (2nd ed., pp. 451–473). New York: John Wiley & Sons.

Linscheid, T.R., Budd, K.S., & Rasnake, L.K. (1995). Pediatric feeding disorders. In M.C. Roberts (Ed.), *Handbook of pediatric psychology* (2nd ed., pp. 501–515). New York: Guilford Press.

Linscheid, T.R., Oliver, J., Blyler, E., & Palmer, S. (1978). Brief hospitalization for the behavioral treatment of feeding problems in the developmentally disabled. *Journal of Pediatric Psychology, 3,* 72–76.

Linscheid, T.R., & Rasnake, L.K. (1985). Behavioral approaches to the treatment of failure to thrive. In D. Drotar (Ed.), *New directions in failure to thrive: Implications for research and practice* (pp. 279–294). New York: Plenum.

Luiselli, J.K. (1993). Training self-feeding skills in children who are deaf and blind. *Behavior Modification, 17,* 457–473.

Luiselli, J.K. (1994). Oral feeding treatment of children with chronic food refusal and multiple developmental disabilities. *American Journal on Mental Retardation, 98,* 646–655.

Macht, J. (1990). *Poor eaters: Helping children who refuse to eat.* New York: Plenum.

Madison, L.S., & Adubato, S.A. (1984). The elimination of ruminative vomiting in a 15-month-old child with gastroesophageal reflux. *Journal of Pediatric Psychology, 9,* 231–239.

Mash, E.J., & Terdal, L.G. (Eds.). (1997). *Assessment of childhood disorders* (3rd ed.). New York: Guilford Press.

Mathisen, B., Skuse, D., Wolke, D., & Reilly, S. (1989). Oral-motor dysfunction and failure to thrive among inner-city infants. *Developmental Medicine and Child Neurology, 31,* 293–302.

McCarthy, D.A. (1972). *Manual for the McCarthy Scales of Children's Abilities.* San Antonio, TX: The Psychological Corporation.

Milner, J.S. (1986). *The Child Abuse Potential Inventory manual* (2nd ed.). Webster, NC: Psytec.

Morris, S.E., & Klein, M.D. (1987). *Pre-feeding skills: A comprehensive resource for feeding development.* Tucson, AZ: Therapy Skill Builders.

Munk, D.D., & Repp, A.C. (1994). Behavioral assessment of feeding problems of individuals with severe disabilities. *Journal of Applied Behavior Analysis, 27,* 241–250.

National Live Stock and Meat Board. (1992). *A food guide for the first five years* [Brochure]. Chicago: Author, Educational Department.

O'Brien, S., Repp, A.C., Williams, G.E., & Christophersen, E.R. (1991). Pediatric feeding disorders. *Behavior Modification, 15,* 394–418.

Palmer, S. (1978). Nutrition and developmental disorders: An overview. In S. Palmer & S. Ekvall (Eds.), *Pediatric nutrition in developmental disorders* (pp. 21–24). Springfield, IL: Charles C Thomas.

Palmer, S., & Horn, S. (1978). Feeding problems in children. In S. Palmer & S. Ekvall (Eds.), *Pediatric nutrition in developmental disorders* (pp. 107–129). Springfield, IL: Charles C Thomas.

Palmer, S., Thompson, R.J., & Linscheid, T.R. (1975). Applied behavior analysis in the treatment of childhood feeding problems. *Developmental Medicine and Child Neurology, 17,* 333–339.

Piers, E.V. (1984). *Piers-Harris Children's Self-Concept Scale* (Rev. manual). Los Angeles: Western Psychological Services.

Pipes, P.L., Bumbalow, J., & Glass, R.P. (1993). Collecting and assessing food intake information. In P.L. Pipes & C.M. Trahms (Eds.), *Nutrition in infancy and childhood* (5th ed., pp. 59–86). St. Louis: C.V. Mosby.

Pipes, P.L., & Glass, R.P. (1993). Developmental disabilities and other special health care needs. In P.L. Pipes & C.M. Trahms (Eds.), *Nutrition in infancy and childhood* (5th ed., pp. 344–373). St. Louis: C.V. Mosby.

Queen, P.M. (1984). The evaluation of nutritional status. In R.B. Howard & H.S. Winter (Eds.), *Nutrition and feeding of infants and toddlers* (pp. 167–208). Boston: Little, Brown.

Reilly, S., Skuse, D., Mathisen, B., & Wolke, D. (1995). The objective rating of oral-motor functions during feeding. *Dysphagia, 10*, 177–191.

Reuter, J., & Bickett, L. (1985). *The Kent Infant Development Scale manual* (2nd ed.). Kent, OH: Kent Developmental Metrics.

Riordan, M.M., Iwata, B.A., Finney, J.W., Wohl, M.K., & Stanley, A.E. (1984). Behavioral assessment and treatment of chronic food refusal in handicapped children. *Journal of Applied Behavior Analysis, 17*, 327–341.

Sanders, M.R., Patel, R.K., Le Grice, B., & Shepherd, R.W. (1993). Children with persistent feeding difficulties: An observational analysis of the feeding interactions of problem and non-problem eaters. *Health Psychology, 12*, 64–73.

Schroeder, C.S., & Gordon, B.N. (1991). *Assessment and treatment of childhood problems: A clinician's guide.* New York: Guilford Press.

Skuse, D., Stevenson, J., Reilly, S., & Mathisen, B. (1995). Schedule for Oral-Motor Assessment (SOMA): Methods of validation. *Dysphagia, 10*, 192–202.

Spanier, G.B. (1989). *Dyadic Adjustment Scale: A manual.* North Tonawanda, NY: Multi-Health Systems.

Sparling, J.W., & Rogers, J.C. (1985). Feeding assessment: Development of a biopsychosocial instrument. *Occupational Therapy Journal of Research, 5*, 3–23.

Sparrow, S.S., Balla, D.A., & Cicchetti, D.V. (1984). *Vineland Adaptive Behavior Scales.* Circle Pines, MN: American Guidance Service.

Stark, L.J., Bowen, A.M., Tyc, V.L., Evans, S., & Passero, M.A. (1990). A behavioral approach to increasing calorie consumption in children with cystic fibrosis. *Journal of Pediatric Psychology, 15*, 309–326.

Stevenson, R.D. (1995). Feeding and nutrition in children with developmental disabilities. *Pediatric Annals, 24*, 255–260.

Stevenson, R.D., & Allaire, J.H. (1991). The development of normal feeding and swallowing. *Pediatric Clinics of North America, 38*, 1439–1453.

Thorndike, R.L., Hagen, E.P., & Sattler, J.M. (1986). *Guide for administering and scoring the Stanford-Binet Intelligence Scale* (4th ed.). Chicago: Riverside.

Turner, K.M.T., Sanders, M.R., & Wall, C.R. (1994). Behavioural parent training versus dietary education in the treatment of children with persistent feeding difficulties. *Behaviour Change, 11*, 242–258.

Walker, C.E., & Roberts, M.C. (Eds.). (1992). *Handbook of clinical child psychology* (2nd ed.). New York: John Wiley & Sons.

Walter, R.S. (1994). The multidisciplinary approach to management of swallowing disorders in the pediatric patient. In D.N. Tuchman & R.S. Walter (Eds.), *Disorders of feeding and swallowing in infants and children: Pathophysiology, diagnosis, and treatment* (pp. 251–257). San Diego: Singular.

Wechsler, D. (1991). *Wechsler Intelligence Scale for Children–Third edition manual.* San Antonio, TX: The Psychological Corporation.

Werle, M.A., Murphy, T.B., & Budd, K.S. (1993). Treating chronic food refusal in young children: Home-based parent training. *Journal of Applied Behavior Analysis, 26,* 421–433.

Woolston, J. (1985). Diagnostic classification: The current challenge in failure to thrive syndrome research. In D. Drotar (Ed.), *New directions in failure to thrive: Implications for research and practice* (pp. 225–233). New York: Plenum.

4

Environmental
Interventions in Feeding

An Overview

When assessment confirms that a feeding disorder exists, biomedical treatment and environmental intervention considerations become salient. Decisions regarding treatment or intervention include whether to proceed at the present time as well as options regarding where to intervene (e.g., in the clinic, in the hospital), how to involve caregivers, and which techniques to use. Biomedical treatments, reviewed in Chapter 2, focus on correcting physical defects or on reducing the impact of organic anomalies using techniques such as surgery, medication, or nutritional supplements. Environmental interventions focus on changing the conditions associated with feeding to influence ongoing behaviors. This chapter introduces the goals and basic features of environmental interventions, and Chapters 5–10 illustrate applications of these interventions to specific types of feeding problems.

Environmental feeding interventions cover a wide array of techniques employed by various disciplinary professionals. In practice, the interventions usually combine several components in a clinical protocol. This chapter organizes environmental interventions into five topical areas: 1) *meal characteristics* (i.e., provision of a developmentally appropriate menu and repeated exposure to varied foods and textures); 2) *schedule of intake* (i.e., frequency and duration of meals); 3) *setting characteristics* (i.e., physical surroundings, feeding position and body support, and activities preceding and following eating); 4) *interactions* (i.e., reciprocity between feeder and child, application of social contingencies using behavior management procedures); and 5) *other interventions* (i.e., nonnutritive sucking, adaptive feeding equipment).

This chapter begins with a discussion of preliminary intervention considerations and then describes the basic features and common ingredients of environmental interventions in the five areas

115

listed in the previous paragraph. Consistent with the behavioral theme of this book, the section on interaction-related interventions contains an overview of learning principles, from which behavior management procedures are derived.

PRELIMINARY INTERVENTION DECISIONS

Before feeding intervention begins, several clinical considerations need to be addressed. These considerations include assessing the feasibility of starting an intervention, determining where to conduct the intervention, and planning for involving the child's caregivers in the intervention.

Feasibility of Beginning Intervention

After initial assessment determines that a feeding disorder exists that is not maintained entirely by organic factors, environmental intervention is clearly an option. The decision to proceed with intervention, however, is not automatic in that an ill-timed or poorly conceived intervention may itself have iatrogenic effects (i.e., adverse consequences of intervention). The decision to proceed rests on consideration of pragmatic issues encompassed in three general questions:

1. Is feeding intervention medically necessary at this time?
2. Are the caregivers receptive to environmental intervention at the present time?
3. Are resources available for intervention to have a reasonable chance of success?

Medical Necessity of Intervention If the child's feeding problem is interfering with nutrient intake or calories required for physical and mental growth (i.e., the answer to the first question above is "yes"), then some form of intervention is medically necessary, in spite of other extenuating conditions. The location and form of intervention will be influenced by the child's particular disorder, as described in subsequent sections. Environmental intervention may be instituted in conjunction with a biomedical treatment, such as when a structured behavioral feeding program is carried out during the day along with non-oral nutritional supplements administered at night. If immediate intervention is not medically essential, then it is possible to consider the other two questions noted above.

Receptiveness of Caregivers Given the dyadic nature of feeding in young children, caregivers' attitudes about the feeding disorder are central to intervention selection. Parents may view a feeding problem as transitory, they may attribute it to causes that are different from those identified by the diagnostic team, or they may attribute the problem to causes that are not remediable by environmental approaches (cf. Sturm & Drotar, 1991). Some parents may fail to view their child's eating patterns or intake as a problem because it fits broadly within family norms, as in cases of childhood obesity. Because of the important role that caregivers play in children's feeding, their receptivity to intervention is a key prerequisite for an intervention's initiation and success.

The importance of parents' attitudes is illustrated by a family referred for assessment of their 3-year-old daughter's finicky eating habits (Werle, Murphy, & Budd, 1994).

■ ■ ■

CASE 4.1. Determining a Family's "Readiness-to-Change"
NAME: Nancy
AGE AT INTERVENTION: 3 years

Nancy's parents were recent immigrants to the United States, and because of language and cultural differences, it was difficult to obtain a thorough picture of their beliefs and feeding practices. According to her mother, Nancy ate approximately one meal or less per day. The meal consisted mostly of rice and meat; the remainder of Nancy's diet consisted of milk and fruit juices. Nancy had been diagnosed with failure to thrive (FTT), displayed little interest in food, frequently refused food, and had no consistent eating location or times. After two sessions with a feeding therapist, it became clear that the parents attributed their daughter's food refusal to ongoing asthma, which medical professionals had ruled out as an explanation. The parents resisted the therapist's suggestions that they interact differently with their daughter during meals, stating that the child was not feeling well and should not be expected to eat. For intervention to succeed, at least one parent, and preferably both parents, would have to have agreed that the child was experiencing a feeding problem and be open to some environmental change.

■ ■ ■

Motivation or "readiness" to engage in intervention is recognized as an important prerequisite for many forms of psychosocial intervention (Kanfer & Schefft, 1988; Prochaska & DiClemente,

1982, 1983). Prochaska and DiClemente (1982) conceptualized four stages of an individual's response to problems: contemplation, determination, action, and maintenance. They also described a fifth stage, *pre*contemplation, in which an individual and/or his or her family is unreceptive to help or denies the existence of problems (Prochaska & DiClemente, 1983). According to Prochaska and DiClemente's model, therapeutic strategies are more likely to succeed when they fit with an individual's and his or her family's current stage of "readiness-to-change."

Applying the readiness-to-change model to childhood feeding problems, one would expect that parents who acknowledge their child's feeding problem and are committed to change (which is reflective of Prochaska and DiClemente's contemplation and determination stages) would be more responsive to action-oriented intervention than parents who do not have these attributes. When parent attitudes or beliefs are not conducive to environmental change, these attitudes and beliefs could be addressed (e.g., through parent-focused counseling, psychotherapy, or educational information) as prerequisites to beginning feeding intervention.

Drotar, Wilson, and Sturm (1989), in discussing the importance of parent receptivity to intervention for children with FTT, emphasized the initial step of developing a working alliance with parents. They noted that clinicians must negotiate a relationship with caregivers rather than simply assume that a relationship exists. Steps that they suggested for facilitating a working alliance include discussing the potential complications that the child's feeding problems could have on later development, focusing on the benefits of parent involvement for the child's intervention, beginning intervention with problems that are of greater concern to the parents, and providing parents with options about the course of intervention. When parents remain unresponsive despite a therapist's best efforts, it may be prudent to withhold intervention and instead recommend monitoring the child's progress over a limited time period, after which the feasibility of intervention can be reassessed.

Availability of Resources The final issue pertinent to intervention decisions concerns the supporting conditions, which include knowledgeable feeding professionals, funding for intervention, and a minimally stable living environment for the child. The first two criteria vary with the type and locale of intervention (see next section on Inpatient versus Outpatient Intervention); the latter criterion, a minimally stable living environment, concerns the caregivers' ability to provide the child with the basic conditions to support change (e.g., safety, regular access to food, supervision of

meals). Feeding problems rarely are resolved in only one or two sessions, so it should be presumed that intervention will continue over
several sessions. The extent of intervention needed will vary with
the type and severity of problem, so it is important to assess
whether resources exist to continue intervention over a reasonable
period of time (at least five or six sessions and often longer) when
deciding whether to initiate intervention. (It should be noted that
before improvement occurs, it is not unusual for feeding patterns to
deteriorate temporarily at the early stages of intervention when familiar eating habits are disrupted.)

Outcome research on intervention for a wide array of child problems has implicated several family factors that predict poorer outcomes (Dumas & Wahler, 1983; Graziano & Diament, 1992; Jackson
& Sikora, 1992; Pekarik & Stephenson, 1988). Poverty, single-parent
status, marital conflict, a history of child abuse or neglect, parental
depression, and changing family circumstances (e.g., an impending
move, birth of a sibling) are among the factors associated with less
successful intervention outcomes. These factors, presumably, also
pose a risk in intervention for children with feeding disorders. In one
of few investigations of familial factors related to feeding interventions, low socioeconomic status and single parenthood were associated marginally with dropout from a behaviorally oriented intervention program for childhood obesity (Israel, Silverman, & Solotar,
1986). The mechanisms linking such family conditions with intervention outcome are not clear; however, it seems likely that they—
directly or indirectly—limit parents' emotional, financial, and/or
time resources for compensatory child care activities.

Thus, in planning feeding interventions, it is important to consider caregivers' understanding of the problem, their motivation to
obtain help, and the resources available to make intervention feasible. Choices about the type of intervention (e.g., nutritional counseling, occupational therapy, behavior management) are influenced
by the nature of the feeding problem, in conjunction with considerations about the family's ability to use various intervention options.
Family circumstances may indicate a need to offer broader support
services as part of feeding intervention. These services may include
home visits; individual, couples, or family therapy; service coordination; advocacy; respite care; or assistance with other family needs
(Alderette & deGraffenried, 1986; Chatoor, Conley, & Dickson,
1988; Drotar, 1995; Graves, Meyers, & Clark, 1988). If family stressors appear highly likely to interfere with feeding intervention, support services should be considered in place of, or as a precursor to,
intervention. The negative consequences of dropping out of inter-

vention prematurely may outweigh the consequences of postponing the start of intervention, and thus discretion in initiating intervention is advised. If professionals have serious concerns about a family's ability to protect the health and welfare of a child with feeding problems, the family will need to be referred to protective services agencies (Drotar, 1995).

Inpatient versus Outpatient Intervention

Assuming that intervention is to proceed, a basic decision concerns *where* to provide intervention. In addition to clinical considerations about the merits of inpatient versus outpatient services, economic realities of the health care industry in the late 1990s exert a major influence on the availability of intervention options.

Linscheid and his colleagues (Linscheid, Oliver, Blyler, & Palmer, 1978; Linscheid & Rasnake, 1985) offered guidelines for evaluating when it may be beneficial to hospitalize a child for feeding intervention. These guidelines are summarized in Table 4.1 along with other related considerations (cf. Frank, 1995). Criteria

Table 4.1.   Criteria for considering inpatient feeding intervention

CHILD AND FAMILY CHARACTERISTICS

Child's feeding disorder is sufficiently severe that it interferes with intake of calories and nutrients needed for physical and mental growth.

Child's weight or height has dropped dramatically, is below the 5th percentile, or is being maintained through food supplements.

Mealtime relationship between caregiver and child is continually being jeopardized and/or is generalizing to other parent–child activities.

Evidence exists for the risk of, or occurrence of, nonaccidental trauma, severe neglect, or conspicuous parental incompetence.

Caregivers are willing to participate in hospital treatment and able to benefit from modeling and training in order to follow through on intervention techniques at home.

Child is already hospitalized for evaluation or treatment of another condition and has stabilized medically.

Previous outpatient feeding intervention has failed.

Family resides too far from trained feeding professionals to make regular outpatient intervention sessions feasible.

HOSPITAL CHARACTERISTICS

Trained feeding therapists are available to conduct and supervise the entire inpatient treatment; ideally, this entails having one to three therapists take full responsibility for feeding treatment to provide consistent coverage.

Resources are available to continue intervention and train caregivers over a period of 1–6 weeks or until feeding improves significantly.

Note: Criteria adapted from Frank (1995), Linscheid et al. (1978), and Linscheid and Rasnake (1985).

proposed by Linscheid and his colleagues focus on the severity of the disorder, the extent to which it interferes with the parent–child relationship, and the caregivers' willingness to participate in the intervention while the child is hospitalized. The guidelines also emphasize the need for a stable team of trained feeding therapists who can consistently implement the intervention on the inpatient ward. Other rationales for hospitalization included in Table 4.1 relate to evidence of serious deficiencies in parental competence, that the child is already hospitalized for a concurrent illness, that prior outpatient feeding treatment or intervention has failed, or that no outpatient services are available within commuting distance of the family's residence.

For each referral, the intervention team must weigh the relative merits of inpatient versus outpatient feeding interventions. Assuming that trained feeding staff are available in the hospital, inpatient treatment offers several potential advantages in terms of greater access to professional help, around-the-clock programming, and ease for parents (Linscheid, Budd, & Rasnake, 1995). Changes, presumably, can be accomplished more quickly when children are hospitalized because greater control is available over who feeds the child; over interactions during meals; and over the schedule, amount, and types of foods offered (Blackman & Nelson, 1985, 1987).

The potential advantages of inpatient intervention, however, need to be weighed against the greater intrusiveness, cost, and artificiality of an inpatient approach as compared with outpatient services. Hospitalization is a significant and often traumatic event for a child that entails separation from family, disruption in child care routines, and loss of familiar experiences (Siegel & Hudson, 1992). Hospitalization also carries an increased risk that the child will be exposed to infections, which can undermine the feeding treatment. Outpatient intervention, by contrast, is far less intrusive and offers greater flexibility for individualizing many clinical aspects of care; for example, the frequency of sessions, the specific professionals involved, and the methods for involving family members can be adapted to an individual family.

Spiraling health care costs mark economics as a decisive factor in many biomedical treatment and environmental intervention deliberations. Bed charges alone on a children's medical ward run approximately $700 per day, to which must be added costs for diagnostic tests and professional therapy (J. Lavigne, personal communication, December 9, 1996). By comparison, outpatient services, which cost $100–$250 per visit, are considerably less expensive. In the late-1990s health care environment, a hospital cannot justify keeping a child long enough to complete a feeding intervention program (e.g., 1–3 weeks) in the absence of other significant medical conditions. Thus, with the exception of a few specialized inpatient feeding units (e.g., Ahearn, Kerwin, Eicher, Shantz, & Swearingin, 1996; Babbitt et al., 1994), hospitalization for feeding problems may not be an option, even when it is viewed as the most therapeutic choice.

Variations on conventional inpatient intervention or treatment are possible in some cases. Brief inpatient treatment, with continued service on an outpatient basis, has been proposed for iatrogenically induced feeding problems, such as those secondary to ventilator support or medical procedures (Ginsberg, 1988). When children do merit admission to inpatient services for feeding problems (for one or more reasons listed in Table 4.1), they may stay only 1–3 days, which is long enough to complete a medical workup, insert a feeding tube, and arrange for caregivers or home health services to carry out supplemental nutrition procedures upon discharge.

Intervention by home health professionals offers a potentially cost-efficient alternative to inpatient treatment. In this model, home health providers plan, introduce, and monitor a feeding program that is implemented by caregivers. Travel time increases the cost of in-home over outpatient visits by a factor of two to three times, but the cost savings of home visits over inpatient fees are still dramatic. The benefits of home visits would be even more compelling if technicians could fill this role under the supervision of professional therapists because home health technicians could provide the service more economically. At present, few clinical feeding programs offer home-based services; however, home-based approaches have been used in applied research (Black, Dubowitz, Hutcheson, Berenson-Howard, & Starr, 1995; Drotar et al., 1985; Werle, Murphy, & Budd, 1993, in press).

The artificiality of an inpatient ward also should be considered in deciding between outpatient and inpatient intervention. From a behavioral standpoint, the ultimate test of effective intervention is the extent to which improved feeding patterns *generalize* (i.e., carry over to conditions beyond those in which training occurs [Stokes & Baer, 1977]). Studies examining the generality of effects following inpatient or outpatient feeding programs have yet to be conducted. Research in other areas indicates that generalization is facilitated by increasing the similarity of stimulus conditions (e.g., people, materials, physical setting) between the training environment and criterion environment (i.e., the eventual location at which behavior change is desired). In addition, transfer (i.e., generalization) can be actively promoted through techniques such as arranging for diversity in training experiences, using naturally occurring reinforcers, and involving family members in intervention (Horner, Dunlap, & Koegel, 1988). Some of these conditions are more amenable to outpatient than inpatient approaches, although outpatient approaches per se do not ensure greater generalization.

In summary, the decision regarding where to intervene should be guided by a combination of service priorities and available health care options. The decision includes determining the location that fits best with the child's health needs and with the family's resources, that is most economically responsible, and that is able to make a significant impact in the child's everyday feeding environment. In the health care climate of the late 1990s, feeding intervention is most likely to occur on an outpatient basis unless clear medical need justifies inpatient services.

Involving Parents as Therapists

The foregoing reference to generalization as an important measure of successful outcome sets the stage for discussion of the role of caregivers in the intervention process. Although it might seem logical that behavior change that is achieved in a hospital or outpatient setting with a therapist would carry over to other environments, the preponderance of research with a diverse range of problems confirms that—in the absence of deliberate efforts—generalization across settings or people is not the rule (Horner et al., 1988; Stokes & Baer, 1977). Likewise, feeding intervention reports occasionally note limitations in the generalization of intervention beyond the training setting (e.g., Babbitt et al., 1994; MacArthur, Ballard, & Artinian, 1986). This is not to say that generalization will not occur but rather that it may be incomplete, transitory, and unpredictable. As Chapter 1 discusses, well-established behavior habits are by nature difficult to change unless the controlling environmental conditions change as well. Thus, for intervention to be successful for children, parents are the key individuals who must change *their* behavior within the criterion environment. Training of parents provides an important connecting link between therapeutic and natural environments.

Thirty years of applied research has contributed data that support the value of a parent training model for modifying diverse child problems (Briesmeister & Schaefer, 1998; Dangel & Polster, 1984; Graziano & Diament, 1992; Lewis & Drabman, 1988; O'Dell, 1985; Schaefer & Briesmeister, 1989). Parents are consistently accessible in children's everyday lives, are major sources of affective and social influence on children, and permit intervention procedures to be individualized to the family's own needs. Feeding specialists often have stressed the importance of including parents in the treatment process (e.g., Bernal, 1972; Drotar et al., 1989; Iwata, Riordan, Wohl, & Finney, 1982; Sanders, Patel, Le Grice, & Shepherd, 1993). Yet in clinical practice, environmental interventions for feeding disorders rarely include *systematic parent training* procedures. Instead, it is as if clinicians view training parents as analogous to writing a pharmaceutical prescription—the parent is given a list of intervention recommendations (e.g., regarding feeding schedules, interaction techniques, menus) on the assumption that they will competently carry them out. Systematic parent training (e.g., use of written training curricula, use of modeling and behavioral rehearsal procedures, use of competency-based assessment of progress) is not the norm in feeding intervention.

Studies that have involved parents in feeding intervention suggest several different training models. In inpatient intervention, parents typically begin by observing a therapist feeding the child and gradually take over more responsibility for feeding after the child begins to show improvement (e.g., Ahearn et al., 1996; Linscheid, Tarnowski, Rasnake, & Brams, 1987; Ramsay & Zelazo, 1988). The model of eventual parent involvement also has been used in outpatient (e.g., Thompson & Palmer, 1974; Thompson, Palmer, & Linscheid, 1977) and school-based feeding interventions (Ives, Harris, & Wolchik, 1978) for behavioral feeding problems. In other models, parents may serve as the primary therapists, in which they receive instructions and guidance from clinicians in how to carry out the treatment procedures themselves (e.g., Madison & Adubato, 1984; Turner, Sanders, & Wall, 1994; Werle et al., 1993, in press).

Feeding intervention involving older children typically consists of sessions directed toward the youth, with concomitant training (either jointly or separately) for parents. The concomitant training model is exemplified in programs to increase caloric intake in children with cystic fibrosis (Stark, Bowen, Tyc, Evans, & Passero, 1990; Stark, Powers, Jelalian, Rape, & Miller, 1994), to decrease food phobia following incidents of choking (Chatoor et al., 1988), and to achieve weight loss (Epstein, Valoski, Wing, & McCurley, 1994; Epstein & Wing, 1987). Reviews of the obesity intervention literature support active parent involvement as a factor contributing to long-term success in weight reduction (Epstein et al., 1994; Kirschenbaum, 1987; Silverman & Israel, 1987). Although the methods of parent training vary, there can be little doubt that systematic parent training enhances the overall positive impact of feeding intervention. Examples of interventions involving parents are included throughout succeeding chapters.

MAJOR AREAS OF FEEDING INTERVENTIONS

Given the range of techniques available for environmental feeding interventions, the selection of intervention strategies for an individual case is based on a combination of factors. These factors include the nature and severity of a child's feeding problem, environmental conditions hypothesized to maintain the problem, the child's developmental and physical capabilities, the acceptability of various procedures to caregivers, previous biomedical treatments and environmental interventions attempted, and areas of professional expertise by the therapist(s). Chapter 3 describes methods of assessing many of these factors. In practice, a clinical protocol usually includes multiple components in an attempt to maximize the effectiveness of treatment and intervention.

This chapter organizes environmental interventions into five major areas, as outlined at the beginning of the chapter: 1) *meal characteristics*, 2) *schedule of intake*, 3) *setting characteristics*, 4) *interactions*, and 5) *other interventions*. Table 4.2 lists examples of intervention procedures in each area, which are described in more detail in the remainder of the chapter.

Meal Characteristics

A fundamental goal of feeding is to provide sufficient calories and nutrients to support growth within normal limits. Interventions focusing on meal characteristics are used when there is evidence of nutritionally inappropriate intake, such as too many or too few calories consumed per day; an unbalanced array of minerals and vitamins; or developmentally inappropriate foods. Meal-related interventions also may be warranted when the diet is sufficiently unusual or restrictive that it results in the child's exclusion from major social eating opportunities, such as failing to eat meals at school or with family members because of finicky eating habits. Two types of meal-related interventions are described in the following paragraphs: 1) developmentally appropriate menus and 2) repeated exposure to new foods and to varied textures.

Developmentally Appropriate Menus Christophersen and Hall (1978), Pipes and Trahms (1993), Satter (1986, 1987), and others have described several general guidelines regarding developmentally appropriate types, quantities, and varieties of food for children at different ages. The guidelines are based on nutritional science

Table 4.2. Sample techniques in major areas of environmental intervention for children's feeding disorders

Topical areas	Sample techniques
Meal characteristics	Offer developmentally appropriate menu (e.g., adjust portion sizes to child).
	Repeatedly offer a new or less preferred food as part of meal.
Schedule of intake	Alter frequency of meals to promote appetite.
	Limit meal length to 10–25 minutes, depending on child's cooperation.
Setting characteristics	Reduce environmental distractors (e.g., television, toys) during feeding.
	Seat child in supported position for meals.
Interactions	Attend and respond to child's hunger and satiety cues.
	Provide pleasant social attention when child is cooperative, and ignore child briefly when disruptive or resistant.
Other interventions	Offer pacifier for nonnutritive sucking during non-oral feedings.
	Provide adaptive eating utensils to facilitate independent feeding skills.

knowledge regarding children's health, dietary needs, and capabilities at different stages of physical maturation, as well as on cultural practices and norms. The guidelines provide a useful starting point for planning meal-related interventions for children who deviate notably from recommended patterns.

The types of foods that children can ingest change greatly across the infant and toddler years. For example, infants should receive breast milk or regular-strength infant formula rather than cow's milk. Semisolid foods are not recommended until around 4–6 months of age, when the child can sit with a support. Iron-fortified cereal is suggested as a first food because of its smooth texture, bland taste, and high nutrient content. Between 6 and 8 months, cooked or soft fruits and vegetables (mashed or chopped) are appropriate, as are finger breads and cereals. Between 9 and 12 months, the child gradually progresses to table foods (e.g., mashed, unseasoned versions of foods served to other family members). For children under age 3, parents are cautioned to avoid serving hard foods or foods on which the child could aspirate, including hot dogs, nuts, grapes, carrots, and round candies. Foods high in salt and sugar should be offered in moderation, as should high-fat foods (e.g., chips and other "junk" foods) without nutritional value (Pipes & Trahms, 1993).

Developmental guidelines also address portion size, food variety, and palatability. To encourage a child to consume a balanced diet, it often is recommended that caregivers offer small portions of various nutritious foods and permit the child to determine what and how much of these items he or she chooses to eat. Parents can capitalize on the emergence of self-feeding skills—normally in the latter half of the first year—by offering finger foods and semisolid items (e.g., yogurt) that can be eaten with a spoon. As chewing skills are developing, meats are easier to handle in bite-size pieces or in ground textures, and small pieces of fruits or vegetables without condiments can be served as finger foods. Toddlers often are more receptive to foods served at room temperature, to foods that are soft and moist, and to foods without strong flavors. Satter (1986) noted that, as a general rule, servings for a preschool-age child are one quarter to one third the size of an adult portion, or approximately 1 tablespoon per year of the child's age.

Many interventions for feeding disorders contain a component directed at offering a developmentally appropriate menu within the treatment recommendations. Providing parents with normative guidelines on children's nutrition constitutes a mild form of preventive or early intervention. Specific educational suggestions (Satter, 1986, 1987) relate to appropriate serving sizes, food choices for introducing new textures, attractive ways to prepare vegetables or other less-preferred items, or nutritional alternatives for nonpreferred foods (e.g., high-protein substitutes for meat, high-calcium substitutes for milk). Caregivers also may benefit from training in food purchasing, budgeting, and using leftovers.

Turner et al. (1994) empirically evaluated the effectiveness of two clinic-based interventions with parents of young children with persistent feeding problems. Turner et al. (1994) compared dietary education (e.g., regarding basic food groups and nutrient requirements, portion sizes, and healthy eating guidelines) and behavioral parent training (e.g., training in child management strategies). Observational data on parent–child interactions, dietary intake records, and growth measures indicated that both dietary education and behavioral parent training were effective in significantly improving feeding patterns, although behavioral parent training resulted in more positive parent–child interactions and was preferred by parents.

Clinicians serving children with nonorganic failure to thrive (NFTT) often encounter parents who have inadequate knowledge about appropriate nutrition. Parents may deliberately overfeed or underfeed children secondary to incorrect beliefs about children's nutritional needs (Pugliese, Weyman-Daum, Moses, & Lifshitz, 1987). Other parents may offer an overly narrow range of foods to support a balanced diet. One parent whom the authors evaluated fed her toddler bologna sandwiches on white bread each day for lunch and fed the toddler a limited array of offerings at other meals, resulting in a diet that was high in sodium and deficient in several vitamins. The child displayed little difficulty with or resistance to eating other foods when offered, which suggested that the child's restricted diet resulted from the mother's inadequate nutrition knowledge. In such instances, intervention should focus on educating parents in the provision of a more varied and balanced diet.

Repeated Exposure to New Foods and Varied Textures   It is apparently quite common for children by the age of 2 years to exhibit neophobia, a preference for familiar foods over novel foods (Birch, 1990). Temporary neophobia is considered an adaptive response, in that unfamiliar foods (as well as nonfood items such as dirt or paint) may be dangerous and should be approached with caution. Parents, however, often interpret a child's initial rejection of an unfamiliar food as reflecting a permanent dislike for the food or as reflecting an allergic reaction to it. Parents respond by removing the item from the child's diet, thereby failing to broaden the variety of foods that the child will accept. In fact, parents so naturally modify their food offerings based on their perceptions of the food's palatability to the child that they may be unaware that they have dropped certain food categories (e.g., vegetables, fish, new fruits) from the child's diet.

The implications of neophobia and parents' common responses to it are especially pertinent to young children with ongoing feeding problems. In addition to not offering previously rejected foods, parents often fail to experiment with new foods, assuming that new foods would only result in food battles. One simple but fundamental technique for countering a child's resistance to new or unfamiliar foods is to repeatedly offer the foods by placing them on the child's plate, even though the child may not be required to eat them. This practice ensures that the child continues to have the opportunity to try the items and will have the opportunity to see them as part of a typical menu.

Birch and Marlin (1982) demonstrated the usefulness of the food presentation technique, which they called repeated exposure, in increasing children's receptivity to foods through repeated tastings. They presented typical 2- to 5-year-olds with one of three versions of an initially novel food (sweetened, salty, or plain tofu). Preferences for the novel food increased markedly after approximately 10 exposures, regardless of whether it was sweet, salty, or plain (Birch & Marlin, 1982). In subsequent research, Birch and colleagues found that children must actually taste the new foods to change preference judgments, rather than simply see or smell the foods (Birch, McPhee, Shoba, Pirok, & Steinberg, 1987).

Analogous to the role of repeated exposure in shaping children's acceptance of new *types* of foods is the presumed importance of experience with respect to food *textures*. Researchers have hypothesized that a *critical or sensitive period* for texture acceptance occurs at around 7–10 months of age, such that children who are not exposed to coarse textures during this period are likely to demonstrate selective refusal of higher textures later. Illingworth and Lister (1964) initially applied this hypothesis to feeding based on clinical observations of children who were medically restricted from eating orally during much of their first years of life. These children thereafter persistently resisted oral intake even after medical problems had been resolved. Additional case reports (e.g., Handen, Mandell, & Russo, 1986; Linscheid & Rasnake, 1985) describe texture sensitivity in children whose medical condition restricted intake during this age period.

The period hypothesis, derived from experimental research on learning processes, has been invoked to explain various instances in which animals or humans show a greater propensity to learn particular phenomena at certain stages of the life cycle than at others. The term *critical period* implies that there is a limited "window of opportunity" for learning, whereas the term *sensitive period* refers to a relatively greater ease or speed of learning during the stage. In the absence of firm data supporting a defined period in which acquisition must take place, the latter term seems more appropriate. One classic example of sensitive periods studied in the animal literature is imprinting, whereby young birds learn to respond socially to a certain class of species, usually their own species (Bateson, 1969). Whereas some researchers have attempted to explain sensitive periods as a purely maturational phenomenon, Bateson's (1969) experiments on imprinting demonstrate the important role of experiences. He showed that organisms develop a preference for conspicuous stimuli as a result of direct, repeated exposure to the conspicuous stimuli and differential consequences and that the timing of this effect could be modified by experimentally manipulating the organisms' exposure to familiar and unfamiliar stimuli.

Extrapolating from experimental research on sensitive periods, it appears that repeated exposure to foods of differing textures is an integral component of developing broad texture preferences. Feeding professionals generally recommend that children receive increasingly textured foods across the latter half of the first year of life, in keeping with developmental guidelines. When texture resistance is encountered in the absence of organic impediments, intervention typically includes gradual but persistent exposure to higher (i.e., coarser) textures (Linscheid et al., 1987; Luiselli, 1994). Christophersen and Hall (1978) cautioned against "backtracking" (i.e., reverting to lower textures) after a child is developmentally ready for higher textures, despite a child's reluctance or initial refusal to accept them. As they noted, health care providers should advise parents that some choking may occur with solid foods, and parents should be shown how to remove particles from a child's mouth.

Provision of a nutritionally balanced, varied, and developmentally appropriate diet sets the stage for a child to form adaptive feeding habits. The timing of a child's intake is considered next.

Schedule of Intake

Because appetite is conditioned by a combination of biological and environmental variables, manipulation of the feeding schedule constitutes one of the most powerful forms of external control available for modifying feeding patterns. By systematically controlling when and how often food is offered, the caregiver can influence a child's appetite. Two major areas of schedule-based interventions relate to the frequency and to the duration of meals.

Frequency of Meals   Just as the types of foods that children consume change dramatically across the first year of life, so does the schedule of intake. Newborns typically eat seven to eight times per day at intervals of 2–4 hours (Pipes & Trahms, 1993). By 2 months of age, intake typically has dropped to five to seven times per day and by 6 months to three meals and four milk feedings per day. As opposed to rigid feeding schedules recommended in the 1950s and 1960s, practice in the 1990s supports the idea of a flexible, demand-feeding schedule (i.e., feeding the infant when he or she is hungry) with most infants (Satter, 1986). As solid foods are introduced in the latter half of a child's first year, the schedule of intake typically decreases to three meals interspersed with one to three light snacks per day. Although children show a good deal of individual variation in appetite, a period of 3–4 hours between meals appears optimal for appetite regulation (Pipes & Trahms, 1993). This time interval results in positive sensations in anticipation of food (presumably through conditioning of pleasant experiences associated with eating and physiological receptivity to food) without the physical discomfort of extreme hunger (Lowenberg, 1993).

In conjunction with the schedule of intake, caloric density and desirability of foods offered also affect appetite. Birch's (1990) research with preschoolers has demonstrated that children compensate for prior high-calorie eating by consuming fewer calories and restricting consumption to preferred foods at the next eating occasion. Thus, interventions directed at the feeding schedule need to control not only *when* but also *what* and *how much* food is offered as part of the intervention protocol.

Schedule interventions for children with irregular appetite or selective eating habits generally involve offering meals and snacks on a consistent schedule from day to day and limiting intake between planned eating occasions (Bernal, 1972; Hatcher, 1979; Linscheid & Rasnake, 1985). To encourage intake of an array of foods, only a small amount of preferred food is offered, at least until after nonpreferred foods are consumed at the meal. Snacks ideally consist of high-nutrient items (e.g., fruits, vegetables, crackers), new foods, or leftovers from the previous meal. Caregivers need to be advised on how to handle nighttime awakenings or other occasions when the child formerly received food or drink. For example, caregivers may be counseled to gradually reduce breast-feedings, eliminate food snacks within 1 hour of meals, and/or offer water or low-calorie liquids instead.

As with other interventions to be implemented by parents, it is important to anticipate problems that may arise and to discuss possible solutions as part of training. Parents often need guidance regarding how long their child can safely forego food if the child initially refuses to eat at scheduled times. Will the child's health tolerate a trial period of as long as 2–3 days without a regular meal, or is more frequent nourishment medically indicated? It is expected that major deviations in the child's intake patterns will be temporary, and it is essential that intervention be carefully monitored by feeding professionals.

If a child has little or no recent experience with oral intake as a result of medical complications, a modified feeding schedule may be more appropriate as an initial intervention strategy. A "mini-meal" format (Azrin & Armstrong, 1973), in which the child is offered a few bites of food 15–20 times across the day, is one option. This schedule gives the child many opportunities to practice food acceptance, without prolonging aversive experiences or satiating the child's appetite. A smaller number of feedings (e.g., 8–10 mini-meals) can be accommodated to the caregiver's schedule. The number of eating occasions is gradually reduced as the child begins to accept food, eventually approximating a typical feeding schedule.

Schedule manipulation also is an integral component of interventions to wean children off non-oral feeding regimens (Handen et al., 1986; Linscheid et al., 1987; Wolf & Glass, 1992). The timing of both the artificial supplement and oral food offerings must be coordinated as part of intervention. When the child's medical condition is stabilized, non-oral supplements often are administered at night or occur 30–60 minutes after oral feeding sessions, to reduce their impact on the child's appetite during oral feedings.

Schedule manipulations also are used in interventions to decrease excessive food intake. Children who are obese often are taught to restrict eating to consistent, planned times within weight reduction programs (Epstein & Wing, 1987). Children are taught to self-monitor (with parent assistance as needed) when and what they eat as one aspect of intervention.

Duration of Meals Meal length is frequently mentioned in clinical descriptions as relevant in evaluating the appropriateness of feeding patterns (Gisel & Patrick, 1988; Linscheid & Rasnake, 1985; Macht, 1990). Clinicians generally recommend that mealtimes for children last between 10 and 25 minutes (or up to 45 minutes for children with physical impairments affecting eating). Within this time frame, longer meals are more likely to be appropriate for children who are able to feed themselves or when mealtimes include other people with whom the child socializes during meals. For children with oral-motor or fine motor impairments, sufficient time is important to facilitate coordination of feeding skills and to reduce fatigue.

Short mealtimes (e.g., shorter than 10 minutes) have been viewed as indicating that the child is being fed in a brusque manner, is rushing through the meal, or is not hungry. Mathisen, Skuse, Wolke, and Reilly (1989) observed parent–child interactions during meals at home for a group of children with NFTT and for a demographically matched control sample. They found substantially shorter meals for NFTT children (mean of 8.5 minutes versus 21 minutes for the control sample). These findings were interpreted to suggest that NFTT children were not receiving sufficient encouragement and social attention for eating.

Long mealtimes (e.g., longer than 20–30 minutes) have been used as a diagnostic sign of a behavioral feeding problem, suggesting that parents are prolonging meals past a constructive point (Linscheid & Rasnake, 1985). To further investigate this issue, Li, Murphy, Werle, and Budd (1993) analyzed patterns of food acceptances (e.g., feeding oneself a bite, taking a bite offered by the feeder) and refusals (e.g., rejecting offered food, saying "no" when instructed to eat, throwing food) across successive minutes of home mealtimes in four preschool-age children undergoing behavioral parent training for selective food refusal. In three cases, Li and colleagues (1993) found a drop in the pace of acceptances at a fairly consistent point across sessions, suggesting that an optimal meal length (ranging between 18 and 25 minutes for individual children) could be determined by observing acceptance patterns. It is interesting to note that they found that the pace of food refusals, which was expected to increase as mealtimes progressed, remained low or even decreased across successive minutes of meals. Parents were allowed to present food as they chose, so the observed pattern of food refusals may be due in part to a reduced rate of food offers by the parents later in meals. Nevertheless, the findings suggest that food refusals may not be a useful indicator of when meals should end, at least for children with selective eating habits.

Interventions to reduce excessive meal length include setting a timer or marking where the hands of a clock will be at the end of the meal to provide a visual reminder of when mealtimes will be over (Linscheid et al., 1987; Luiselli, Evans, & Boyce, 1985). Extended food battles can be avoided by terminating the meal based on the child's behavior, such as ending the meal when the child indicates that he or she is finished or when he or she begins to engage in disruptive behavior. To avoid inadvertently reinforcing disruptive behavior, however, the child should be excused contingent on cooperative (as opposed to oppositional) mealtime behavior. Cooperative responses to be requested could include eating one to two more bites, wiping one's hands on a napkin, or complying with a simple parental request. Once the meal is ended, it is important that caregivers not provide children with dessert, leftovers, or other snacks for a period of at least 1–2 hours, in order to establish a clear discrimination between eating and noneating occasions.

Although clinical interventions for meal length frequently target children with undereating or food selectivity problems, procedures also have been designed to extend meal length in cases of overly rapid eating. Kirschenbaum (1987) noted that children who are obese tend to exhibit a "high-density eating style" characterized by eating quickly, taking big spoonfuls of food, and gulping food by chewing relatively little before swallowing. Similar eating habits often are reported in children with moderate to severe mental retardation (Sisson & Van Hasselt, 1989). Intervention goals for overly rapid eating include deliberate elongation of the eating chain, in which a child is taught to set down the fork or spoon after each bite to slow the rate of food intake (Knapczyk, 1983). Children who tend to "pack" food in their mouths rather than swallow it, or those with choking problems, often are prompted to chew and swallow each bite or to take a drink of liquid between bites, thereby extending meal length.

Setting Characteristics

In addition to meal composition and scheduling characteristics, the setting in which eating occurs exerts an influence over intake. Relevant aspects of the physical setting include the immediate surroundings of the eating area and the child's position and body support during meals. Activity-related characteristics include events preceding or following meals. Setting characteristics may have a direct impact on the feeding environment, and/or they may affect feeding through a history of being paired with a child's learning experiences. In behavioral terms, these paired setting events are described as exerting *stimulus control* over feeding behavior (Bijou, 1993; Bijou & Baer, 1965; Wahler & Hann, 1986). For example, a young girl who typically is fed in a high chair learns to associate the high chair with eating. The chair provides a confined, supported location for the child to eat, but it also constitutes a salient cue for eating because it has been paired repeatedly with feeding. Based on these experiences, the child expects that she will be fed when put in the high chair, and she may go to the high chair when she is hungry to communicate her readiness to eat.

Setting characteristics can exert facilitative or detrimental effects on children's behavior (Rogers-Warren & Warren, 1977; Wahler & Hann, 1986). Little research has investigated setting variables associated with feeding disorders, and therapists rarely get a first-hand look at the child's home feeding environment to pinpoint potential setting problems. A few studies (Drotar, Eckerle, Satola, Pallotta, & Wyatt, 1990; Mathisen et al., 1989), however, have investigated naturalistic feeding environments. These studies, together with the clinical advice of experienced feeding therapists, suggest several potentially important attributes of the feeding setting—physical surroundings, feeding position and body support, and activities preceding and following eating.

Physical Surroundings of Eating A facilitative physical context for feeding depends on the nature of feeding problems. If a child is resistant to virtually all oral foods or has severe attention deficits, a solitary location devoid of visual or auditory distractions may be most conducive to eating (e.g., Handen et al., 1986). For other feeding problems, an environment that permits the child to concentrate on eating and yet includes some attractive features may make mealtimes more pleasant. Caregivers of finicky eaters typically are advised to serve meals in a consistent eating area (e.g., kitchen, dining room), to restrict the people present to those who are eating, and to allow toys or activities (e.g., Peekaboo, television) only if they do not disrupt eating. In addition, clinicians intervening with children who are underweight or with selective eaters often recommend limiting the number of feeders—especially early in intervention—to one or two people who are trained in the feeding procedures (e.g., Linscheid et al., 1987).

Arranging the child's physical environment so that it is conducive to eating makes intuitive sense from a clinical perspective; however, studies examining environmental differences between problem and nonproblem feeders reveal inconsistent results. For example, Drotar and colleagues (1990) found no differences among environmental characteristics such as noise level, number of people present, and mealtime distractions in homes of children with FTT and in homes of comparison children with normal growth. These findings are in contrast to the findings of Mathisen et al. (1989), who reported that infants with FTT were more often fed in a living room than in a kitchen or dining area, and they less often sat in a high chair than did comparison children with normal growth.

The concept of stimulus control with regard to feeding environments also applies to intervention for overeating (Epstein & Wing, 1987). It is recommended that children who are overweight eat in a defined location (e.g., a kitchen table) and avoid eating while engaging in other activities. Eating is discouraged while watching television, reading, or playing games because of the difficulty restricting the amount eaten at these times and because the practice strengthens the association between leisure activities and food intake.

Feeding Position and Body Support A secure, well-balanced posture during meals enhances a child's motor coordination and attention to feeding. The standard feeding position for infants is to be cradled in a caregiver's arms or to be held securely on the caregiver's lap. Older children typically are seated upright in a chair or high chair, which allows maximal use of the hands for self-feeding and reduces the likelihood of choking. Parents of a child with inadequate intake often allow their child to eat in many different positions (e.g., held atop a counter, seated on the floor or in the parent's lap, wandering around the room). As part of intervention, these parents often are told to seat the child securely for meals.

Muscle tone and posture are interrelated with a child's state, physiological control, and oral-motor coordination (Lewis, 1982; Wolf & Glass, 1992). Children with physical disabilities often need modifications in feeding positions to provide for optimal alignment of head, neck, and trunk. For a child with swallowing difficulties, it is important that the head remain upright or slightly flexed forward (5–10 degrees) to guard against aspirating food. Atypical tone and persistent underdeveloped reflexes accompanying cerebral palsy make it difficult for the feeder to control an infant in one's arms during feeding. Instead, it may be recommended that the child be placed on a pillow or infant seat that is propped against a table edge and supported on the feeder's lap. The goal of positioning is to provide postural control in a manner so that the child does not resort to abnormal postures (e.g., head hyperextension, shoulder retraction) to compensate for lack of control (Lewis, 1982; Morris & Klein, 1987).

Activities Preceding and Following Eating The type of activity immediately preceding meals may influence children's behavior during mealtimes, particularly when the reinforcement attributes of the prefeeding period contrast with those during feeding. For example, premeal activities that are fast paced and stimulating or those that provide high-rate adult attention may result in uncooperative behavior by the child during meals as a function of the shift from a rewarding activity to one with fewer reinforcers. Likewise, routinely providing a preferred activity immediately after meals could result in a child's rushing through the meal or failing to eat the recommended amount.

Little research has directly examined the effects of pre- or postmeal activities for children with feeding problems. Research in other areas, however, has shown that the sequence of activities influences children's on-task behavior, sleep routines, and other behavior patterns (Risley, 1977). The sequence of activities around mealtimes has been incorporated as a component in feeding interventions. For example, Handen et al. (1986) included modification of the premeal schedule as part of a multicomponent protocol with seven feeding-resistant children, six of whom were treated as inpatients. Handen et al. instructed staff to avoid social stimulation of the children prior to meals, and the study reported successful results, although the function of individual components of the program was not evaluated. Postmealtime schedules also have been incorporated into feeding interventions. Preferred activities, such as playing a game or watching a favorite videotape, have been arranged to follow desired eating during mealtimes, using behavior management procedures as described in the section entitled Positive Reinforcement Procedures.

The unique features of hospital environments may inadvertently contribute to making mealtimes less reinforcing for some children. Unstructured times (e.g., in child-life recreational programs, playrooms, during family visits) occurring before and after meals often provide more opportunities for positive attention than during hospital mealtimes. For example, the authors evaluated a toddler who was hospitalized for an extended period for bone marrow treatment of leukemia, secondary to which the child displayed diminished appetite and food selectivity. Upon evaluation on the ward, it was noted that the child spent much of the time between meals cuddled in the arms of hospital staff, a condition that contrasted sharply with the structured format imposed during meals. In addition to activity-related factors, inpatient meals often are served in patients' rooms rather than in a dining area (a physical setting variable) and occur on a different schedule than the children are accustomed to eating at home (a scheduling variable). If a child's appetite is already reduced secondary to illness or medical treatment, these hospital conditions may exacerbate feeding difficulties.

Interactions

Social interchanges between the feeder and the child are fundamental to mealtimes for young children. Two general aspects of dyadic interactions have been studied as potential contributors to the etiology of and intervention for feeding disorders: 1) the *reciprocity* in feeder–child interchanges (i.e., the mutual responsivity of the feeder and child to each other's behavior), and 2) the *contingencies* of interactions (i.e., the learning function of social antecedents and consequences to feeder and child responses). Although the two areas overlap in some respects, they reflect differences in the presumed underlying problems and in the intervention strategies implicated. Each area is described further in the next sections, along with an overview of illustrative feeding interventions. Relevant learning principles are reviewed as they relate to specific behavior management procedures.

Reciprocity in Feeder–Child Interactions Developmental research suggests that adaptive feeding interactions are characterized by reciprocity or synchrony—that is, by mutual attentiveness and responsivity to behavioral cues emitted by the feeder and by the child (Barnard et al., 1989; Bornstein, 1995; Brazelton, Koslowski, & Main, 1974). A sensitive caregiver notices when the child is hungry, picks up and cradles the infant while he or she sucks, verbalizes to and gently strokes the infant during feeding, pauses when the infant averts his or her eyes or pulls away, and terminates feeding when the infant repeatedly shows disinterest. A communicative infant cries when hungry, is alert at the beginning of feeding, gazes at the caregiver in response to stimulation, settles when repositioned, and signals satiation by falling asleep or resisting food offered.

Ainsworth and Bell (1969), in a classic observational study of mother–infant feeding interactions during the first 3 months of life, found that the most effective feeding patterns involved the infant as an active participant in determining the timing of feeding, pacing of feeding, and amount ingested during feedings. Termed "demand" or "flexible-schedule" feeding patterns, the styles were associated with less infant crying and more positive parent perceptions at initial assessment. Furthermore, these feeding styles were related to more secure mother–infant attachment patterns at 1 year of age. The researchers hypothesized that early feeding experiences provide a model of parent responsivity and accessibility in other interactional contexts, which shapes the child's confidence in his or her ability to influence events.

In some cases, attachment problems have been attributed to inexperienced, arbitrary, or deprived parenting (Ainsworth, 1979). In other cases, neurological disorganization, temperament difficulties, ongoing health conditions, or other child characteristics are presumed to interfere with the formation of reciprocal parent–child interactions (Field, 1977). Parental psychological problems, particularly depression, also have been implicated (Drotar, 1995). Interventions directed at strengthening parent–child attachment focus mainly on teaching caregivers to more accurately read the child's signals and respond accordingly. This training may occur within a program of psychotherapy for the parent, or it may be conceptualized primarily as an educational intervention.

Interactional coaching is a technique often used to provide caregivers with in vivo training to learn how to "match" the child's behavior through appropriate reciprocal responses (e.g., McDonough, 1995). The trainer observes ongoing interactions and points out specific child behaviors that are purposeful and voluntary; the goal is to help the caregiver notice, interpret, and predict child responses. The trainer often models behaviors and encourages the parent to respond immediately to meaningful child behavior with vocalizations (e.g., soothing responses, encouragement, descriptions of the child's behavior) or actions consistent with the child's cues (e.g., offering a preferred food, repositioning the child). Interactional coaching is useful in increasing the overall level of parent–child stimulation and for altering the quality and timing of the caregiver's responses to child behavior. If reciprocity problems exist across several dimensions of interaction, training may incorporate other child care activities such as bathing, dressing, and playing, as well as feeding. Interactional coaching often is combined with other intervention components to address issues of parental distress or family disharmony (e.g., Chatoor, Dickson, Schaeffer, & Egan, 1985; Drotar et al., 1985).

Behavior Management Procedures in Feeder–Child Interactions Behavior management procedures consist of a body of techniques based on learning principles that can be applied to socially relevant problems to strengthen adaptive behaviors and to weaken maladaptive behaviors. Learning principles describe the ways that antecedent and consequent events influence the future probability of designated target behaviors (Skinner, 1953). Of particular interest in clinical feeding interventions are 1) aspects of the feeder's responses that have an inadvertent impact on feeding patterns and 2) planned techniques for "unlearning" or modifying maladaptive feeding patterns by rearranging social and environmental concomitants to feeding. For example, a child's rejection of new foods could be strengthened accidentally if the parent responds frequently by withdrawing the new food and offering familiar foods instead. In such a case, behavioral intervention might entail teaching the parent to consistently offer a neutral or nonpreferred item at each meal, deliver praise and preferred food immediately on child acceptance of a bite of less preferred food, ignore refusals briefly, and reoffer rejected food in a matter-of-fact manner.

As the preceding example illustrates, behavior management procedures may encompass a wide range of environmental aspects related to a child's feeding. In addition to specifying the timing and nature of feeder–child social interactions, behavior management procedures often include specific menu items, feeding schedules, and setting characteristics. The critical variable in defining an intervention as a behavior management procedure is that it involves systematic application of environmental events contingent on (i.e., in immediate relation to) specific child behavior. Because social interaction is integral to most behavior management procedures, it is appropriate to review behavioral techniques in this section.

Clinical reports describe various forms of parental mismanagement in response to children's feeding problems (e.g., Bernal, 1972; Butterfield & Parson, 1973; Chatoor et al., 1988; Sanders et al., 1993), suggesting that parents' misplaced social contingencies play a role in some feeding disorders. Even when feeding problems did not originally develop because of maladaptive parent–child interactions, however, behavior management techniques often are incorporated into feeding intervention. Feeding problems rarely develop from a single cause, and, unless corrected quickly, underlying etiological factors may be superseded by the effects of learning experiences (Iwata et al., 1982; Palmer & Horn, 1978). Behavioral intervention offers a strategy for initiating desired changes by capitalizing on the influence of environmental contingencies. Linscheid (1992) recommended behavior management procedures particularly for problems relating to food selectivity, mealtime conduct problems, and delays in self-feeding, as opposed to problems with quantity of intake, which may be more affected by appetitive variables.

The major techniques used in behavioral feeding interventions are described briefly in the next few paragraphs. To highlight the empirical underpinnings of the behavioral approach, techniques are organized according to the operant and respondent conditioning principles from which they are derived (Bijou, 1993; Bijou & Baer, 1965; Skinner, 1953). Most behavioral techniques used in feeding interventions are based on operant learning principles, and these are described first. *Operant principles* emphasize control of voluntary behaviors by events that predictably follow the behaviors, sometimes in conjunction with antecedent stimuli that set the occasion for voluntary behaviors. By contrast, *respondent principles* emphasize control of reflexive behaviors or internal states by antecedent, eliciting stimuli. Table 4.3 summarizes the most common behavioral techniques and examples of applications to feeding treatment.

Positive Reinforcement Procedures *Positive reinforcement* is defined as the delivery of a desired stimulus (e.g., praise, preferred food), contingent on performance of a target behavior (e.g., taking a sip of milk), that strengthens the probability that the target behavior will occur in the future. A ubiquitous stimulus that usually functions as a reinforcer for children is adult attention, particularly affectionate or approving forms of attention. Thus, an integral component of most behavioral intervention programs is social approval contingent on (i.e., immediately following) desired feeding behavior. Both discrete praise (e.g., "good girl," "you did it all by yourself!" clapping for the child) and other forms of attention that show interest in the child (e.g., including the child in conversation, describing the child's actions) appear to function as positive reinforcement for most children. Training in positive reinforcement emphasizes precise delivery of attention while the child is cooperating, rather than the more natural tendency of responding to the child's inappropriate or disruptive behavior.

Table 4.3. Overview of behavior management principles and applications to feeding interventions

Underlying principle	Description of application	Examples
To increase desired behaviors		
Positive reinforcement	Provide positive consequences for desired behavior.	Give praise, physical affection, preferred foods, or tangible rewards.
Negative reinforcement	Terminate aversive stimulus contingent on desired behavior.	Release physical restraint (for food expulsion) when child accepts food.
Discrimination	Reinforce target behavior in presence of defined stimulus.	Praise modeled behavior of eating. Reward cooperation with feeding requests.
Shaping	Reinforce successive approximations toward desired response.	Praise 1) looking at food, then 2) allowing food to touch lips, then 3) opening mouth, then 4) accepting food.
Fading	Gradually remove assistance and reinforcement needed to maintain behavior.	Decrease extent of guidance and rewards as child gains self-feeding skills.
To decrease undesired behaviors		
Extinction	Withhold rewarding stimulus contingent on target response.	Ignore mild inappropriate behavior. Continue prompts during escape behavior.
Satiation	Continually present desired stimulus until it loses its reinforcing value.	Offer unlimited portions of food to reduce rumination.
Punishment	Present aversive stimulus or remove rewarding stimulus contingent on undesired behavior.	Use time-out. Give verbal reprimand. Restrict toys. Use overcorrection.
Desensitization	Pair conditioned aversive stimulus with absence of aversive events or with presence of positive events.	Distract child during fearful procedure. Use gentle massage to promote acceptance of touch.

Next to social attention, the most common consequence in behavioral feeding programs probably is preferred food (e.g., Hatcher, 1979). The technique, based on a variation of the principle of positive reinforcement called the Premack Principle, uses a high-probability behavior (eating preferred food) to reinforce a low-probability behavior (eating new or nonpreferred food) (Premack, 1959). Delivery of social attention and/or preferred food often is combined with tangible forms of reinforcement, such as the opportunity to play with toys, sensory stimulation (e.g., music) (Larson, Ayllon, & Barrett, 1987), the opportunity to watch television (Bernal, 1972), the opportunity to gain tokens redeemable for items of value (Linscheid et al., 1987), or the opportunity to gain access to other preferred activities.

Because the rewarding values of particular consequences vary across children, it is necessary to determine which consequences serve as positive reinforces for particular children. Reinforcement value also is subject to change based on prior exposure and consumption, such that a reward that has been present continuously loses its positive value, an effect known as *satiation*. Because satiation is a predictable phenomenon following excessive exposure to a stimulus, some intervention programs have successfully decreased unwanted behaviors (e.g., rumination) by providing individuals with large quantities of the presumed reward (e.g., food) (Rast, Johnston, Drum, & Conrin, 1981).

Extinction Procedures   Just as contingent delivery of a positive reinforcer strengthens the reinforced behavior, systematically discontinuing a reward following a response reduces the future probability of the response occurring—a technique called *extinction.* The most common example of extinction in behavioral feeding programs is to ignore undesired child behaviors such as refusals or tantrums. Ignoring is a deliberate act in which the feeder turns his or her head and eyes away from the child and provides no verbal or physical attention for a brief period (usually 5–10 seconds) or until the undesired behavior ceases. *Differential social attention* involves combining the techniques of providing positive social attention contingent on cooperative behavior and ignoring the child briefly contingent on misbehavior, which presumably maximizes the child's opportunity to learn the behaviors that are desired by the feeder. A variation called *differential reinforcement of other behavior (DRO)* refers to delivery of rewarding stimuli contingent on any response except the target behavior one wishes to decrease. Several feeding programs have employed differential social attention as an intervention component (e.g., Butterfield & Parson, 1973; Palmer, Thompson, & Linscheid, 1975; Stark et al., 1993).

Although extinction procedures are simple to explain, they are much more difficult to execute consistently, particularly when a child is resistant or disruptive (Bernal, 1972; Linscheid, 1992). Thus, parent training in differential attention procedures often needs to include modeling, behavior rehearsal, and practice to refine care-givers' skills and to provide emotional support during intervention. Research outside the feeding literature documents cases in which some children with conduct or developmental disorders display an apparent paradoxical reaction to differential attention procedures, resulting in persistent increased levels of negative behavior (Budd, Green, & Baer, 1976; Herbert et al., 1973). This reaction appears more likely when there is a history of high-rate parental attention to child behavior and high pre-intervention levels of negative child behavior, such that differential attention results in a precipitous drop in the overall rate of parent attention (Budd et al., 1976). To avoid this problem, other behavior management procedures often are combined with social contingencies to provide parents with greater control over the child's behavior.

Another form of extinction that appears in the behavioral feeding literature is called *escape extinction*. This term is somewhat difficult to interpret because it assumes a functional role of the child's behavior. When a child engages in an "escape behavior" (e.g., fussing, refusing food)—presumably to avoid eating—an escape extinction can be applied. Escape extinction involves discontinuing a reward for the hypothesized escape behavior, with the result of decreasing the strength of the escape response. For example, if a child turns away (the escape response) when a cracker is offered to her lips, escape extinction involves holding the cracker up to the child's mouth until she accepts it. Hoch, Babbitt, Coe, Krell, and Hackbert (1994) used the term "contingency contacting" to describe the application of escape extinction following refusals, together with positive reinforcement for acceptances. They found that contingency contacting dramatically increased acceptances in two children with severe feeding problems after a prior intervention using positive attention procedures was ineffective. Cooper et al. (1995) also found escape extinction to be a necessary component of feeding intervention for four children with serious food refusal. Because of the similarity of escape extinction to negative reinforcement, described next, the two procedures are considered together.

Negative Reinforcement and Punishment Procedures   Behavioral techniques that are generally viewed as disciplinary strategies are based on the principles of negative reinforcement and punishment. *Negative reinforcement* involves terminating or withholding an aversive stimulus contingent on performance of a desired behavior, with the result that it strengthens the probability that the desired behavior will occur in the future. Negative reinforcement is exemplified in the use of *physical guidance* (also called jaw prompting or in its more intrusive form, forced feeding) to induce a child to accept or swallow a bite of food. Riordan, Iwata, Finney, Wohl, and Stanley (1984), for example, incorporated negative reinforcement into an intervention protocol that effectively reduced food refusal. A child is offered a bite of food; if he or she fails to accept it after a few seconds, the feeder physically guides the food into the child's mouth and holds the jaw until the child accepts the bite. Termination of physical guidance (the aversive stimulus) when the child accepts the food (the desired behavior) presumably reinforces food acceptance.

Physical guidance is a more intensive strategy than escape extinction because the former entails actively inserting food into the child's mouth, whereas the latter involves waiting for the child to accept it. Both procedures result in negative reinforcement for acceptances. Ahearn et al. (1996) systematically compared the effects of physical guidance and escape extinction—each of which were paired with positive reinforcement for acceptances—in treating three young children hospitalized with severe feeding problems. Both procedures were effective in reducing food refusals and increasing acceptances; however, it is interesting to note that physical guidance was associated with somewhat fewer maladaptive behaviors, shorter meal durations, and parental preference.

These research demonstrations provide a rationale for considering either physical guidance or escape extinction in cases of serious food refusal, and the latter study suggests that physical guidance may be more acceptable to caregivers. Both procedures, however, have potential aversive effects on children and feeders, and thus, application of the procedures must be carefully supervised by feeding professionals.

The term punishment has a different meaning with respect to operant principles of behavior than its lay connotation of pain or retribution. *Punishment* is defined as delivery of an aversive stimulus or removal of a rewarding stimulus contingent on undesired behavior that weakens the probability that the response will occur. A widely used punishment technique in feeding intervention is *time-out* from reinforcement, which entails removing the child's access to food, adult attention, and other reinforcing stimuli for a brief period (e.g., between 5 and 60 seconds) (MacArthur et al., 1986). Time-out is commonly used as a disciplinary option because it is safe, effective, and less intrusive than many other forms of punishment. To accomplish time-out, the child may actually be turned or moved away from the table or his or her plate may be removed to preclude eating for the duration of time-out (Linscheid, 1992; Sisson & Dixon, 1986).

In addition to time-out, other forms of punishment have been used in feeding intervention. For example, Madison and Adubato (1984) taught parents to use verbal disapproval (a firm "no") and noise (a clicker), followed by 10 seconds of attention withdrawal, contingent on their young child's ruminative responses. As with positive reinforcement techniques, it is essential to monitor the effects of delivering aversive stimuli to determine whether they actually function to decrease the target behavior. Negative verbal attention may, in fact, serve as a positive reinforcer for some children. Response-contingent withdrawal of positive reinforcement is another form of punishment. It is exemplified by withdrawing toys, music, or other preferred stimuli during a meal as a consequence for misbehavior (Larson et al., 1987). In conjunction with contingent removal, the child should have the opportunity to again earn access to the favored materials and activities by engaging in cooperative behavior.

In cases of serious maladaptive feeding behaviors (e.g., persistent rumination, psychogenic vomiting), more extreme aversive consequences such as electric shock or lemon juice (squirted into the child's mouth or dabbed on the child's lips) have been effectively applied as punishment techniques (e.g., Cunningham & Linscheid, 1976). *Overcorrection*, a procedure in which the child is physically directed through a series of repetitive, presumably unpleasant acts (e.g., "cleaning up" after intentionally spilling food), is another form of punishment (Duker, 1981). Punishment procedures involving highly aversive stimuli are recommended only when less intrusive procedures are not successful, the target behavior is damaging to the child or others, and when carefully monitored by trained personnel.

Discrimination Training Techniques   The behavior management techniques described in the previous paragraphs, based on operant learning principles, illustrate the use of consequences in a contingent fashion to increase or decrease target behaviors. Another aspect of operant learning concerns the stimulus conditions that precede or occur concomitant with the target response. The principle of *discrimination* refers to the increased probability of a specific behavior in the presence of an antecedent stimulus that has been paired with positive or negative reinforcement for the behavior. In behavioral intervention, the feeder's instructions and physical assistance often acquire a discriminative function as a result of being paired with contingent consequences. For example, the feeder may verbally prompt the child to eat when presenting a bite of food (Werle et al., 1993). Over repeated occasions, the child learns that when the feeder says, "Take a bite," it is highly likely that food acceptance will be followed by praise or access to preferred food and that refusal will be followed by ignoring or disapproval. As a result, the feeder's instructions become discriminative cues for appropriate eating. When a child displays a certain class of operant responses in close conjunction with a class of discriminative stimuli, stimulus control is demonstrated.

Discrimination training techniques have several applications in feeding. One example is *observational learning*, also called *modeling*, in which the discriminative stimulus is the behavior of another person (e.g., parent, sibling, peer), which the child imitates (Bandura, 1969). Often, imitated responses that match the model are differentially reinforced, which presumably strengthens the child's imitative repertoire. Observational learning accounts for an enormous amount of learning in the course of normal development, and it serves as a primary mechanism for the transmission of cultural practices. In addition to the natural role of modeling, in feeding intervention, people who eat with the child can be enlisted as models of appropriate feeding behavior. By making the modeled behavior salient to the child and by providing consistent consequences to the model, the child learns to imitate the modeled behavior (Greer, Dorow, Williams, McCorkle, & Asnes, 1991).

Other forms of discriminative stimuli used in feeding interventions are exemplified by a kitchen timer and color-coded cues to control eating. For children who dawdle during meals, a timer can be set to go off after a predetermined length of time, after which the child receives dessert if his or her meal is finished. In this case, the presence of the timer serves to notify the child that eating at a sufficient pace will lead to reinforcement (Christophersen & Hall, 1978). Epstein and Squires (1988) developed a "stoplight" system of foods as part of a behavioral intervention program for childhood obesity, in which color-coded symbols teach children the rules for consumption within the program: nutritious foods with no limitations (green symbol), foods that can be eaten in moderation (yellow), and foods to be avoided (red). The objective of intervention is that the color symbols exert discriminative control overeating by guiding the children's choice and consumption of foods.

Progressive Training Techniques   Two behavioral techniques, shaping and fading, refer to progressive changes in the criteria for delivery of antecedents and consequences in relation to child behavior. *Shaping* involves reinforcing successive approximations toward the desired response criterion to establish new combinations or more complex series of behaviors. For example, to develop texture acceptance, a child might initially receive reinforcement for taking liquids, next the child would be required to try puréed foods, then semisolid foods, and later would need to eat food with small chewable chunks to receive reinforcement (Johnson & Babbitt, 1993; Luiselli & Gleason, 1987). Shaping also is exemplified over the course of intervention by progressively increasing the number of bites a child needs to eat before receiving a preferred consequence. As Bijou (1993) noted, shaping is one of the most useful tools generated by the behavioral approach because it provides a strategy for producing novel response combinations from existing behavioral repertoires.

Fading is defined as the gradual removal of prompts, assistance, or reinforcement needed to establish independent performance of the behavior. For example, Leibowitz and Holcer (1974) taught a child with developmental delays to use a spoon by gradually fading instructions, motor assistance, and reinforcement as the child acquired more control over self-feeding. Lamm and Greer (1988) systematically faded physical cues in an intervention program that successfully induced swallowing responses in infants with dysphagia. Shaping and fading are integral components of programs for training adaptive feeding skills in children with physical/sensory impairments or developmental delays. Tasks are broken into small steps, and contingencies are gradually changed to require more independent performance as the child learns successive steps in the chain (Luiselli, 1993; Sisson & Van Hasselt, 1989).

The techniques and principles described thus far concern control of voluntary behaviors (e.g., eating, talking, throwing food) through contingent consequences and antecedent stimulus cues, as embodied in operant conditioning principles. By contrast, respondent conditioning principles emphasize control of reflexive behaviors, internal body functions, or feeling states through eliciting stimuli. Some feeding problems consist of conditioned respondent behaviors such as gagging, vomiting, or hypersensitive reactions to oral touch that initially may have been elicited by unconditioned aversive stimuli such as choking, nausea, or painful sensations, respectively.

Aversive Conditioning Techniques Aversive conditioning, a form of respondent conditioning, can be influential in maintaining avoidance of certain foods and in eliciting physiological responses (e.g., vomiting, gag reflex) to the foods. Aversive conditioning occurs when a neutral stimulus acquires some of the negative properties of an aversive event through a history of being paired with the event. For example, a person who chokes (the aversive event) on a piece of hard candy (the neutral stimulus) may come to associate candy with the negative experience of choking and thereafter find hard candy aversive (Chatoor et al., 1988). Similarly, strong taste aversions can develop following a single pairing of a food with nausea or vomiting after eating (Rozin, 1984). Thus, respondent learning provides an etiological explanation for the development of some problematic feeding behaviors.

Desensitization Procedures   To reverse the effects of aversive conditioning on feeding patterns, *desensitization* procedures often are used. Desensitization is accomplished by repeatedly pairing the conditioned aversive stimulus with the absence of aversive events or with delivery of positive reinforcement for an alternative, adaptive response. Siegel (1982) described use of desensitization in intervention for a 6-year-old boy who refused most solid foods. The boy showed signs of anticipatory nausea, anxiety, and gagging when presented with solid food (the conditioned aversive stimulus), presumably secondary to illness following an overdose of medication. The desensitization component involved having the child watch television to serve as a distracting activity while eating, which was combined with delivery of reinforcement for gradual steps toward eating. The combination of procedures effectively reduced gagging and increased intake of a wide variety of table foods. In a related example, Stark et al. (1993) taught children with cystic fibrosis to use relaxation skills to ease abdominal pain after food intake.

Desensitization procedures also are used to weaken aversive reactions during feeding in children secondary to neuromuscular incompetence, invasive oral procedures, or artificial feeding histories. Children with central nervous system dysfunction may exhibit problems such as oral hypersensitivity or sensory defensiveness, in which ordinary stimuli such as food, a spoon, or noise occasion exaggerated responses that interfere with feeding. One component of therapy involves graduated exposure to the stimuli in nonthreatening conditions (e.g., through play activities, with a gentle massage, with a brief warning cue to prepare the child) (Morris & Klein, 1987). Intervention for behavioral resistance to oral feeding often includes desensitization procedures prior to attempting feeding, such as stroking the child's cheeks and lips while providing pleasant social attention (Geertsma, Hyams, Pelletier, & Reiter, 1985).

Luiselli and his colleagues also have demonstrated the effectiveness of an intervention package that includes a desensitization phase for children with highly selective feeding patterns and multiple developmental disabilities (Luiselli, 1994; Luiselli & Gleason, 1987). In this approach, the child receives noncontingent, pleasurable stimulation in the feeding setting for several sessions, in the absence of any feeding demands. This phase presumably blurs the association between the feeding environment and previous aversive conditioning experiences around feeding. In the second phase, feeding demands are gradually introduced, and pleasurable stimuli are provided contingent on appropriate behavior. Intervention resulted in marked improvements in food acceptance, although the role of individual intervention components was not evaluated.

It should be noted that the therapeutic techniques described here under the rubric of desensitization also are used by allied health clinicians who do not conceptualize the techniques within a respondent conditioning paradigm. Occupational and physical therapists, as well as speech-language pathologists, frequently treat children with neuromuscular incompetence or invasive feeding histories using oral facilitation techniques (Morris & Klein, 1987). For example, oral sensorimotor treatment was shown to be effective in improving eating skills in children with moderate cerebral palsy (Gisel, Applegate-Ferrante, Benson, & Bosma, 1996). Although the techniques are topographically similar across disciplinary professionals, the conceptual basis on which the procedures are used affects therapists' decisions regarding which specific techniques to apply, how to respond to positive versus negative child reactions, and when to change aspects of the intervention procedures.

Other Interventions

To complete the survey of environmental feeding interventions, it is important to include additional techniques that do not fit neatly within the broad categories described in preceding sections. A miscellaneous section has been created for these conceptually disparate but clinically relevant feeding interventions. Two examples of such interventions are nonnutritive sucking and adaptive feeding equipment.

Nonnutritive Sucking In contrast to nutritive sucking, nonnutritive sucking is a pattern of sucking on a pacifier, nipple, or other object as a means of regulating the child's state of alertness or to provide oral-motor experiences rather than to obtain nourishment (Wolf & Glass, 1992). When physical immaturity or medical factors prevent a child from being able to take in food orally, nonnutritive sucking sometimes is recommended, usually concomitant with artificial feedings. Premature infants often are given the opportunity to engage in nonnutritive sucking while in neonatal intensive care units, in an attempt to ease the transition to oral feedings. This approach has resulted in faster weight gain and earlier hospital discharge for premature infants in some studies, as described further in Chapter 7.

Use of Adaptive Feeding Equipment An integral aspect of mealtimes is eating-related equipment such as spoons, cups, and bottles. To become independent feeders, children inevitably go through a period of messy eating as they develop coordination in use of utensils and learn the social amenities of mealtimes. The developmental progression, however, is complicated for children with motor impairments. An array of adaptive feeding utensils, such as bottles with enlarged nipple holes, Tippy cups, and spoons with specialized handle and/or bowl shapes can influence children's success at feeding. Appropriately designed equipment helps to regulate the amount of food taken in, reduce spillage, and decrease fatigue in self-feeding efforts (Morris & Klein, 1987; Singer, Nofer, Benson-Szekely, & Brooks, 1991).

SUMMARY

This chapter covers key issues in determining whether to begin feeding intervention, and it introduces the major components of environmental intervention programs. Preliminary issues include deciding whether feeding intervention is medically necessary, whether caregivers are receptive to the use of environmental techniques, and whether resources are available to enact and support change. Environmental interventions are organized into five major areas: meal characteristics, schedule of intake, setting characteristics, interactions, and other interventions. Learning theory principles, involving operant and respondent conditioning, underlie behavior management intervention.

In practice, several intervention components often are combined within clinical recommendations, and many variations of each component can be found in research and clinical accounts of interventions. The remaining chapters describe applications of environmental approaches to specific feeding disorders; evidence regarding their effectiveness with different feeding problems; and issues involved in training, generalization, and ongoing evaluation of intervention and treatment progress.

REFERENCES

Ahearn, W.H., Kerwin, M.E., Eicher, P.S., Shantz, J., & Swearingin, W. (1996). An alternating treatments comparison of two intensive interventions for food refusal. *Journal of Applied Behavior Analysis, 29,* 321–332.
Ainsworth, M.D.S. (1979). Infant–mother attachment. *American Psychologist, 34,* 932–937.
Ainsworth, M.D.S., & Bell, S.M. (1969). Some contemporary patterns of mother–infant interaction in the feeding situation. In A. Ambrose (Ed.), *Stimulation in early infancy* (pp. 133–170). New York: Academic Press.

Alderette, P., & deGraffenried, D.F. (1986, May–June). Nonorganic failure-to-thrive syndrome and the family system. *Social Work*, 207–211.

Azrin, N.H., & Armstrong, P.M. (1973). The "mini meal"—A method for teaching eating skills to the profoundly retarded. *Mental Retardation, 11,* 9–13.

Babbitt, R.L., Hoch, T.A., Coe, D.A., Cataldo, M.F., Kelly, K.J., Stackhouse, C., & Perman, J.A. (1994). Behavioral assessment and treatment of pediatric feeding disorders. *Journal of Developmental and Behavioral Pediatrics, 15,* 278–291.

Bandura, A. (1969). Modeling and vicarious processes. *Principles of behavior modification* (pp. 118–216). New York: Holt, Rinehart & Winston.

Barnard, K.E., Hammond, M.A., Booth, C.L., Bee, H.L., Mitchell, S.K., & Spieker, S.J. (1989). Measurement and meaning of parent–child interaction. In F. Morrison, C. Lord, & D. Keating (Eds.), *Applied developmental psychology* (Vol. III, pp. 40–76). New York: Academic Press.

Bateson, P.P.G. (1969). Imprinting and the development of preferences. In A. Ambrose (Ed.), *Stimulation in early infancy* (pp. 109–132). New York: Academic Press.

Bernal, M.E. (1972). Behavioral treatment of a child's eating problem. *Journal of Behavior Therapy and Experimental Psychiatry, 3,* 43–50.

Bijou, S.W. (1993). *Behavior analysis of child development* (2nd Rev. ed.). Reno, NV: Context.

Bijou, S.W., & Baer, D.M. (1965). *Child development: I. A systematic and empirical theory.* Englewood Cliffs, NJ: Prentice Hall.

Birch, L.L. (1990). The control of food intake by young children: The role of learning. In E.D. Capaldi & T.L. Powley (Eds.), *Taste, experience, and feeding* (pp. 116–135). Washington, DC: American Psychological Association.

Birch, L.L., & Marlin, D.W. (1982). I don't like it; I never tried it: Effects of exposure on two-year-old children's food preferences. *Appetite, 3,* 353–360.

Birch, L.L., McPhee, L., Shoba, B.C., Pirok, E., & Steinberg, L. (1987). What kind of exposure reduces children's food neophobia? Looking versus tasting. *Appetite, 9,* 171–178.

Black, M.M., Dubowitz, H., Hutcheson, J., Berenson-Howard, J., & Starr, R.H. (1995). A randomized clinical trial of home intervention for children with failure to thrive. *Pediatrics, 95,* 807–814.

Blackman, J.A., & Nelson, C.L.A. (1985). Reinstituting oral feedings in children fed by gastrostomy tube. *Clinical Pediatrics, 24,* 434–438.

Blackman, J.A., & Nelson, C.L.A. (1987). Rapid introduction of oral feedings to tube-fed patients. *Journal of Developmental and Behavioral Pediatrics, 8,* 63–67.

Bornstein, M.H. (1995). Parenting infants. In M.H. Bornstein (Ed.), *Handbook of parenting: Vol. 1. Children and parenting* (pp. 3–39). Hillsdale, NJ: Lawrence Erlbaum Associates.

Brazelton, T.B., Koslowski, B., & Main, M. (1974). The origins of reciprocity: The early mother–infant interaction. In M. Lewis & L.A. Rosenblum (Eds.), *The effect of the infant on its caregiver* (pp. 49–78). New York: John Wiley & Sons.

Briesmeister, J.M., & Schaefer, C.E. (1998). *Handbook of parent training: Parents as co-therapists for children's behavior problems* (2nd ed.). New York: John Wiley & Sons.

Budd, K.S., Green, D.R., & Baer, D.M. (1976). An analysis of multiple mis-placed parental social contingencies. *Journal of Applied Behavior Analysis, 9,* 459–470.

Butterfield, W.H., & Parson, R. (1973). Modeling and shaping by parents to develop chewing behavior in their retarded child. *Journal of Behavior Therapy and Experimental Psychiatry, 4,* 285–287.

Chatoor, I., Conley, C., & Dickson, L. (1988). Food refusal after an incident of choking: A posttraumatic eating disorder. *Journal of the American Academy of Child and Adolescent Psychiatry, 27,* 105–110.

Chatoor, I., Dickson, L., Schaeffer, S., & Egan, J. (1985). A developmental classification of feeding disorders associated with failure to thrive: Diagnosis and treatment. In D. Drotar (Ed.), *New directions in failure to thrive: Implications for research and practice* (pp. 235–258). New York: Plenum.

Christophersen, E., & Hall, C.L. (1978). Eating patterns and associated problems encountered in normal children. *Issues in Comprehensive Pediatric Nursing, 3,* 1–16.

Cooper, L.J., Wacker, D.P., McComas, J.J., Brown, K., Peck, S.M., Richman, D., Drew, J., Frischmeyer, P., & Millard, T. (1995). Use of component analyses to identify active variables in treatment packages for children with feeding disorders. *Journal of Applied Behavior Analysis, 28,* 139–153.

Cunningham, C.E., & Linscheid, T.R. (1976). Elimination of chronic infant rumination by electric shock. *Behavior Therapy, 7,* 231–234.

Dangel, R.F., & Polster, R.A. (Eds.). (1984). *Parent training: Foundations of research and practice.* New York: Guilford Press.

Drotar, D. (1995). Failure to thrive (growth deficiency). In M. Roberts (Ed.), *Handbook of pediatric psychology* (2nd ed., pp. 516–536). New York: Guilford Press.

Drotar, D., Eckerle, D., Satola, J., Pallotta, J., & Wyatt, B. (1990). Maternal interactional behavior with nonorganic failure-to-thrive infants: A case comparison study. *Child Abuse and Neglect, 14,* 41–51.

Drotar, D., Malone, C.A., Devost, L., Brickell, C., Mantz-Clumpner, C., Negray, J., Wallace, M., Woychik, J., Wyatt, B., Eckerle, D., Bush, M., Finlon, M.A., El-Amin, D., Nowak, M., Satola, J., & Pallotta, J. (1985). Early preventive intervention in failure to thrive: Methods and preliminary outcome. In D. Drotar (Ed.), *New directions in failure to thrive: Implications for research and practice* (pp. 119–138). New York: Plenum.

Drotar, D., Wilson, F., & Sturm, L. (1989). Parent intervention in failure-to-thrive. In C.E. Schaefer & J.M. Briesmeister (Eds.), *Handbook of parent training* (pp. 364–391). New York: John Wiley & Sons.

Duker, P.C. (1981). Treatment of food refusal by the overcorrective functional movement training method. *Journal of Behavior Therapy and Experimental Psychiatry, 12,* 337–340.

Dumas, J.E., & Wahler, R.G. (1983). Predictors of treatment outcome in parent training: Mother insularity and socioeconomic disadvantage. *Behavioral Assessment, 5,* 301–313.

Epstein, L.H., & Squires, S. (1988). *The stoplight diet for children.* Boston: Little, Brown.

Epstein, L.H., Valoski, A., Wing, R.R., & McCurley, J. (1994). Ten-year outcomes of behavioral family-based treatment for childhood obesity. *Health Psychology, 13,* 373–383.

Epstein, L.H., & Wing, R.R. (1987). Behavioral treatment of childhood obesity. *Psychological Bulletin, 101*, 91–95.

Field, T. (1977). Maternal stimulation during infant feeding. *Developmental Psychology, 13*, 539–540.

Frank, D. (1995). Failure to thrive. In S. Parker & B. Zuckerman (Eds.), *Behavioral and developmental pediatrics: A handbook for primary care* (pp. 134–139). Boston: Little, Brown.

Geertsma, M.A., Hyams, J.S., Pelletier, J.M., & Reiter, S. (1985). Feeding resistance after parenteral hyperalimentation. *American Journal of Diseases of Children, 139*, 255–256.

Ginsberg, A.J. (1988). Feeding disorders in the developmentally disabled population. In D.C. Russo & J.H. Kedesdy (Eds.), *Behavioral medicine with the developmentally disabled* (pp. 21–41). New York: Plenum.

Gisel, E.G., Applegate-Ferrante, T., Benson, J., & Bosma, J.F. (1996). Oral-motor skills following sensorimotor therapy in two groups of moderately dysphagic children with cerebral palsy: Aspiration vs nonaspiration. *Dysphagia, 11*, 59–71.

Gisel, E.G., & Patrick, J. (1988, February 6). Identification of children with cerebral palsy unable to maintain a normal nutritional state. *Lancet,* 283–286.

Graves, T., Meyers, A.W., & Clark, L. (1988). An evaluation of parental problem-solving training in the behavioral treatment of childhood obesity. *Journal of Consulting and Clinical Psychology, 56*, 246–250.

Graziano, A.M., & Diament, D.M. (1992). Parent behavioral training: An examination of the paradigm. *Behavior Modification, 16*, 3–38.

Greer, R.D., Dorow, L., Williams, G., McCorkle, N., & Asnes, R. (1991). Peer-mediated procedures to induce swallowing and food acceptance in young children. *Journal of Applied Behavior Analysis, 24*, 783–790.

Handen, B.L., Mandell, F., & Russo, D.C. (1986). Feeding induction in children who refuse to eat. *American Journal of Diseases of Children, 140*, 52–54.

Hatcher, R.P. (1979). Treatment of food refusal in a two-year-old child. *Journal of Behavior Therapy and Experimental Psychiatry, 10*, 363–367.

Herbert, E.W., Pinkston, E.M., Hayden, M.L., Sajwaj, T.E., Pinkston, S., Cordua, G., & Jackson, C. (1973). Adverse effects of differential parental attention. *Journal of Applied Behavior Analysis, 6*, 15–30.

Hoch, T.A., Babbitt, R.L., Coe, D.A., Krell, D.M., & Hackbert, L. (1994). Contingency contacting: Combining positive reinforcement and escape extinction procedures to treat persistent food refusal. *Behavior Modification, 18*, 106–128.

Horner, R.H., Dunlap, G., & Koegel, R.L. (Eds.). (1988). *Generalization and maintenance: Life-style changes in applied settings.* Baltimore: Paul H. Brookes Publishing Co.

Illingworth, R.S., & Lister, J. (1964). The critical or sensitive period, with special reference to certain feeding problems in infants and children. *Journal of Pediatrics, 65*, 839–848.

Israel, A.C., Silverman, W.K., & Solotar, L.C. (1986). An investigation of family influences on initial weight status, attrition, and treatment outcome in a childhood obesity program. *Behavior Therapy, 17*, 131–143.

Ives, C.C., Harris, S.L., & Wolchik, S.A. (1978). Food refusal in an autistic type child treated by a multi-component forced feeding procedure. *Journal of Behavior Therapy and Experimental Psychiatry, 9*, 61–64.

Iwata, B.A., Riordan, M.M., Wohl, M.K., & Finney, J.W. (1982). Pediatric feeding disorders: Behavioral analysis and treatment. In P.J. Accardo (Ed.), *Failure to thrive in infancy and early childhood: A multidisciplinary team approach* (pp. 297–329). Baltimore: University Park Press.

Jackson, R.H., & Sikora, D. (1992). Parenting: The child in the context of the family. In C.E. Walker & M.C. Roberts (Eds.), *Handbook of clinical child psychology* (2nd ed., pp. 727–747). New York: John Wiley & Sons.

Johnson, C.R., & Babbitt, R.L. (1993). Antecedent manipulation in the treatment of primary solid food refusal. *Behavior Modification, 17,* 510–521.

Kanfer, F.H., & Schefft, B.K. (1988). *Guiding the process of therapeutic change.* Champaign, IL: Research Press.

Kirschenbaum, D.S. (1987). Elements of success in the treatment of childhood and adolescent obesity. *Advances in Eating Disorders, 1,* 235–251.

Knapczyk, D.R. (1983). Use of teacher-paced instruction in developing and maintaining independent self-feeding. *Journal of The Association for the Severely Handicapped, 8,* 10–16.

Lamm, N., & Greer, R.D. (1988). Induction and maintenance of swallowing responses in infants with dysphagia. *Journal of Applied Behavior Analysis, 21,* 143–156.

Larson, K.L., Ayllon, T., & Barrett, D.H. (1987). A behavioral feeding program for failure-to-thrive infants. *Behaviour Research and Therapy, 25,* 39–47.

Leibowitz, J.M., & Holcer, P. (1974). Increasing food variety and texture: Building and maintaining self-feeding skills in a retarded child. *American Journal of Occupational Therapy, 28,* 545–548.

Lewis, C., & Drabman, R.S. (1988). Training parents in behavioral medicine techniques for the chronic care of their developmentally disabled children. In D.C. Russo & J.H. Kedesdy (Eds.), *Behavioral medicine with the developmentally disabled* (pp. 211–228). New York: Plenum.

Lewis, J.A. (1982). Oral motor assessment and treatment of feeding difficulties. In P.J. Accardo (Ed.), *Failure to thrive in infancy and early childhood: A multidisciplinary team approach* (pp. 265–295). Baltimore: University Park Press.

Li, N.N., Murphy, T.B., Werle, M.A., & Budd, K.S. (1993, April). *Temporal and pacing factors during parent–child mealtime interactions for children with selective food refusal.* Paper presented at the meeting of Florida Conference on Child Health Psychology, Gainesville.

Linscheid, T.R. (1992). Eating problems in children. In C.E. Walker & M.C. Roberts (Eds.), *Handbook of clinical child psychology* (2nd ed., pp. 451–473). New York: John Wiley & Sons.

Linscheid, T.R., Budd, K.S., & Rasnake, L.K. (1995). Pediatric feeding disorders. In M.C. Roberts (Ed.), *Handbook of pediatric psychology* (2nd ed., pp. 501–515). New York: Guilford Press.

Linscheid, T.R., Oliver, J., Blyler, E., & Palmer, S. (1978). Brief hospitalization for the behavioral treatment of feeding problems in the developmentally disabled. *Journal of Pediatric Psychology, 3,* 72–76.

Linscheid, T.R., & Rasnake, L.K. (1985). Behavioral approaches to the treatment of failure to thrive. In D. Drotar (Ed.), *New directions in failure to thrive: Implications for research and practice* (pp. 279–294). New York: Plenum.

Linscheid, T.R., Tarnowski, K.J., Rasnake, L.K., & Brams, J.S. (1987). Behavioral treatment of food refusal in a child with short-gut syndrome. *Journal of Pediatric Psychology, 12,* 451–459.

Lowenberg, M.E. (1993). Development of food patterns in young children. In P.L. Pipes & C.L. Trahms (Eds.), *Nutrition in infancy and early childhood* (5th ed., pp. 165–180). St. Louis: C.V. Mosby.

Luiselli, J.K. (1993). Training self-feeding skills in children who are deaf and blind. *Behavior Modification, 17,* 457–473.

Luiselli, J.K. (1994). Oral feeding treatment of children with chronic food refusal and multiple developmental disabilities. *American Journal on Mental Retardation, 98,* 646–655.

Luiselli, J.K., Evans, T.P., & Boyce, D.A. (1985). Contingency management of food selectivity and oppositional eating in a multiply handicapped child. *Journal of Clinical Child Psychology, 14,* 153–156.

Luiselli, J.K., & Gleason, D.J. (1987). Combining sensory reinforcement and texture fading procedures to overcome chronic food refusal. *Journal of Behavior Therapy and Experimental Psychology, 18,* 149–155.

MacArthur, J., Ballard, K.D., & Artinian, M. (1986). Teaching independent eating to a developmentally handicapped child showing chronic food refusal and disruption at mealtimes. *Australia and New Zealand Journal of Developmental Disabilities, 12,* 203–210.

Macht, J. (1990). *Poor eaters: Helping children who refuse to eat.* New York: Plenum.

Madison, L.S., & Adubato, S.A. (1984). The elimination of ruminative vomiting in a 15-month-old child with gastroesophageal reflux. *Journal of Pediatric Psychology, 9,* 231–239.

Mathisen, B., Skuse, D., Wolke, D., & Reilly, S. (1989). Oral-motor dysfunction and failure to thrive among inner-city infants. *Developmental Medicine and Child Neurology, 31,* 293–302.

McDonough, S.C. (1995). Promoting positive early parent–infant relationships through interaction guidance. *Child and Adolescent Psychiatric Clinics of North America, 4,* 661–672.

Morris, S.E., & Klein, M.D. (1987). *Pre-feeding skills: A comprehensive resource for feeding development.* Tucson, AZ: Therapy Skill Builders.

O'Dell, S.L. (1985). Progress in parent training. *Progress in Behavior Modification, 19,* 57–107.

Palmer, S., & Horn, S. (1978). Feeding problems in children. In S. Palmer & S. Ekvall (Eds.), *Pediatric nutrition in developmental disorders* (pp. 107–129). Springfield, IL: Charles C Thomas.

Palmer, S., Thompson, R.J., & Linscheid, T.R. (1975). Applied behavior analysis in the treatment of childhood feeding problems. *Developmental Medicine and Child Neurology, 17,* 333–339.

Pekarik, G., & Stephenson, L.A. (1988). Adult and child client differences in therapy outcome research. *Journal of Clinical Child Psychology, 17,* 316–321.

Pipes, P.L., & Trahms, C.L. (Eds.). (1993). *Nutrition in infancy and childhood* (5th ed.). St. Louis: C.V. Mosby.

Premack, D. (1959). Toward empirical behavior laws: I. Positive reinforcement. *Psychological Review, 66,* 219–233.

Prochaska, J.O., & DiClemente, C.C. (1982). Transtheoretical therapy: Toward a more integrative model of change. *Psychotherapy Theory, Research and Practice, 19,* 276–288.

Prochaska, J.O., & DiClemente, C.C. (1983). Stages and processes of self-change in smoking: Toward an integrative model of change. *Journal of Consulting and Clinical Psychology, 51*, 390–395.

Pugliese, M.T., Weyman-Daum, M., Moses, N., & Lifshitz, M. (1987). Parental health beliefs as a cause of nonorganic failure to thrive. *Pediatrics, 80*, 185–192.

Ramsay, M., & Zelazo, P.R. (1988). Food refusal in failure-to-thrive infants: Nasogastric feeding combined with interactive behavioral treatment. *Journal of Pediatric Psychology, 13*, 329–347.

Rast, J., Johnston, J.M., Drum, C., & Conrin, J. (1981). The relation of food quantity to rumination behavior. *Journal of Applied Behavior Analysis, 14*, 121–130.

Riordan, M.M., Iwata, B.A., Finney, J.W., Wohl, M.K., & Stanley, A.E. (1984). Behavioral assessment and treatment of chronic food refusal in handicapped children. *Journal of Applied Behavior Analysis, 17*, 327–341.

Risley, T.R. (1977). The ecology of applied behavior analysis. In A. Rogers-Warren & S.F. Warren (Eds.), *Ecological perspectives in behavior analysis* (pp. 149–163). Baltimore: University Park Press.

Rogers-Warren, A., & Warren, S.F. (1977). *Ecological perspectives in behavior analysis.* Baltimore: University Park Press.

Rozin, P. (1984). The acquisition of food habits and preferences. In J.D. Matarazzo, S.M. Weiss, J.A. Herd, N.E. Miller, & S.M. Weiss (Eds.), *Behavioral health: A handbook of health enhancement and disease prevention* (pp. 590–607). New York: John Wiley & Sons.

Sanders, M.R., Patel, R.K., Le Grice, B., & Shepherd, R.W. (1993). Children with persistent feeding difficulties: An observational analysis of the feeding interactions of problem and non-problem eaters. *Health Psychology, 12*, 64–73.

Satter, E. (1986). *Child of mine: Feeding with love and good sense.* Palo Alto, CA: Bull.

Satter, E. (1987). *How to get your kid to eat . . . but not too much.* Palo Alto, CA: Bull.

Schaefer, C.E., & Briesmeister, J.M. (Eds.). (1989). *Handbook of parent training.* New York: John Wiley & Sons.

Siegel, L.J. (1982). Classical and operant procedures in the treatment of a case of food aversion in a young child. *Journal of Clinical Child Psychology, 11*, 167–172.

Siegel, L.J., & Hudson, B.O. (1992). Hospitalization and medical care of children. In C.E. Walker & M.C. Roberts (Eds.), *Handbook of clinical child psychology* (2nd ed., pp. 845–858). New York: John Wiley & Sons.

Silverman, W.K., & Israel, A.C. (1987). The development and treatment of childhood obesity: Parental and family factors. *The Behavior Therapist, 10*, 197–201.

Singer, L.T., Nofer, J.A., Benson-Szekely, L.J., & Brooks, L.J. (1991). Behavioral assessment and management of food refusal in children with cystic fibrosis. *Journal of Developmental and Behavioral Pediatrics, 12*, 115–120.

Sisson, L.A., & Dixon, M.J. (1986). A behavioral approach to the training and assessment of feeding skills in multihandicapped children. *Applied Research in Mental Retardation, 7*, 149–163.

Sisson, L.A., & Van Hasselt, V.B. (1989). Feeding disorders. In J.K. Luiselli (Ed.), *Behavioral medicine and developmental disabilities* (pp. 45–73). New York: Springer-Verlag.

Skinner, B.F. (1953). *Science and human behavior.* New York: Free Press.

Stark, L.J., Bowen, A.M., Tyc, V.L., Evans, S., & Passero, M.A. (1990). A behavioral approach to increasing calorie consumption in children with cystic fibrosis. *Journal of Pediatric Psychology, 15,* 309–326.

Stark, L.J., Knapp, L.G., Bowen, A.M., Powers, S.W., Jelalian, E., Evans, S., Passero, M.A., Mulvihill, M.M., & Hovell, M. (1993). Increasing calorie consumption in children with cystic fibrosis: Replication with 2-year follow-up. *Journal of Applied Behavior Analysis, 26,* 435–450.

Stark, L.J., Powers, S.W., Jelalian, E., Rape, R.N., & Miller, D.L. (1994). Modifying problematic mealtime interactions of children with cystic fibrosis and their parents via behavioral parent training. *Journal of Pediatric Psychology, 19,* 751–768.

Stokes, R.F., & Baer, D.M. (1977). An implicit technology of generalization. *Journal of Applied Behavior Analysis, 10,* 349–367.

Sturm, L., & Drotar, D. (1991). Maternal attributions of etiology in nonorganic failure to thrive. *Family Systems Medicine, 9,* 53–63.

Thompson, R.J., & Palmer, S. (1974). Treatment of feeding problems—a behavioral approach. *Journal of Nutrition Education, 6,* 63–66.

Thompson, R.J., Palmer, S., & Linscheid, T.R. (1977). Single-subject design and interaction analysis in the behavioral treatment of a child with a feeding problem. *Child Psychiatry and Human Development, 8,* 43–53.

Turner, K.M.T., Sanders, M.R., & Wall, C.R. (1994). Behavioural parent training versus dietary education in the treatment of children with persistent feeding difficulties. *Behaviour Change, 11,* 242–258.

Wahler, R.G., & Hann, D.M. (1986). A behavioral systems perspective in childhood psychopathology: Expanding the three-term operant contingency. In N.A. Krasnegor, J.A. Arasteh, & M.F. Cataldo (Eds.), *Child health behavior: A behavioral pediatrics perspective* (pp. 146–167). New York: John Wiley & Sons.

Werle, M.A., Murphy, T.B., & Budd, K.S. (1993). Treating chronic food refusal in young children: Home-based parent training. *Journal of Applied Behavior Analysis, 26,* 421–433.

Werle, M.A., Murphy, T.B., & Budd, K.S. (1994, May). *Behavioral parent training in the treatment of selective food refusal: An ecological analysis.* Paper presented at the meeting of the Association for Behavior Analysis, Atlanta, GA.

Werle, M.A., Murphy, T.B., & Budd, K.S. (in press). Broadening the parameters of investigation in treating young children's chronic food refusal. *Behavior Therapy.*

Wolf, L.S., & Glass, R.P. (1992). *Feeding and swallowing disorders in infancy: Assessment and management.* Tucson, AZ: Therapy Skill Builders.

5 | Children Who Eat Too Little
From Mild to Extreme Selectivity

For most people, eating is one of the great pleasures of life. Across cultures, food figures prominently into valued occasions such as religious and ethnic celebrations, social gatherings with friends and family, and gift giving (DeGarine, 1972). The positive connotations usually associated with food contrast sharply with oft-observed patterns of selective eating in childhood. Indeed, the inherent hedonic value of eating is so strong that overeating represents a far greater problem than does undereating for most adults and for many children (see Chapter 10). This chapter considers two types of undereating in children—mild and extreme selectivity—and includes discussion of the prevalence, etiology, and consequences of selectivity, as well as a review of interventions for undereating. The initial part of the chapter discusses criteria for distinguishing mild from extreme selectivity and reviews prevalence studies on selective eating and related feeding problems in children. The remainder of the chapter is divided into sections on children with mild selectivity and children with more extreme selectivity. Children with problems of undereating resulting in poor growth, who also carry the diagnosis of failure to thrive (FTT), are discussed in Chapter 6.

DEFINITION

Selective eating is defined as self-restriction of type, texture, or amount of food available to the child. The term "self-restriction" is used to distinguish voluntary selectivity on the child's part from dietary restrictions attributable to factors outside the child's control. The terms "mild" and "extreme" define two ends of a continuum of childhood undereating. The presence of a continuum implies that many feeding problems lie between these end points at a level of moderate or intermediate severity. Various issues enter into the judgment of whether selective eating is mild, moderate, or severe. Quantitative aspects of selectivity (e.g., the number of available foods accepted by the child), developmental expectations, the degree of child and family distress, and health implications all play a role in this decision. Some of the factors that typically differentiate mild from extremely selective eating are summarized in Table 5.1 and further discussed in the following paragraphs.

Mild selectivity includes those common feeding problems often described with phrases such as "picky eating," "finicky eating," and "poor appetite." These terms are not always used consistently by parents, clinicians, or researchers. Children can place restrictions on the types of foods they will accept, have strong flavor preferences, be texture selective, or eat smaller portions than expected. No consensual quantitative criteria are available to apply to these different types of selectivity.

Furthermore, the term "feeding problem" often is extended to behaviors that may accompany and complicate feeding. In infancy, mild selectivity may be associated with irritability, frequent crying, spitting up, formula intolerance, and colic. When these occur in conjunction with feeding, they often (but not always) are included under the term "feeding problem." In early childhood, mealtime behavior problems (e.g., throwing food) can be associated with mild selectivity (in this case, if the child throws nonpreferred foods). Mealtime behavior problems, however, may not be related to any dimension of eating, per se, but rather may be a reflection of more general problems with child discipline.

Mild selectivity and its associated feeding problems often are correlated with developmental stages and do not have significant social, developmental, or health consequences. For this reason, mild selectivity is usually regarded as a subclinical feeding problem.

By contrast, selective eating can be described as extreme when self-restriction on the variety or type of dietary intake results in significant health, developmental, or social problems. Children with extreme selectivity may consume only one or two types of food (e.g., milk and peanut butter sandwiches), may self-restrict diet to particular textures (e.g., liquids, puréed foods), or may select on the basis of taste (e.g., exclusive acceptance of sweet foods). The terms "partial food refusal," "chronic food refusal," "conditioned dysphagia," and "feeding aversion" sometimes are applied to these children. Extreme selectivity very often is accompanied by strong negative emotional reactions to the introduction of novel foods as well as socially stigmatizing mealtime behavior problems.

Table 5.1. Mild versus extreme selectivity: Typical features

Mild (subclinical)	Extreme
Degree of self-restriction	
Type/taste	
• May have strong preferences within food groups (e.g., eats chicken and pork, refuses beef) • May refuse all members of single food group (e.g., vegetables) • May have strong flavor preference (usually sweets)	• Frequently rejects all members of several food groups (e.g., may consume milk and peanut butter sandwiches exclusively) • May refuse all unsweetened foods
Texture	
• May prefer liquids • May have some difficulty making transition to advanced textures	• Chronic resistance to developmentally appropriate textures • May have exclusive preference for single texture (e.g., liquids, puréed)
Volume	
• Meal portion size frequently small • Caloric intake may be highly variable but is satisfactory over time	• May refuse to eat entirely (e.g., sustained by tube feeding) • Caloric intake often suboptimal over time
Associated problems	
• Recurrent mealtime struggles	• Significant child and caregiver distress • Strong emotional (often phobic) reactions to introduction of novel foods
Persistence/response to intervention	
• Often developmentally correlated • Feeding problems managed with parent guidance or short-term professional intervention	• Usually chronic • Resistant to brief interventions • Requires intensive, sustained, professional intervention
Consequences	
• No health or developmental consequences • Limited social consequences	• High risk of health problems (e.g., suboptimal nutrition, increased vulnerability to infection, poor growth) • Significant developmental consequences (e.g., limited opportunity to practice oral-motor skills) • Significant social consequences (e.g., unable to eat with family and peers)

As noted previously, some selective eating patterns fall midway between mild and extreme levels or may show features of both types. Designating selectivity as mild or extreme is useful chiefly as a means of organizing what is known about etiology and interventions, topics that are covered following the section entitled Prevalence.

PREVALENCE

As noted in Chapter 1, many early childhood feeding problems are considered to be quite common, although prevalence estimates are clouded by inconsistent definitions, by unrepresentative or small samples, and by reliance on parent reports to identify feeding problems. To highlight what is known about selective feeding difficulties in the general population, a closer look at some of the prevalence studies is warranted. These studies are most pertinent to estimating the occurrence of mild selectivity and associated subclinical feeding problems.

Bentovim's (1970) classic review of several early studies reported rates of variable or finicky eating or feeding disturbances of 30%–45% in the general child population. Bentovim (1970) distinguished three types of feeding problems: 1) feeding mismanagement problems associated with initial establishment of infant feeding patterns, which showed a peak occurrence during the first 6 months of life; 2) feeding problems, presumably due to issues of children's developing autonomy, which showed a peak occurrence during the second to fourth years of life; and 3) obesity, which had a peak occurrence in years 8–12.

A study by Forsyth, Leventhal, and McCarthy (1985) of maternal reports of infant crying and feeding-related problems during the first 4 months of life further investigated the initial peak period noted by Bentovim (1970). Forsyth and colleagues (1985) studied 373 healthy-born infants—half of whom were initially breast-fed and the remainder were formula-fed—in the New Haven, Connecticut, area. Mothers of the two groups of children reported moderate to severe difficulties at 4 months of age for the following behaviors: excessive crying, 24% for breast-fed infants and 22% for formula-fed infants; spitting, 10% and 18%, respectively; colic, 12% and 10%; and other feeding difficulties, 7% and 4%. These findings suggest relatively frequent crying- and feeding-related problems in early infancy, with spitting and colic reported more frequently than other feeding difficulties. Furthermore, Forsyth and colleagues (1985) indicated that the method of infant feeding was not related to the likelihood of behavior difficulties.

A large-scale study of a birth cohort of 1,265 children in urban New Zealand (Beautrais, Fergusson, & Shannon, 1982) provided more information about the second peak period suggested by Bentovim (1970)—feeding problems. The study tracked reported rates of several child-rearing problems, one of which was eating or feeding problems (including finicky eating, picking at food, and refusal to eat unless assisted) in toddlers and preschool-age children. Based on structured interviews with mothers when their children were 2, 3, and 4 years of age, eating or feeding problems were reported for 24%, 19%, and 18% of the children at each age level, respectively. Two other areas of child-rearing problems that showed comparable prevalence rates to eating and feeding problems were "difficult to manage or control" and "temper tantrums, breath-holding." The reported rates of feeding problems suggest that mothers often experience feeding difficulties as well as other child-management problems with young children. Despite reports of frequent occurrence, only 3% of the mothers annually reported seeking medical or other professional advice for any of the problems, which suggests that the difficulties were rarely considered severe.

A study of 281 healthy, full-term infants and toddlers who were followed in Chicago-area pediatric practices (Reau, Senturia, Lebailly, & Christoffel, 1996) also identified a high rate of parent-reported feeding problems. Some of the data from this study are shown in Table 5.2. Parents in this study completed questionnaires during well-care visits. Rates of feeding-related problems in this study appear to increase with age, with toddlers more frequently identified as problem feeders than are infants. Sixty-two percent of the parents of toddlers in this study reported at least one feeding problem. This is an uncharacteristically high prevalence of reported feeding problems, but parents were not asked to rate the severity of problems or to express their degree of concern. This study of 130 infants and 151 toddlers also provides percentile distributions for feeding times (not shown in Table 5.2). Picky eating in toddlers was significantly related to longer feeding times.

Two prospective longitudinal studies provide information about the patterns of feeding problems over time. Marchi and Cohen (1990) compared data from maternal interviews at three points over a 10-year span for a randomly selected sample of 659 children in upstate New York. Table 5.3 shows selective findings from Marchi and Cohen's study regarding two clusters of eating behaviors: 1) prevalence of pickiness (in which parents endorsed at least three of four of the following items: The child does not eat enough, often or very often is choosy about food, usually eats slowly,

Table 5.2.   Parent-reported feeding problems in infants and toddlers

Problem	Infants (%)	Toddlers (%)
Is not always hungry at mealtimes	33	54
Does not always enjoy a feeding	9	33
Has strong food preferences	12	34
Refuses to eat a meal		26
Requests specific foods, then refuses them		21
Tries to end meal after a few bites		42
Picky eating		36

Adapted from Reau, Senturia, Lebailly, & Christoffel (1996).

Note: Parents of toddlers reporting one or more problem: 62%

and usually is not interested in food); 2) prevalence of problem meals (in which parents endorsed both of the following items: Meals are hardly ever pleasant, and there are frequent struggles about eating.)

Consistent with Bentovim (1970) and Beautrais et al.'s (1982) findings, Marchi and Cohen (1990) found that pickiness about food was reported for 27%–29% of children. By contrast, "problem meals," which reflect the negative impact of children's eating habits on family mealtime interactions, were reported for a substantially smaller proportion of children. Rates of both behavior clusters were significantly correlated across time periods, suggesting that children showing eating problems in early childhood are at increased risk of showing parallel problems in later childhood and adolescence. In addition, pickiness about food in early childhood was associated with higher incidence of symptoms of anorexia

Table 5.3.   Prevalence of feeding problems in a normal sample across a 10-year time span

Feeding problem	Interview 1 1–10[a] (6)[b]	Interview 2 9–18[a] (14)[b]	Interview 3 11–21[a] (16)[b]
Frequency of pickiness	29%	28%	27%
Frequency of problem meals	3.8%	2.6%	2.4%

Source: Marchi and Cohen (1990).

[a] Age range.

[b] Mean age.

nervosa in the 9- to 18-year-old group, indicating a possible link between early feeding problems and adolescent eating disorders.

Dahl (1987) and her colleagues (Dahl & Kristiansson, 1987; Dahl & Sundelin, 1986, 1992) conducted an impressive series of investigations on early childhood feeding problems. Initial review of 2,472 infants (representing virtually every birth in the Uppsula area of Sweden during the study period) identified 50 children at ages 3–12 months meeting fairly stringent criteria for feeding problems: 1) Both the parents and a child health center nurse considered that the child had a feeding problem, 2) the feeding problem had continued without interruption for at least 1 month, and 3) the problem had not responded to medical or psychological advice or treatment (Dahl & Sundelin, 1986). Three main problem categories were distinguished: 1) refusal to eat (child regularly and distinctly refuses offered food), 2) colic (daily recurring episodes of screaming for at least 2 hours without obvious cause), and 3) vomiting (daily episodes of ejecting stomach contents). The 50 cases represent a 2% prevalence rate of infant feeding problems, with an identification rate of 1.4% per year. Eight of the fifty infants had significant medical disorders (e.g., congenital heart disease, cerebral palsy, milk allergy); seven of those eight infants' feeding problems could be explained by their medical disorders.

In subsequent studies, the 42 children without obvious medical problems were followed to determine the impact of early-onset feeding problems on behavior and growth 2 years later and, for a smaller subgroup, 4 years later. After 2 years, feeding problems persisted in 50% of the cases; however, although most problems in the colic and vomiting groups had resolved, 76% of children in the refusal-to-eat group still had feeding problems (Dahl, 1987). When the 24 refusal-to-eat cases were reexamined at 4 years, 70% continued to show feeding problems, although the severity of problems had lessened from major to minor in most cases (Dahl & Sundelin, 1992).

Dahl and colleagues also studied a carefully matched control group of 42 children without early-onset feeding problems to compare the course of development for the two groups. At 2 years, 14% of the control children had developed feeding problems, specifically, refusal-to-eat problems (Dahl, 1987). By 4 years, 21% of the control group had feeding problems (Dahl & Sundelin, 1992), a level that approaches the prevalence rates reported in other normative samples (Beautrais et al., 1982; Bentovim, 1970; Marchi & Cohen, 1990).

Comparisons between the refusal-to-eat and control children indicated that, by 4-year follow-up, several differences that had favored the control group at 2-year follow-up were now either less pronounced or absent (Dahl & Kristiansson, 1987; Dahl & Sundelin, 1992). For example, group differences were no longer present with respect to significant health problems or the use of medical services. Growth indices showed that the refusal-to-eat children were significantly smaller than control children from birth and remained so throughout the study; however, at 4 years, all but one of the refusal-to-eat children were within normal growth parameters, and none were considered nutritionally impaired.

By contrast, behavioral differences between the two groups persisted over time. Parents of refusal-to-eat children reported significantly more overall behavior problems than parents of control children at 4-year follow-up (Dahl & Sundelin, 1992). It is interesting to note that the investigators also found that control children with feeding problems after 4 years had significantly more "other behavior problems" (e.g., regarding sleep, shyness, tantrums) according to parent report than controls without feeding problems. This finding suggests a relationship between feeding problems and other behavioral difficulties, irrespective of when feeding problems begin.

Taken together, the prevalence studies suggest several generalizations, which include the following: 1) Maternal reports of feeding problems (e.g., finickiness, colic, vomiting) are indeed fairly common (i.e., 20%–50%) in infancy and early childhood; 2) when more stringent criteria are applied to exclude transitory feeding problems (cf. Dahl & Sundelin, 1986), reported frequencies of feeding problems are lower—at least in early infancy—but show an increasing trend during ages 2–4 years; 3) whereas colic and vomiting are usually time-limited problems, selective eating tends to persist for 2 or more years and may be associated with other behavior problems as well; and 4) although food refusal can be associated with reduced growth rates, most children without other medical disorders remain grossly within normal limits (i.e., within 2 standard deviations of the mean for weight and height).

MILD SELECTIVITY: FINICKY EATING AND OTHER COMMON MEALTIME PROBLEMS

Based on the prevalence studies discussed in the previous section, the problem of mild selectivity, or "finickiness," appears to be a common and relatively persistent parental feeding concern of otherwise typically developing children. Finickiness includes eating small amounts, choosiness or pickiness about food, eating slowly, and showing low interest in food (e.g., Marchi & Cohen, 1990). Most children with finicky eating habits, however, are not self-restricting to the extent of severely deleterious growth or nutrition consequences.

Etiology

Clinical feeding specialists from diverse professions (e.g., Finney, 1986; Macht, 1990; Pridham, 1990; Satter, 1987; Skuse, 1993) have related a variety of causal factors to common childhood feeding problems. These factors are, for the most part, clinically derived and can be characterized using the causal constructs on the etiological dimension of the bidimensional classification system proposed in Chapter 1. Factors often found to be associated with common feeding problems include 1) diet (e.g., failure to match diet to developmental stage), 2) appetite (e.g., meal scheduling issues), 3) interaction/management (e.g., parent feeding styles, physical/structural aspects of the feeding situation), 4) child constitution (e.g., difficult temperament), 5) caregiver competence variables (e.g., the parent's own history of feeding difficulty, caregiver naiveté about appropriate foods and child consumption styles), and 6) systemic variables (e.g., family financial status). Diminished physical competence and chronic illness are less frequently postulated as causes of mild selectivity but are thought to play an increasingly significant role in the emergence of moderate to extreme selectivity.

Research on the causes of mild selectivity is not extensive but lends some support to clinical impressions regarding etiology. Studies by Dahl and her associates, described next, have shed some light on the possible precursors of mild selectivity by comparing groups of children with and without early-onset feeding problems. Hagekull and Dahl (1987) found several psychosocial and environmental differences between a group of 42 infants with early-onset feeding problems and a control group with no reported problems, based on maternal interviews during the first year of life. Mothers of infants with feeding problems described their infants as more irritated, tense, and sensitive to disturbances, suggesting possible temperament differences. Mothers of infants with feeding problems reported having more negative feelings toward the feeding situation and their infants, suggesting interactional differences. Problem-group mothers also had more feedings per day and spent more time during meals, suggesting possible meal schedule variables. It is unclear from this study, however, whether the psychosocial and environmental differences preceded or resulted from feeding difficulties. With regard to biological factors, Dahl and Sundelin (1992) found that children who were identified at 3–12 months of age with refusal-to-eat problems were smaller physically from birth than a matched control sample. This suggests that normal variations in health status, growth parameters, or appetite may predispose some children to mealtime problems.

In a related study of factors that predated the onset of feeding problems, parents' own histories of experiencing feeding problems in infancy emerged as a strong predictor of their child's feeding problems (Dahl, Eklund, & Sundelin, 1986). This finding, which was corroborated through interviews with grandparents, hints at a possible familial link for the development of feeding problems. In the same study, mothers of children with feeding problems reported greater anxiety during pregnancy, experienced more breast-feeding problems, and acknowledged more personal health problems than mothers of control children. Nevertheless, given the number of between-group differences found and plausible alternative explanations, it is premature to conclude that any of these variables indeed cause common feeding problems.

A study using a different sample of healthy, full-term, Swedish children with feeding problems (Lindberg, Bohlin, Hagekull, & Thunstrom, 1994) found that early childhood food refusal was associated with difficult infant temperament, less positive perception of parenting, weaning problems, lower caloric intake, higher prevalence of breast-feeding, a larger number of meals, and more psychosocial family problems as compared with a matched group of children without food refusal. This is also one of the few studies that shows early food refusal to be associated with lower relative weight when comparison groups are matched on birth weight.

The strong clinical impression that parent feeding practices are an important factor in the etiology of common feeding problems was examined in an observational study comparing feeding interactions in matched groups of children with and without persistent feeding difficulties (Sanders, Patel, Le Grice, & Shepherd, 1993). Parents of children with feeding difficulties were more negative and coercive, engaged in higher levels of aversive instruction giving, aversive prompting, and negative eating-related comments.

The preceding paragraphs summarize research that characterizes specific child and caregiver variables with potential etiological importance. Two broader, contextual variables with significance for feeding are discussed in the following sections.

Developmental Issues   Early childhood feeding occurs in the context of complex anatomical, physiological, cognitive, and social developmental processes. From an etiological perspective, a child's physical competence and other constitutional characteristics change and assume evolving functional significance across the first years of life. The developmental context can influence the emergence of feeding problems in at least three ways. First, the physical maturation of the child's feeding skills (see, e.g., Figure 3.1 in Chapter 3) represents a clear biological constraint on the utility of specific feeding practices (Stevenson & Allaire, 1991). For example, an infant's oral-motor skills include a reflexive vertical bite before 5 months, but coordinated biting and chewing emerge later, with rotary chewing beginning at about 12 months. Parents who misinterpret the reflexive bite may introduce inappropriate foods, a practice that may result in gagging and infant distress. Second, there may be an increased risk of particular types of feeding problems during specific developmental periods. For example, "messy eating" between 8 and 12 months, picky eating between 18 and 24 months, and pica between 24 and 36 months may represent developmentally specific challenges to parent tolerance (Nelson, 1995). Dietary neophobia (resistance to trying new foods) is typical in children (Birch & Fischer, 1995) and may be especially evident during the preschool years. Developmental stages also have played a prominent role in the classification of more severe feeding dysfunction in FTT (Chatoor, Dickson, Schaeffer, & Egan, 1985).

Third, there has been considerable speculation regarding the etiological significance of developmental "sensitive periods," during which children are receptive to the introduction of textures and tastes. The sensitive, or "critical," period for accepting solid textures has been postulated to occur around 7–10 months of age (Illingworth & Lister, 1964). Skuse (1993) reviewed research suggesting that a related sensitive period for acceptance of novel tastes occurs at about 4–6 months of age. The period hypothesis proposes that children who are not exposed to varied textures or tastes during these "windows of opportunity" are at increased risk to become intolerant of novel textures or tastes. Indirect support for the period hypothesis comes from case studies of clinical feeding problems in children with chronic health conditions who were precluded from exposure to varied textures for a prolonged time period (see Chapter 7). For practical and ethical reasons, prospective studies with humans have not investigated this issue, yet the period hypothesis remains a useful heuristic to account for the development of some feeding problems.

Sociocultural Practices Sociocultural factors also represent important, often underappreciated, systemic variables to consider in the emergence of common feeding problems (cf. Skuse, 1993). Sociocultural practices refer to shared expectations, beliefs, values, and actions specific to particular ethnic, regional, religious, or class subgroups (Messer, 1984). Sociocultural conventions influence the types, textures, and combinations of foods offered to infants and young children; for example, in Malaysia, the presence of cooked rice defines a "meal," and all food eaten without cooked rice is considered a "snack" (Messer, 1984), whereas in the United States, snacks generally consist of sweets, finger foods, or small bits of leftovers. Cultural practices also reflect the accepted methods by which parents influence what children eat. Dettwyler (1989) described a continuum of caregiver-control tactics that range from maternal force-feeding (e.g., pinching an infant's nose while depositing food) as a routine tactic in some societies to progressively greater laxity (e.g., walking the child around to distract him or her while eating, relying on the child to dictate the eating schedule). Dettwyler noted that, in most Western cultures, parents tend toward more control-oriented tactics, using structured mealtimes and persuasive interactional strategies to encourage children to "clean their plates."

The role of sociocultural norms in the development of common feeding problems is unclear, in part because it is difficult to isolate their impact from other variables affecting feeding problems. Skuse (1993) has suggested that sociocultural and developmental influences may act in combination to increase the risk of finicky eating in toddlers who have been offered a culturally normative bland or limited diet during the first several months of life. In any case, variations in sociocultural practices should be factored into judgments about the clinical significance of common feeding problems and into the professional evaluation of parent feeding styles.

Intervention

As noted previously, Beautrais et al. (1982) found that only a small fraction of parents reported their young children's feeding or other common behavior problems to pediatricians or other professionals. In some cases, the lack of professional attention may be of little consequence because some feeding problems resolve on their own. In other cases, however, feeding difficulties are persistent topics of concern to parents, even if the problems do not threaten the child's health or development (e.g., Dahl & Sundelin, 1992; Marchi & Cohen, 1990). Also, a substantial number of first-time parents have questions about how to feed their child, what to expect at different developmental points, and how best to promote their child's healthy eating. Thus, there is a role for preventive, educative, or supportive assistance for families regarding common feeding issues, as well as for short-term intervention for managing feeding problems.

Information for parents regarding mild selectivity and other common feeding problems can be broadly categorized into three types: 1) anticipatory guidance to support adaptive feeding practices offered during health care visits, 2) bibliographic materials to educate parents about feeding and management of common feeding problems, and 3) parent training by allied health professionals to address identified problems. Further description of these three approaches is offered next.

Anticipatory Guidance   The most logical setting for prevention or early management of mild selectivity and other common feeding problems would seem to be during routine primary care visits. During these periodic visits—recommended at 2–4 weeks, 2 months, 4 months, 6 months, 9 months, and 12 months during the first year (American Academy of Pediatrics, 1988)—physicians usually obtain basic measures of growth status, inquire about the child's food intake, and provide some anticipatory guidance (i.e., practical suggestions for promoting healthy child development) (Brazelton, 1995). Particularly with infants and toddlers, physicians typically offer recommendations about feeding practices (e.g., appropriate foods, serving amounts, methods of encouraging intake).

Although the logic of anticipatory guidance is compelling, the brevity of routine health care visits limits the actual delivery of educational information in practice. Reisinger and Bires (1980) found that well-child pediatric visits last an average of only 10 minutes, less than 10% of which is devoted to anticipatory guidance issues. Pediatricians are encouraged to cover many different topics (e.g., gross motor development, psychosocial development, child safety issues) during the time allotted to anticipatory guidance during well-care visits. On average, less than 50% of the approximately 60 seconds devoted to anticipatory guidance is spent on feeding issues. Parents also may be reticent to ask questions or bring up minor problems during these brief appointments, and some parents prefer other methods (e.g., telephone, newsletters) for gaining child care information (Pridham, 1990). Furthermore, not all parents accept professional advice on feeding issues, especially when it conflicts with family or cultural beliefs (Pridham, 1990). Whether anticipatory guidance reduces the likelihood of early childhood feeding problems is unknown. Anticipatory guidance during well-care visits potentially can be supplemented with written materials. Bibliographic materials are discussed next.

Bibliographic Materials   A wealth of written resources are available to inform parents about healthy feeding practices with children. Pamphlets containing general information about childhood feeding are published by the American Academy of Pediatrics, the American Dietetic Association, and food-related organizations such as the National Live Stock and Meat Board (1992) and Kellogg Company (Kellogg's Food and Nutrition Communications, 1991). These pamphlets outline basic food groups, age-appropriate serving sizes, and tips for increasing the attractiveness of foods to children. A variety of magazines devoted to child care also are available. *Healthy Kids*, for example, is a magazine published by the American Academy of Pediatrics and is freely available in many waiting rooms.

Written feeding guidelines have been developed expressly to supplement the health care provider's anticipatory guidance regarding feeding practices for children of different ages (Finney, 1986). These guidelines would seem to be a valuable addition to primary health care visits, regardless of whether parents express concerns about feeding. For more detailed information, the parent can consult one of the many useful books devoted to child care issues and nutrition. There are also several books devoted exclusively to feeding issues, designed especially for parents (e.g., Macht, 1990; Satter, 1986, 1987). These books provide potentially valuable resources for parents on a variety of feeding and child nutrition issues.

Although little research has investigated parents' ability to translate the information from bibliographic sources to managing their own children's feeding, a few studies suggest that written materials can be a viable teaching tool for at least some parents. For example, McMahon and Forehand (1978) prepared a $2^1/_2$-page brochure for parents of preschool children describing behavioral techniques (specifically, differential social attention and time-out) for reducing children's disruptive mealtime behavior. Using a single-subject experimental design with three families, McMahon and Forehand (1978) demonstrated systematic reductions in inappropriate mealtime behaviors at home after parents received the brochures.

Another investigation of bibliographic materials targeted children's inappropriate behavior while dining out at restaurants. Bauman, Reiss, Rogers, and Bailey (1983) showed that a written advice package was effective in reducing children's crying, noncompliance, and other inappropriate behaviors and was effective in decreasing parents' disapproving statements during meals at restaurants. The advice package included several practical recommendations for structuring the dining environment and for using parental attention to improve mealtime behavior, such as 1) preparing children for dining out by reviewing the behaviors expected of them; 2) seating children against the wall, preferably in a booth, in a less busy area of the restaurant; 3) keeping children within an arm's reach of a parent;

4) bringing crackers to eat while waiting for the meal to be served; 5) allowing children to order foods they like; and 6) praising appropriate mealtime behavior. This study, which involved children ages 3–8 years of age, suggests that bibliographic interventions can successfully increase parents' skills in managing common mealtime issues. Whether the same methods would be sufficient with parents of children exhibiting mild selectivity has yet to be established. Moreover, parent literacy and reading skill level place some constraints on the general application of bibliographic interventions.

Parent Training Most research involving parents as intervention agents for their children's feeding problems has involved children with clinical feeding disorders. The intervention procedures prescribed for clinical feeding problems, however, overlap considerably with those appropriate for use with subclinical feeding problems. In general, common feeding problems would be expected to respond to naturalistic or "low-key" strategies such as providing a nutritious, developmentally appropriate menu, arranging mealtime surroundings to support feeding, and providing pleasant social interactions during meals. Negative reinforcement, punishment, and desensitization procedures (as described further in Chapter 4) are rarely needed or appropriate for children with mild selectivity. Table 5.4 outlines feeding techniques most appropriate for use with mild selectivity or other common feeding problems. Case 5.1 illustrates a parent training program using behavior management procedures to modify a child's finicky eating habits.

■ ■ ■

CASE 5.1. FINICKY EATING HABITS
NAME: Ellen
AGE AT INTERVENTION: 3 years

BACKGROUND

Ellen was one of three children who participated with their mothers in a home-based feeding intervention study (Werle, Murphy, & Budd, in press). Ellen had a history of selective eating patterns, which had become of increasing concern to her mother.

Ellen's feeding difficulties were first noted after she was ill with the flu at about 3 months of age. Medical workups had revealed no organic explanation for her feeding problems, although she reportedly remained a finicky eater. On referral for the current project, her weight was slightly below the 50th percentile and her height was at the 33rd

Table 5.4. Clinical guidelines for mild selectivity interventions

EVALUATION

Screen for possible medical or developmental correlates of the feeding problem.
Screen for significant nutrition issues.
Assess parental concern.
Assess specific factors that may contribute to or co-occur with the problem:
- Parent naiveté about appropriate nutrition, child development, or feeding techniques
- Maladaptive meal schedules
- Child constitutional factors (e.g., fussy or passive feeder)
- Social attention and reinforcement of finicky habits
- Missed opportunities for exposure to novel tastes and textures during optimal developmental periods
- Parent stress from other problems

INTERVENTION

Educate parents about the following:
- Expectations regarding normal variation in child's daily intake
- Expectations regarding age-appropriate portion sizes
- Developmental feeding issues (e.g., neophobia, "readiness" for taste and texture, autonomy issues)

Counsel parents to do the following:
- Rely on the child's capacity for self-regulation of energy intake
- Avoid overwhelming social interactions and criticism during meals
- Avoid pressured, coercive, or forced feeding
- Avoid unnecessary interruptions (e.g., frequent burping), especially when feeding infants
- Offer a developmentally appropriate menu
- Systematically offer novel foods and textures
- Schedule meals and snacks to preserve or promote appetite (e.g., no eating or drinking 1 hour before meals)
- Serve meals seated at table or high chair
- Provide pleasant social interaction during meals
- Tolerate age-appropriate messiness
- Model sampling and enjoyment of novel foods
- Encourage child's independence during meals (e.g., finger-feeding, use of spoon, selection of drink)

Counsel parents to consider the following mild behavioral contingencies (if needed):
- Set limits on child's access to sweets and "empty" junk foods
- Limit length of meal (20–30 minutes is usually ample)
- Reduce environmental distractions during feeding
- Define consequences for mealtime disruption (e.g., time-out)
- Reinforce sampling of novel foods

percentile. Ellen's diet consisted of grains, fruits, a few meats, and a large quantity of liquids, in particular milk and fruit juices. When asked to eat vegetables or many meats, Ellen frequently ignored her mother's requests, left the table, cried, or attempted to bargain with her mother by asking how many bites she had to take. Ellen lived with her mother and two siblings, neither of whom had a history of feeding difficulties. Her parents were separated, and Ellen's mother attended a community college full time.

FORMULATION

Ellen's selective eating habits originated from unknown causes, possibly associated with negative experiences when she was ill. Because Ellen consumed enough food to maintain normal weight gain, her selectivity was not seen as a clinical problem until her mother reported it in the context of dealing with the stresses of marital separation. Baseline observations in the home showed that the mother attempted to reason with Ellen about why foods were good for her, and she provided pleasant but noncontingent social attention during meals. Thus, behavioral intervention was designed to broaden Ellen's food choices by increasing her intake of nonpreferred foods, particularly vegetables. In addition, because Ellen frequently left the table during meals, her out-of-seat behavior was monitored for possible intervention at a later date.

INTERVENTION

Systematic parent training was provided to teach behavior management skills to Ellen's mother for use during mealtimes. Training sessions took place in the home, and videotapes of home mealtimes were used to monitor progress. Training methods included instruction, discussion, handouts, role plays, behavior rehearsal during mealtimes, and verbal feedback after meals. The key intervention ingredients were as follows:

1. Educational information on child nutrition (e.g., expected types and amounts of different food groups at different ages)
2. Suggestions on how to introduce nonpreferred foods in small quantities (e.g., offering only one or two bites of vegetables at first, then gradually increasing the amount as Ellen began to eat more)
3. Use of preferred menu items, specifically liquids, as reinforcers for nonpreferred items (e.g., having Ellen eat a bite of corn or green beans, then providing her access to fruit juice at meals)
4. Use of clear, specific prompts if Ellen fails to eat any vegetables or if she requests a drink (e.g., "Try a spoon of peas, and then I'll give you some milk")
5. Provision of pleasant social conversation with Ellen as long as she cooperates with eating; disruptive behaviors (e.g., crying, refusing) were ignored

OUTCOME

Parent training was successful in increasing both Ellen's intake of vegetables and the mother's behavior management skills. Ellen ate an average of 2 bites of vegetables during baseline observations, which increased to an average of 10 bites during intervention. The mother's use of trained procedures increased from 33% before training to 80% of total parent behaviors after training. Furthermore, Ellen's out-of-seat behavior decreased without special procedures over the course of intervention, reducing from 22% of the time prior to parent training to 10% after training. Follow-up observations conducted every 2 weeks for 12 weeks after intervention showed that these improvements were maintained.

■ ■ ■

EXTREME SELECTIVITY: FOOD REFUSAL AND FOOD PHOBIA

Food selectivity can be described as extreme when self-restriction on the type, texture, or volume of dietary intake results in significant health, developmental, or social problems. Associated conditions and consequences of extreme selectivity are described in the next section.

Consequences of Extreme Selectivity and Associated Conditions

Nutritional Consequences Ingestion of appropriate amounts and proportions of proteins, fats, carbohydrates, water, vitamins, and trace minerals is necessary to support growth and optimal development. Making a variety of healthful foods available to children is generally sufficient to ensure balanced nutrition, but children with extreme selectivity can be an exception to this rule. A dramatic example of severe nutritional consequences of extreme selectivity is described by Clark, Rhoden, and Turner (1993). An 8-year-old boy with autism had a long history of food selectivity with a more recent 2-year history of extreme selectivity characterized by consumption of french fries and water, exclusively. Although his weight for age and weight for height were just within normal limits, his diet was severely deficient, especially in calcium and vitamins A and D. He presented with a limp and with preorbital swelling and was found to have hypocalcemia and rickets, as well as xerophthalmia (conjunctival dryness) and corneal erosions. These symptoms of hypocalcemia and vitamin deficiency were reversed with dietary supplementation in the form of nasogastric Pediasure

(a nutritionally balanced liquid supplement), as well as with therapeutic doses of calcium and vitamin A. Although not all highly
selective diets result in malnutrition, this risk needs to be considered. A careful nutritional assessment is therefore warranted for all
children referred for extreme selectivity.

Developmental Consequences Extreme dietary selectivity
can be associated with and contribute to developmental feeding delays. Refusal to eat textured foods, for example, may have minimal
nutritional significance (if appropriate dietary supplements are prescribed) but can compromise attainment of developmental oral-
motor milestones by reducing opportunities to practice chewing
and other oral-motor skills.

Social Consequences Extremely selective eating generally
has adverse social consequences. Sharing food is a common setting
event for other forms of social sharing and learning. The implied
rejection of this form of shared experience can arouse anger and anxiety in parents, caregivers, extended family, and friends. During
preschool and school years, children with restrictive eating habits
may find themselves socially isolated during snack periods and
at lunch times. In rare cases, extreme selectivity characterized by
food phobia (see Interventions) has been accompanied by refusal to
attend school (Chatoor, Conley, & Dickson, 1988).

Etiology

Any of the causal factors related to mild selectivity could potentially contribute to extreme selectivity as well. Because there is a
dearth of either epidemiological or case comparison studies, inferences about the etiology of extreme selectivity tend to be drawn
from case studies. Reviews of the available studies (see, e.g., Babbitt
et al., 1994; O'Brien, Repp, Williams, & Christophersen, 1991) suggest that children with extreme selectivity frequently, but not invariably, have histories that include significant illness and diminished physical, intellectual, and social competence. Clinical
explanatory accounts of extreme selectivity have emphasized the
causal role of physical competence (primarily oral-motor and neurodevelopmental dysfunction), interaction/management (primarily
misplaced social contingencies), acute and chronic illness (primarily as it affects appetite or motivation to eat), or some combination
of each.

Physical Competence The physical ability to consume textured food (e.g., ground, chopped, regular table foods) is dependent on
the complex coordination of oral-motor and swallowing skills. When
a child is incapable of processing these textures, or when eating tex-

tured food induces fatigue or discomfort, the child may become texture selective. In the face of persistent child resistance, the parent may fail to offer textured foods, thereby removing the opportunity to develop more mature oral-motor skills. Diminished or immature oral-motor competence should be strongly suspected in cases in which a child presents with primary extreme texture selectivity.

When selectivity is characterized by an aversion to a broad class of stimulation, in the absence of oral-motor dysfunction, a neurological basis is sometimes assumed. For example, aversion to strong tastes or advanced food textures may be attributed to lowered sensory threshold (Morris & Klein, 1987) or, in the case of premature infants, to neurological immaturity (Wolf & Glass, 1992). The "critical period" hypothesis (Illingworth & Lister, 1964) that is discussed previously in the chapter is another hypothetical neurodevelopmental construct frequently invoked to account for extreme selectivity. One problem with these types of explanations is that they are often circular. For example, an oral aversion may be "explained" by lowered sensory thresholds, but there may be no evidence for the presence of the causal factor other than the phenomenon (oral aversion) that it is intended to explain.

Interaction/Management   As described in Chapter 4, feeding can become selective as a function of misplaced social reinforcement contingencies. For example, children with relatively mild food preferences and aversions may become increasingly selective 1) if refusing less preferred foods leads to more parental attention than accepting highly preferred foods or 2) if refusing less preferred foods causes the parent to provide highly preferred foods more frequently to compensate for the child's inadequate intake of less preferred foods.

Extreme selectivity also can evolve from the mismanagement of developmentally expected neophobia. Children between the ages of 2 and 5 are known to show a strong preference for familiar over novel foods (Birch, 1990). As Birch pointed out, parents often interpret a child's rejection of a food as immutable, and then they fail to offer that food again. When this happens repeatedly, the range of foods to which the child is exposed can narrow significantly.

Finally, when the range of accepted foods is limited to only highly palatable foods (e.g., sweets), the palatability of nonpreferred foods may be further reduced. This phenomenon, known as "negative contrast," has been demonstrated in a number of studies, including a well-designed study of infants who were shown to consume less plain water when it was preceded by an opportunity to consume sweetened water (Kobre & Lipsitt, 1972).

Illness   The multiple effects of acute and chronic illness, and their treatment, on feeding are provided detailed coverage in Chapter 7. For the present discussion, let it suffice to note that traumatic or aversive experiences with eating (e.g., choking) have been reported to result in extreme selectivity in otherwise healthy children. This type of selectivity, also characterized as a "food phobia," "conditioned dysphagia," or "posttraumatic eating disorder" (Chatoor et al., 1988; DiScipio & Kaslon, 1982) often is marked by refusal to consume solid foods of any kind. Food phobia is frequently, but not invariably, a form of secondary selectivity; that is, extreme selectivity emerging after an unremarkable feeding history. Food phobias are discussed further in the Interventions section.

Multiple etiological factors often interact to produce an ongoing selective feeding problem of considerable clinical significance. This is illustrated in the case of Mark, the selective eater described in Case 5.2.

■ ■ ■

CASE 5.2. A CHILD WITH EXTREME SELECTIVITY
NAME: Mark
AGE AT INTERVENTION: 24 months

BACKGROUND

Mark was a 24-month-old child with mild to moderate global developmental delays of unknown etiology, ectodermal anomalies, and a history of chronic otitis media (middle-ear infections). His weight and height were slightly above the 5th percentile, and his weight-for-height was slightly above the 10th percentile. Mark was enrolled in an early intervention program at which he received individual speech-language, occupational, and physical therapies.

He was seen as an outpatient for an interdisciplinary feeding evaluation, with the chief concern of extremely selective eating. Mark's diet at initial evaluation was self-limited to Pediasure, sweetened dry cereal, and cookies. Mark's early feeding history was unremarkable. He had started on infant formula, which he had taken without difficulty, and had made an uneventful transition to whole milk at 12 months of age before being changed to Pediasure by his pediatrician. He had started puréed infant foods at about 6 months of age, but, for unknown reasons, he abruptly stopped accepting these at 9 months of age.

During the evaluation, he became extremely distressed when the speech-language therapist attempted an oral examination; but he would accept chewable vitamins provided orally by his mother. Despite his oral aversion, his oral-motor skills were judged functional for biting and chewing, and there was no historical or current evidence for swallowing difficulties. He would periodically drink Pediasure from a cup but often insisted on a bottle. He refused apple juice by cup but accepted apple juice by bottle. He refused all food by spoon, becoming distressed when the spoon was brought close to his mouth, but he was able to hold a spoon and mimic self-feeding. He readily finger-fed sweetened dry cereal, as well as candy mints. His mother was aware that these were not nutritious foods but informed the team that "it's sweets or nothing." Although his parents would periodically try to offer novel foods, these attempts were unpredictable and always ended with Mark's vehement refusal.

Mark's extreme selectivity set the occasion for frequent mealtime struggles and ongoing parental stress related to his feeding and resulted in Mark's gradual tacit exclusion from family meals. Most of his eating and drinking occurred in brief bouts during the day, and he seldom sat for meals. Mark would frequently wake at night, demanding a bottle. During the evaluation, Mark was induced to accept a small amount of peanut butter placed on a piece of dry cereal, apparently a "first" for him.

FORMULATION

Despite an early history of gradual growth deceleration, Mark's diet of Pediasure and sweet snacks now kept him on a growth trajectory above the 5th percentile, and he no longer met diagnostic criteria for FTT. Predisposing child constitutional factors, developmental delays, and chronic illnesses had complicated the introduction of solid foods. His initial acceptance of puréed foods, as well as his marked aversion to feeding utensils (i.e., spoon, cup) suggested a selective feeding aversion acquired during the transition to solid foods, possibly as a result of overly insistent parent feeding attempts. Aversion to being fed with utensils also contributed to self-feeding delays. His willingness and ability to chew cookies and candy ruled out selectivity based on texture aversion. Mark's initial preference for sweet foods had become an exclusive preference, most likely as a result of parental concessions and the decreased palatability of nonsweet foods. The deterioration of any semblance of mealtime structure and indiscriminate "grazing" undermined normal hunger–satiety cycles. These factors, as well as increasing parental discouragement, resulted in infrequent exposure to novel foods.

INTERVENTION

A parent-mediated outpatient intervention plan was negotiated with Mark's mother, which included systematic graduated exposure to novel foods and textures, restrictions of sweets, differential reinforcement of food acceptance, and clearly defined mealtime structure. Mark's progress was monitored during the course of biweekly sessions with a pediatric psychologist and a clinical nutritionist. Essential features of the initial plan are outlined in Table 5.5.

OUTCOME

After 6 months of parent-mediated, outpatient intervention, Mark was consuming up to 2 ounces of peanut butter, served on small crackers, per meal, and was sampling small amounts of cream cheese, strawberries, and sunflower seeds, while continuing to follow his growth curve. Both the variety and the quality of his diet had improved, and consumption of sweet foods with little nutritional value had been significantly reduced. Mark was still a very selective eater, however, and he relied heavily on Pediasure to meet his nutritional needs. Mealtime struggles, although less frequent, had not abated entirely. Progress was compromised by several factors: frequent setbacks due to recurrent illness—chiefly chronic ear infections—as well as by multiple systemic stressors including family financial and marital difficulties.

■ ■ ■

Mark's case illustrates several characteristic features of extreme selectivity: a self-restricted diet with a narrow range of foods (in this case, dictated primarily by taste selectivity), differential intake patterns across feeders or feeding utensils (aversion to spoon feeding), strong preference for sweet tastes, narrowing of range of preferences over time, and the negative influence of frequent recurrent illness.

Interventions

Children with extreme selectivity have generally failed to benefit from exposure to the natural social contingencies that encourage nonselective eating in most children. Observational learning, frequency of exposure, and favorable adult information about the tastes of unfamiliar foods appear to be factors that mitigate a child's natural reluctance to try new foods. Adult modeling has been shown to increase acceptance of unfamiliar foods in children ages 14–48 months (Harper & Sanders, 1975). Birch and Marlin (1982) found that 10 exposures to novel foods, if they were tasted, were sufficient to increase preference for novel foods in a nonclinical population of 2-year-old children. Informing children that a novel food "tastes good" also has been shown to increase sampling of unfamiliar foods in children ages 3–8 years (Pelchat & Pliner, 1995). Al-

Table 5.5. Mealtime guidelines for Mark

Meal pattern
- Serve five evenly distributed mini-meals (Do not allow any other snacks [drinks or solids] between meals).

Types of food
- Offer finger foods: peanut butter on crackers and unsweetened dry cereals but not cookies or other sweets. Try to mix very small amounts of cheese or other foods into peanut butter. Introduce at least one new finger food each week.
- Serve Pediasure by cup, offered *after* solids.
- Serve Pediasure by bottle, only in the morning.

Meal setting
- Offer all meals in his high chair, including morning bottle.
- Continue with family-style meal at dinner.

Utensils
- Use both cup and bottle for formula, as above. (Do not attempt spoon feeding at this point in the program, but do encourage Mark to eat his peanut butter with a spoon. Modeling utensil use seems to be useful.)

Mealtime behavior
- Always praise *acceptance* of food.
- Ignore food refusals.
- Ignore throwing of food or utensils.
- Use a 5-minute time-out and start the meal over if Mark has a tantrum during the first half of the meal. If he has a tantrum during the second half of the meal, use a 5-minute time-out, but do not re-start the meal.
- Refocus attention on eating if Mark plays with food. (Brief playing with food is OK, but Mark is no longer at the stage at which sustained food play is useful.)

Other suggestions
- Limit solid meal to 10 minutes.
- Limit bottle/cup part of meal to 20 minutes.
- Offer drink *before* bed but not *in* bed.
- Offer water if Mark wakes up at night and requests a drink.

though adult modeling, instruction, and systematic exposure can be important components of a therapeutic intervention, they have not, by themselves, been demonstrated to be effective in the treatment of extremely selective children.

It is not uncommon for children with extreme selectivity to have failed to respond to anticipatory guidance, parent counseling, and other therapies. The failure of less intensive interventions may reflect a greater chronicity of selectivity, the convergence of more risk factors, or simply the more definitive influence of a single risk factor (e.g., oral-motor dysfunction, neurological immaturity, obsessive temperament). It is also possible that successfully resisting previous interventions strengthens a child's resistance to subsequent interventions.

Empirically validated interventions for extreme selectivity have emphasized the use of structured behavior modification procedures, including differential reinforcement of oral intake, successive approximation, ignoring food refusal, and time-out or other defined consequences for disruptive behavior. A schedule of frequent meals or feeding sessions, trained caregivers or professional feeders, minimally distracting feeding environments, appetite manipulation, and timed meals are also common features of behavior modification interventions. Several useful and detailed reviews of interventions for extreme selectivity are available (Babbitt et al., 1994; Linscheid, Budd, & Rasnake, 1995; O'Brien et al., 1991). The ensuing discussion provides an overview of the most common features of behavioral interventions for extreme selectivity, with somewhat more extended coverage of selected techniques and related issues.

In a typical behavioral intervention, the selective child is initially reinforced for sampling very small amounts of a novel food type or texture. Reinforcers usually are chosen on the basis of an individualized behavioral child assessment (see Chapter 3); but differential social attention, praise, activity rewards (e.g., gaining access to toys or television), tokens, and sensory reinforcers (e.g., rocking, massage) often are used. Another common feature of interventions for extreme selectivity is to reinforce the child's intake of a new or less favored food with a highly preferred food. The amount and variety of novel food intake required for reinforcement is then gradually increased. Table 5.6 lists some representative studies that used preferred foods to reinforce ingestion of novel foods.

Although contingent use of preferred food is a common intervention technique for extreme selectivity, inspection of Table 5.6 shows that this technique usually is employed in a multi-element intervention package that includes other potentially active components. The separate role of each intervention component is rarely evaluated. It is also important to note that using a preferred food as a reinforcer requires that the child's access to the preferred food be restricted. Because favored foods usually constitute a major portion of a selective child's diet, reinforcer restriction also may substantially decrease caloric (and sometimes fluid) intake. Thus, relative deprivation and appetite manipulation may contribute as much to the success of these interventions as does the contingent relationship established between favored and unfavored foods. This also means that interventions using preferred foods may involve some

Table 5.6. Studies using preferred foods as reinforcers in interventions for extreme selectivity

Study	Participants	Diet before intervention	Target foods	Additional interventions
Bernal (1972)	4-year-old girl	Strained foods	Table foods: cupcakes, french fries, cookies, peanut butter bread, and so forth. 50 new foods	Reinforced successive approximations, using a variety of reinforcers, including praise and contingent television, ignoring tantrums
Hatcher (1979)	2-year-old girl	Milk, juice, a few strained foods	A variety of solid foods	Praising, ignoring, peer reinforcement, time-limited meals
Linscheid, Oliver, Blyler, & Palmer (1978)	4- to 7-year-old girls	Case 1: Peanut butter sandwich, chocolate milk, french fries	Meats, vegetables, fruits	Praise, time-out, access to toys/television
	2- to 10-year-old boys	Case 2: Formula by bottle	Meats, vegetables, fruits	Praise, time-out
Luiselli, Evans, & Boyce (1985)	11-year-old boy	Bread, macaroni, bananas, peanut butter and jelly sandwiches, milk	"Regular" meals	Timed meals, ignoring, reinforcer menu
Palmer, Thompson, & Linscheid (1975)	6-year-old boy	Puréed foods, milk, pudding	Minced and "bite-size" foods	Praising, ignoring

(continued)

Table 5.6. *(continued)*

Study	Participants	Diet before intervention	Target foods	Additional interventions
Riordan, Iwata, Wohl, & Finney (1980)	16- and 23-month-old girls 40-month-old boy	Case 1: Milk, dry cereal, graham crackers Case 2: Canned fruits, ice cream Case 3: Milk, yogurt	Meats, vegetables, fruits, starch	Praising, ignoring
Riordan, Iwata, Finney, Wohl, & Stanley (1984)	6- and 9-year-old girls	Primarily liquids	Vegetables, meats, fruits	Praising
Thompson, Palmer, & Linscheid (1977)	30-month old boy	Dry cereal, cookies, candy, milk	"Regular" meals	Praising, ignoring, snack restriction

degree of short-term health risk and must be closely monitored, especially when the child's weight gain is also a concern.

Some feeding specialists expressly advise against using preferred foods to reinforce a child's acceptance of nonpreferred foods (e.g., Harris, 1993; Satter, 1987). Support for this caution often is derived from experimental studies with healthy children (Birch & Marlin, 1982; Newman & Taylor, 1992). These studies seem to show that when foods serve as the instrumental part of a means–ends contingency ("eat your spinach, then you can have dessert"), they come to be less preferred as a result of this relationship. It appears that children in these experiments conclude that foods that they are required to eat in order to gain access to other foods must be inferior in value. Whether these findings apply to the treatment of children with extreme selectivity is unclear. First, these studies were conducted with healthy children, who differ in many respects from children with extreme selectivity. Second, there are important differences in the initial value of the foods to each group of children: The foods in the means–ends experiments are of neutral and equal value prior to being assigned to either the means or the end condition, whereas the foods involved in selectivity interventions differ greatly in value from the start. Third, it is not clear whether differences in preference of the degree measured in means–end experiments have any ecological or clinical significance. Finally, none of the means–end experiments include follow-up studies to determine whether children do, in fact, avoid foods that they have been reinforced for eating over any meaningful period of time. Until the clinical relevance of these studies is clarified, it seems imprudent to discard a technique with demonstrated clinical efficacy in the intervention for extreme selectivity.

When children are extremely selective on the basis of texture rather than taste, texture fading is sometimes employed (e.g., Luiselli & Gleason, 1987). For example, the texture of pudding might be gradually increased by adding very small amounts of cream of wheat or cracker crumbs. The amounts of these additives are increased gradually, as tolerated by the child. Texture fading often is used in combination with differential reinforcement procedures. Behavioral intervention for a child with texture selectivity and self-feeding impairments is described in Chapter 8.

A study with extremely selective children that combines differential reinforcement with observational learning contingencies was reported by Greer, Dorow, Williams, McCorkle, and Asnes (1991). This study is unusual both in the use of peer-mediated reinforcement and in the location of treatment, a preschool lunch room. In peer-mediated reinforcement, the child with extreme selectivity is paired with a nonselective child. Each child is successively offered a bite of food and reinforced (e.g., with praise or a token) if food is consumed within a specified period of time. The procedure was used successfully in the intervention for two young children, one of whom refused to swallow, and another, an extremely selective 2-year, 5-month-old boy with an almost exclusively liquid diet. Peer-mediated reinforcement shows promise and merits further study for use with extremely selective eaters.

Some children with extreme selectivity fail to respond to structured behavioral interventions that rely entirely on positive reinforcement techniques. Children with the most severe forms of selectivity may vehemently refuse to accept even the small amounts of novel food or the barely discernible increments in texture that are required to meet the initial criteria for reinforcement. Children with severe selectivity may persistently turn their faces away from the spoon or bottle, may push utensils away, may attempt to leave the chair or feeding area, and may spit out any foods that the feeder manages to introduce. These children may benefit from the use of escape extinction or negative reinforcement techniques (see Chapter 4) in combination with positive reinforcement of oral intake (Hoch, Babbitt, Coe, Krell, & Hackbert, 1994; Riordan, Iwata, Finney, Wohl, & Stanley, 1984). These techniques usually are used only by highly trained therapists and are implemented most often in the context of inpatient treatment programs.

Interventions based exclusively on the use of differential reinforcement may not be effective or appropriate for some children with extreme food aversions. This may be especially true in the case of children characterized as having "food phobias," that is, extreme selectivity accompanied by strong negative affect (e.g., crying, verbal expressions of fear of eating or choking, psychogenic gagging) associated with caregiver attempts to feed a typical diet. Older, physically competent children, especially, may effectively resist contingency management procedures. Representative studies of children with food phobias are summarized in Table 5.7 and are described further in the next section.

Siegel (1982) described a case of chronic food aversion in a 6-year-old boy whose intervention involved systematic desensitization after differential reinforcement procedures had proved largely ineffective. This child had a normal developmental course and had accepted all foods until he accidentally received an overdose of paregoric at age 2 years. After the overdose, he consumed only a very nar-

Table 5.7. Children with extreme selectivity and food phobia: Associated factors

Study	Case	Age (in years)	Sex	Acute trauma	Tube feeds	Acute weight loss/FTT
Chatoor, Conley, & Dickson (1988)	1	8	F	Y	N	Y/N
	2	9	F	Y	N	Y/N
	3	10	M	Y	N	Y/N
	4	10	M	Y	N	?/N
	5	11	F	Y	Y	Y/N
Culbert, Kajander, Kohen, & Reaney (1996)	1	6	M	Y	N	?/N
	2	10	F	N	N	?/N
	4	7.5	M	N	N	N/N
Linscheid, Tarnowski, Rasnake, & Brams (1987)	1	6	M	N	Y	N/?
Siegel (1982)	1	6	M	Y	N	?/N
Singer, Ambuel, Wade, & Jaffe (1992)	1	8	M	Y	N	Y/N
	2	6	M	N	N	Y/?
	3	7.5	M	N	N	N/Y

Key: Y, yes; N, no; ?, unclear.

row range of foods, and he would gag and vomit when he attempted
to sample new foods. A variety of interventions, including withholding favored foods for up to 3 days, had been tried and found ineffective. At the time of intervention, his diet consisted largely of
cold cereal and milk, chocolate milk, orange juice, and sweets. A
contingency management program that specified differential consequences for sampling new foods was minimally effective, resulting
in the addition of only one new food (bacon) to the diet. Attempts to
sample other new foods continued to elicit reflexive gagging and
vomiting. A systematic desensitization program then was added to
the contingency management program. This provided for a graded
exposure to novel foods, with progressive steps defined as 1) smelling
the novel food, 2) touching the food to his lips, 3) placing food in his
mouth and then removing it, and 4) swallowing the food. Each phase
lasted from 1 to 2 weeks, and the child received rewards for completing the task required in each step. After 7 weeks of systematic
desensitization, gradual increases in the amount of food eaten were
required to obtain rewards. A 6-month follow-up assessment indicated that the boy had eaten more than 90 different table foods.

Similar techniques were used by Singer, Ambuel, Wade, and
Jaffe (1992) in the intervention for three children with acquired food
phobias. The three boys in this study were of average intelligence
and were hospitalized subsequent to a relatively recent onset of extreme selectivity. Selectivity of food type and texture were accompanied by verbalizations of fear, somatic complaints, and in one
case, vomiting. In addition to behavioral contingencies (e.g., gaining
contingent access to ward privileges), children were taught relaxation skills and cognitive coping skills to help them cope with anxiety aroused by eating feared foods.

Chatoor et al. (1988) described interventions for five cases of
food refusal and extreme selectivity resulting from traumatic
episodes of choking. The children in the study, ranging in age from
8 to 11 years, refused solid foods, sustained acute weight loss, and
survived on primarily liquid diets. They expressed fears of choking,
somatic complaints, and fears of dying. Systematic desensitization,
including relaxation therapy, was a common feature in intervention
for these children, as was psychoeducation (e.g., about the anatomy
of the esophagus, the trachea, and the lungs), family therapy, and in
some cases, pharmacotherapy.

Culbert, Kajander, Kohen, and Reaney (1996) described a series
of children with functional dysphagia and food aversion treated
with "hypnobehavioral" techniques, without the explicit inclusion
of contingency management or traditional psychotherapies. Three
of the five children described in this series meet the criteria for extreme selectivity, and these cases are included in Table 5.7. These

children expressed fears of choking and dying, and one presented with a "hyperactive gag reflex" and a tendency to become nauseated when undesired foods were discussed or were in proximity. Hypnobehavioral techniques included relaxation therapies, mental imagery, and systematic desensitization. Posthypnotic suggestions linking positive feelings with eating and swallowing also were used, as were cognitive-behavioral techniques such as positive self-talk. These interventions were remarkable for their brevity, with significant symptom resolution often accomplished in a matter of days.

It is notable that most of the children in the cases summarized in Table 5.7 are older and physically and verbally capable. It may be that a child with advanced verbal skills is more likely to be described as "phobic." Also, all but one of these children (a child with short gut syndrome described by Linscheid, Tarnowski, Rasnake, & Brams, [1987]) have "secondary" extreme selectivity—that is, they became extremely selective after having had a normal feeding history. This may partially account for the relatively rapid response to intervention that is sometimes reported (Culbert et al., 1996).

The foregoing discussion appears to encompass two very different types of children who benefit from two very different types of intervention. Children of the first type are younger and have physical and intellectual impairments, often have complex medical histories, have primary selectivity, and their behavior is described with terms such as "chronic food refusal." Children of the other type are older, generally healthy children of average intelligence, with secondary selectivity, and their behavior is described with terms such as "food phobia" and "conditioned dysphagia." Effective interventions for the former group tend to utilize highly structured behavioral procedures that emphasize differential reinforcement; effective interventions for the latter group tend to utilize procedures that emphasize systematic desensitization, relaxation therapy, and cognitive therapy techniques. Although the distinctions are certainly salient, two points of possible similarity should be noted. First, the extreme distress and desperate behavioral evasions of the young child with "chronic food refusal" may not be entirely dissimilar to the "fears" expressed by older, more articulate children. Second, there are functional psychological similarities between seemingly different techniques such as systematic desensitization and escape extinction and between what may be achieved by using activity or sensory reinforcers and what is achieved by relaxation therapies. In both cases, planned exposure to the object of fear is coupled with a countervailing psychophysiological state.

Clinical guidelines for interventions with children with extreme selectivity are summarized in Table 5.8. When extreme selectivity results in chronically poor weight gain, children may qual-

Table 5.8. Clinical guidelines for extreme selectivity interventions

EVALUATION

Rule out mild selectivity (extreme selectivity is usually associated with significant social, developmental, or health consequences).

Conduct medical evaluation to assess possible organic contributors and immediate and long-term health risks of the child's selectivity.

Conduct thorough assessment of nutritional status:
- Is intake adequate for optimal growth?
- Are there any micronutrient deficiencies?

Assess for specific factors that may contribute to the problem:
- Misplaced social contingencies
- Neurological immaturity
- Oral-motor problems
- Developmental neophobia
- Learned aversion (e.g., traumatic events, forced feeding)
- Sensory factors (e.g., negative contrast)
- Reduced dietary offering by caregiver
- Caregiver competence issues

Determine where and how intervention should be delivered (e.g., outpatient, inpatient, by therapist, by parent [see Chapter 4 for discussion of these considerations]).

INTERVENTION

If there are significant health risks, secure all necessary services to address risks.

When possible, optimize nutritional value of the baseline self-restricted diet (e.g., whole milk rather than skim, multivitamin).

Secure specific therapies for oral/motor problems if these contribute to or accompany selectivity.

Secure other developmental interventions, as needed.

Develop an individualized behavioral feeding program derived from evaluation of contributory factors. Most interventions will include the following:
- Systematic, graded exposure to novel foods or increasing food textures (texture fading)
- Contingent use of preferred foods
- Identification and use of other effective reinforcers (e.g., praise, activity rewards)
- Consistent mealtime structure (e.g., predictable meals/snacks/feeding sessions)
- Defined consequences (e.g., ignoring, time-out) for refusal and disruptive mealtime behavior
- Training all feeders to promote consistency

Some interventions will include the following:
- Structured observational learning component
- Escape extinction
- Systematic desensitization
- Relaxation therapies, hypnotherapy, and other cognitive-behavioral therapies for older (6–7 years old and older) children
- Appetite modification (e.g., limiting child's access to preferred foods)
- Interaction counseling/family therapy (see Chapter 6 for additional discussion of psychosocial interventions)

ify for a diagnosis of FTT. These children are discussed in the next chapter.

SUMMARY

Mild selectivity is common in early childhood. Finicky eating and other common feeding problems are consistently reported in 20%–50% of children during infancy and preschool years. Etiological variables are not well understood but probably include many of the same child, environmental, developmental, and sociocultural conditions that presage more serious feeding problems. Because mild selectivity and related feeding problems lack the adverse developmental and health sequelae of more severe feeding problems, the problems often escape formal attention by health professionals. Intervention approaches for mild feeding problems consist of anticipatory guidance to prevent or ameliorate difficulties, bibliographic materials, and parent training programs using low-key behavior management strategies.

Extreme food selectivity usually is characterized by a narrower range of food acceptance, persistent refusal to sample novel foods, and strong emotional reactions to the introduction of new foods. Adverse health, developmental, and social sequelae are common, even when extreme selectivity does not result in growth deficiency. Extreme selectivity is unlikely to respond to the low-key strategies used to manage mild selectivity. Use of structured behavioral interventions, systematic desensitization, and relaxation and cognitive behavior therapies, as well as more comprehensive mental health interventions often are required to treat extreme food selectivity.

REFERENCES

American Academy of Pediatrics. (1988). *Guidelines for health supervision.* Elk Grove Village, IL: Author.

Babbitt, R.L., Hoch, T.A., Coe, D.A., Cataldo, M.F., Kelly, K.J., Stackhouse, C., & Perman, J.A. (1994). Behavioral assessment and treatment of pediatric feeding disorders. *Journal of Developmental and Behavioral Pediatrics, 15,* 278–291.

Bauman, K.E., Reiss, M.L., Rogers, R.W., & Bailey, J.S. (1983). Dining out with children: Effectiveness of a parent advice package on pre-meal inappropriate behavior. *Journal of Applied Behavior Analysis, 16,* 55–68.

Beautrais, A.L., Fergusson, D.M., & Shannon, F.T. (1982). Family life events and behavioral problems in preschool-aged children. *Pediatrics, 70,* 774–779.

Bentovim, A. (1970). The clinical approach to feeding disorders of childhood. *Journal of Psychosomatic Research, 14,* 267–276.

Bernal, M.E. (1972). Behavioral treatment of a child's eating problem. *Journal of Behavior Therapy and Experimental Psychiatry, 3,* 43–50.

Birch, L.L. (1990). The control of food intake by young children: The role of learning. In E.D. Capaldi & T.L. Powley (Eds.), *Taste, experience, and feeding* (pp. 116–135). Washington, DC: American Psychological Association.

Birch, L.L., & Fischer, J.A. (1995). Appetite and eating behavior in children. *Pediatric Clinics of North America, 42,* 931–953.

Birch, L.L., & Marlin, D.W. (1982). I don't like it; I never tried it: Effects of exposure on two-year-old children's food preferences. *Appetite, 3,* 353–360.

Brazelton, T.B. (1995). Touchpoints for anticipatory guidance in the first three years. In S. Parker & B. Zuckerman (Eds.), *Behavioral and developmental pediatrics* (pp. 10–14). Boston: Little, Brown.

Chatoor, I., Conley, C., & Dickson, L. (1988). Food refusal after an incident of choking: A posttraumatic eating disorder. *Journal of the American Academy of Child and Adolescent Psychiatry, 27,* 105–110.

Chatoor, I., Dickson, L., Schaeffer, S., & Egan, J. (1985). A developmental classification of feeding disorders associated with failure to thrive: Diagnosis and treatment. In D. Drotar (Ed.), *New directions in failure to thrive* (pp. 235–258). New York: Plenum.

Clark, J.H., Rhoden, D.K., & Turner, D.S. (1993). Symptomatic vitamin A and D deficiencies in an eight-year old boy with autism. *Journal of Parenteral and Enteral Nutrition, 17,* 284–286.

Culbert, T.P., Kajander, R.L., Kohen, D.P., & Reaney, J.B. (1996). Hypnobehavioral approaches for school-age children with dysphagia and food aversion: A case series. *Journal of Developmental and Behavioral Pediatrics, 17,* 335–341.

Dahl, M. (1987). Early feeding problems in an affluent society: III. Follow-up at two years: Natural course, health, behaviour and development. *Acta Paediatrica Scandinavia, 76,* 872–880.

Dahl, M., Eklund, G., & Sundelin, C. (1986). Early feeding problems in an affluent society: II. Determinants. *Acta Paediatrica Scandinavia, 75,* 380–387.

Dahl, M., & Kristiansson, B. (1987). Early feeding problems in an affluent society. IV. Impact on growth up to two years of age. *Acta Paediatrica Scandinavia, 76,* 881–888.

Dahl, M., & Sundelin, C. (1986). Early feeding problems in an affluent society: I. Categories and clinical signs. *Acta Paediatrica Scandinavia, 75,* 370–379.

Dahl, M., & Sundelin, C. (1992). Feeding problems in an affluent society. Follow-up at four years of age in children with early refusal to eat. *Acta Paediatrica, 81,* 575–579.

DeGarine, I. (1972). The socio-cultural aspects of nutrition. *Ecology of Food and Nutrition, 1,* 143–163.

Dettwyler, K.A. (1989). Styles of infant feeding: Parental/caretaker control of food consumption in young children. *American Anthropologist, 91,* 696–703.

DiScipio, W.J., & Kaslon, K. (1982). Conditioned dysphagia in cleft palate children after pharyngeal flap surgery. *Psychosomatic Medicine, 44,* 247–257.

Finney, J.W. (1986). Preventing common feeding problems in infants and young children. *Pediatric Clinics of North America, 33,* 775–788.

Forsyth, B.W.C., Leventhal, J.M., & McCarthy, P.L. (1985). Mothers' perceptions of problems of feeding and crying behaviors: A prospective study. *American Journal of Diseases of Children, 139,* 269–272.

Greer, R.D., Dorow, L., Williams, G., McCorkle, N., & Asnes, R. (1991). Peer-mediated procedures to induce swallowing and food acceptance in young children. *Journal of Applied Behavior Analysis, 24,* 783–790.

Hagekull, B., & Dahl, M. (1987). Infants with and without feeding difficulties: Maternal experiences. *International Journal of Eating Disorders, 6,* 83–98.

Harper, L.V., & Sanders, K.M. (1975). The effects of adults' eating on young children's acceptance of unfamiliar foods. *Journal of Experimental Child Psychology, 20,* 206–214.

Harris, G. (1993). Feeding problems and their treatment. In I. St. James, G. Harris, & D. Messer (Eds.), *Infant crying, feeding, and sleeping* (pp. 118–132). London: Harvester Wheatsheaf.

Hatcher, R.P. (1979). Treatment of food refusal in a two-year-old child. *Journal of Behavior Therapy and Experimental Psychiatry, 10,* 363–367.

Hoch, T.A., Babbitt, R.L., Coe, D.A., Krell, D.M., & Hackbert, L. (1994). Contingency contracting: Combining positive reinforcement and escape extinction procedures to treat persistent food refusal. *Behavior Modification, 18,* 106–128.

Illingworth, R.S., & Lister, J. (1964). The critical or sensitive period, with special reference to certain feeding problems in infants and children. *Journal of Pediatrics, 65,* 839–848.

Kellogg's Food and Nutrition Communications. (1991). *Nutrition knowhow: For children ages 1–5 years old* [Brochure]. Battle Creek, MI: Kellogg Company.

Kobre, K.R., & Lipsitt, L.P. (1972). A negative contrast effect in newborns. *Journal of Experimental Child Psychology, 14,* 81–91.

Lindberg, L., Bohlin, G., Hagekull, B., & Thunstrom, M. (1994). Early food refusal: Infant and family characteristics. *Infant Mental Health Journal, 15,* 262–277.

Linscheid, T.R., Budd, K.S., & Rasnake, L.K. (1995). Pediatric feeding disorders. In M.C. Roberts (Ed.), *Handbook of pediatric psychology* (2nd ed., pp. 501–515). New York: Guilford Press.

Linscheid, T.R., Oliver, J., Blyler, E., & Palmer, S. (1978). Brief hospitalization for the behavioral treatment of feeding problems in the developmentally disabled. *Journal of Pediatric Psychology, 3,* 72–76.

Linscheid, T.R., Tarnowski, K.J., Rasnake, L.K., & Brams, J. (1987). Behavioral treatment of food refusal in a child with short-gut syndrome. *Journal of Pediatric Psychology, 12,* 451–459.

Luiselli, J.K., Evans, T.P., & Boyce, D.A. (1985). Contingency management of food selectivity and oppositional eating in a multiply handicapped child. *Journal of Clinical Child Psychology, 14,* 153–156.

Luiselli, J.K., & Gleason, D.J. (1987). Combining sensory reinforcement and texture fading procedures to overcome chronic food refusal. *Journal of Behaviour Therapy and Experimental Psychology, 18,* 149–155.

Macht, J. (1990). *Poor eaters: Helping children who refuse to eat.* New York: Plenum.

Marchi, M., & Cohen, P. (1990). Early childhood eating behaviors and adolescent eating disorders. *Journal of the American Academy of Child and Adolescent Psychiatry, 29,* 112–117.

McMahon, R.J., & Forehand, R. (1978). Nonprescription behavior therapy: Effectiveness of a brochure in teaching mothers to correct their children's inappropriate mealtime behaviors. *Behavior Therapy, 9,* 814–820.

Messer, E. (1984). Sociocultural aspects of nutrient intake and behavioral responses to nutrition. In J.R. Galler (Ed.), *Nutrition and behavior* (pp. 417–471). New York: Plenum.

Morris, S.E., & Klein, M.D. (1987). *Pre-feeding skills: A comprehensive resource for feeding development.* Tucson, AZ: Therapy Skill Builders.

National Live Stock and Meat Board. (1992). *A food guide for the first five years* [Brochure]. Chicago: National Live Stock and Meat Board, Educational Department.

Nelson, K. (1995). Feeding problems. In S. Parker & B. Zuckerman (Eds.), *Behavioral and developmental pediatrics* (pp. 143–148). Boston: Little, Brown.

Newman, J., & Taylor, A. (1992). Effects of a means–end contingency on young children's food preferences. *Journal of Experimental Child Psychology, 64,* 200–216.

O'Brien, S., Repp, A.C., Williams, G.E., & Christophersen, E.R. (1991). Pediatric feeding disorders. *Behavior Modification, 15,* 394–418.

Palmer, S., Thompson, R.J., & Linscheid, T.R. (1975). Applied behavior analysis in the treatment of childhood feeding problems. *Developmental Medicine and Child Neurology, 17,* 333–339.

Pelchat, M.L., & Pliner, P. (1995). "Try it. You'll like it." Effects of information on willingness to try new foods. *Appetite, 24,* 153–166.

Pridham, K.F. (1990). Feeding behavior of 6- to 12-month-old infants: Assessment and sources of parental information. *Journal of Pediatrics, 117*(Suppl.), S174–S180.

Reau, N.R., Senturia, Y.D., Lebailly, S.A., & Christoffel, K.K. (1996). Infant and toddler feeding patterns and problems: Normative data and a new direction. *Journal of Developmental and Behavioral Pediatrics, 17,* 149–153.

Reisinger, K.S., & Bires, J.A. (1980). Anticipatory guidance in pediatric practice. *Pediatrics, 66,* 889–892.

Riordan, M.M., Iwata, B.A., Finney, J.W., Wohl, M.K., & Stanley, A.E. (1984). Behavioral assessment and treatment of chronic food refusal in handicapped children. *Journal of Applied Behavior Analysis, 17,* 327–341.

Riordan, M.M., Iwata, B.A., Wohl, M.K., & Finney, J.W. (1980). Behavioral treatment of food refusal and selectivity in developmentally disabled children. *Applied Research in Mental Retardation, 1,* 95–112.

Sanders, M.R., Patel, R.K., Le Grice, B., & Shepherd, R.W. (1993). Children with persistent feeding difficulties: An observational analysis of the feeding interactions of problem and non-problem eaters. *Health Psychology, 12,* 64–73.

Satter, E. (1986). *Child of mine: Feeding with love and good sense* (Expanded ed.). Palo Alto, CA: Bull.

Satter, E. (1987). *How to get your kid to eat . . . but not too much.* Palo Alto, CA: Bull.

Siegel, L.J. (1982). Classical and operant procedures in the treatment of a case of food aversion in a young child. *Journal of Clinical Child Psychology, 11,* 167–172.

Singer, L.T., Ambuel, B., Wade, S., & Jaffe, A.C. (1992). Cognitive-behavioral treatment of health-impairing food phobias in children. *Journal of the American Academy of Child and Adolescent Psychiatry, 31,* 847–852.

Skuse, D. (1993). Identification and management of problem eaters. *Archives of Disease in Childhood, 69,* 604–608.

Stevenson, R.D., & Allaire, J.H. (1991). The development of normal feeding and swallowing. *Pediatric Clinics of North America, 38,* 1439–1453.

Thompson, R.J., Palmer, S., & Linscheid, T.R. (1977). Single-subject design and interaction analysis in the behavioral treatment of a child with a feeding problem. *Child Psychiatry and Human Development, 8,* 43–53.

Werle, M.A., Murphy, T.B., & Budd, K.S. (in press). Broadening the parameters of investigation in treating young children's chronic food refusal. *Behavior Therapy.*

Wolf, L.S., & Glass, R.P. (1992). *Feeding and swallowing disorders in infancy.* Tucson, AZ: Therapy Skill Builders.

6

Undereating with Growth Deficiency

Failure to Thrive
and Related Disorders

Children who eat too little may not grow adequately. As Chapter 5 discusses, mildly selective eating rarely has significant health consequences, and even extremely selective eating may not result in growth failure. It is equally true that not all growth failure results from undereating. The first section of this chapter considers failure to thrive (FTT) from a general perspective, but it emphasizes the co-occurrence of growth deficiency and undereating. The reader also is referred to Chapter 2, which discusses in more detail many of the medical issues raised by growth failure. This chapter concludes with a brief overview of two other, far less common, childhood disorders of undereating: nutritional dwarfing and prepubertal anorexia nervosa. The chapter's final section discusses psychosocial dwarfism, a growth disorder not related to undereating but often confused with FTT.

FAILURE TO THRIVE

Definition

FTT is usually defined by deficient somatic growth for age as indicated by a weight, height, or weight-for-height relationship that falls below the 5th percentile on growth charts of the National Center for Health Statistics (NCHS) (Hamill et al., 1979; see Figure 2.2 in Chapter 2); the 3rd percentile is used as a cutoff in some older studies. The term "FTT" also may be applied to children who evidence weight loss across more than two major percentile groups on the NCHS charts (e.g., falling from the 50th to the 10th percentile) over a sustained period of time (e.g., for 3 months in infants, 6 or more months in children older than 12 months of age). This velocity-based definition also is referred to as "growth faltering" (Peterson, Rathbun, & Herrera, 1985). Although the use of objective anthropometric measures lends an apparent precision to the term, consensus on a definition of FTT continues to be elusive (Bithoney & Dubowitz, 1985; Wilcox, Nieburg, & Miller, 1989; Wright, Ashenburg, & Whitaker, 1994).

Complete unanimity on a definition of FTT has been slow to develop for several reasons. First, the term was used historically to designate a growth disorder that was thought to coexist with developmental impairments and/or behavior problems in a child. When these growth, developmental, and behavior problems could not be attributed to a clear organic cause (termed "organic FTT"), FTT was presumed to be secondary to extreme psychosocial or maternal deprivation. These historical connotations continue to haunt contemporary practice, especially in the expression "nonorganic" failure to thrive (NFTT), the term still commonly used to designate those growth problems for which no clear organic cause has been identified. Because FTT may continue to elicit these superfluous associations, it has been suggested that the term be jettisoned and replaced by "growth deficiency" (Bithoney & Dubowitz, 1985; Drotar, 1995) or "failure to gain weight" (Villee, 1989). The terms "FTT" and "growth deficiency" will be used interchangeably in this chapter. Issues related to possible developmental impairments or behavior problems in children with FTT receive additional consideration in the following section, and the causal significance of maternal competence is discussed in the Etiology section.

Second, the diagnosis of FTT is not as simple as obtaining an accurate weight and height. Low weight-for-age, height-for-age, and weight–height relationships each have different clinical implications, which can be understood only when a *pattern* of growth, not merely a single set of growth parameters, is considered. The relationship between weight gain velocity and linear growth velocity in childhood is complex and must be carefully delineated to differentiate FTT from other forms of growth variation, including familial short stature, constitutional growth delay, intrauterine growth retardation (IUGR), and variation in growth due to breast-feeding (Maggioni & Lifshitz, 1995).

For example, a child may have short stature (a length-for-age below the 5th percentile) because 1) both parents are short (familial short stature), 2) his or her growth is delayed (constitutional short stature), 3) the child is born small (e.g., IUGR), or 4) the child has a chronic history of undernutrition resulting in stunting. A child may have a weight-for-age below the 5th percentile because 1) this is consistent with short stature, due to any of the above; or 2) the child is undernourished. Children with a weight-for-height relationship below the 5th percentile are always diagnosed with FTT, but a normal weight-for-height relationship does not rule out FTT because short stature may be the result of stunting. In the latter instance, a history of malnutrition can be hidden by a "normal" weight–height relationship. Sustained weight gain deceleration, relative to linear growth velocity, is probably the most reliable clinical indicator of FTT, but studies of children with FTT have not consistently used sustained weight gain deceleration to define FTT (Wilcox et al., 1989).

Third, even when patterns of growth are considered, using a percentile (usually the 5th) as a criterion for FTT/growth deficiency does not address the important issue of the degree or severity of growth failure. The severity of FTT usually is scaled using conventions (see Table 2.2 in Chapter 2) for describing degrees of malnutrition, which are based on the parameter of percentage of the median value for age (i.e., the 50th percentile for age on the NCHS growth charts). For example, a 3-year-old boy with a weight of 12 kilograms (26.4 pounds) falls just below the 5th percentile and is approximately 80% of the median weight on standardized growth charts. This child would be characterized as "mildly" malnourished, whereas a boy of the same age with a weight of 10 kilograms (22 pounds) is approximately 68% of the median and would be considered "moderately" malnourished. Although both boys are diagnosed with "FTT," the severity of their conditions differs and would likely lead to different clinical interventions. An added complication is that different methods may be used to categorize degree of undernutrition and that the same child may be classified as normal or as mildly or severely malnourished depending on the method used (Wright et al., 1994).

Conditions Associated with Growth Deficiency

Poor growth often is associated with other child health problems as well as with developmental or behavioral problems. It is usually difficult to determine whether these additional problems result from malnutrition, cause it, or both. In any case, associated health, developmental, and behavioral problems require clinical attention when assessing and intervening with children who have growth deficiencies. Some, but not all, of these non–growth-related problems may resolve when the child's growth failure is effectively treated, whereas other conditions require additional concurrent and ongoing intervention.

Health Problems Malnutrition compromises a child's ability to resist and to respond to infection. In turn, infection increases a child's energy requirements and reduces the child's ability to utilize nutrients, a synergism known as the infection–malnutrition cycle. Children who are malnourished are at increased risk for infection, especially for otitis media and for gastrointestinal and respiratory infections, and are also more susceptible to lead toxicity (Frank & Drotar, 1994). In developing countries, even mild to moderate malnutrition is associated with elevated child mortality (Pelletier, 1994).

Developmental Problems   A history of malnutrition has been associated with intellectual impairment in a number of studies, chiefly in children who were severely malnourished who lived in developing countries. For example, Galler, Ramsey, Solimano, Lowell, and Mason (1983) found that children with histories of moderate to severe protein-energy malnutrition in the first year of life had significantly lower IQ scores (an average difference of 12 points) at ages 5–11 years, compared with a matched group of children who had not been malnourished. Children in the Galler et al. (1983) study did not have intellectual assessments during the first year of life, so it is unclear whether IQ differences that existed in infancy may have contributed to follow-up findings.

In a study of children with NFTT, Drotar and Sturm (1988) found a decline in cognitive development in children assessed at diagnosis (average age of 5 months) and later at 36 months of age. The decline in cognitive development (from a Bayley Mental Development Index of 99.6 to a Stanford-Binet IQ of 85.4) was not, however, related directly to initial nutritional status (as measured by weight-for-height) but rather to environmental factors such as family income and maternal education. The finding that malnutrition itself plays a relatively minor role in predicting cognitive decline is consistent with other outcome studies of children with FTT (Drotar, 1995).

Behavior Problems   Various behavior problems have been reported to coexist with FTT and, in some studies, have been reported to differentiate children with nonorganic FTT from children with organic FTT. In some studies, hospitalized children with FTT have been found to prefer distal over proximal stimulation, to be less active, to show less facial expression, and to demonstrate flexed hips and knees, as well as to show gaze abnormalities (Powell, Low, & Speers, 1987; Rosenn, Loeb, & Jura, 1980). Behavioral differences among children with FTT and normally growing children also have been observed in other settings. In a study of infants observed in the home, Wolke, Skuse, and Mathisen (1989) found that, compared with matched controls, children with NFTT were more irritable, fussy, and demanding; had a shorter attention span; were less task oriented; vocalized less; and used less mature verbal signaling. Using a standardized observation procedure, Polan et al. (1990)

assessed affect expression in 6- to 36-month-old children with FTT who were recruited from primary care and subspecialty practices. Polan and colleagues (1990) compared children with FTT with normally growing children in both feeding and nonfeeding situations. Children with FTT had significantly less positive affect in both feeding and nonfeeding situations and had significantly more negative affect in the feeding situation. Severity of malnutrition was associated with expression of negative affect during feeding. Affect expression did not distinguish children with NFTT from children with organic FTT.

Taken together, these studies suggest that some children with FTT also may exhibit behavior and/or affective disturbances, although no single behavior, or set of behaviors, has been found to characterize all children with FTT (Drotar, 1989). Whether these disturbances are causally related to growth deficiency, either by increasing the likelihood of undernutrition or by occurring as sequelae of malnutrition, is not clear. Behavior disturbance often is assessed or observed during feeding. The relationship between growth deficiency and feeding disorders is treated later in this chapter in the section entitled Etiology.

PREVALENCE

As is the case with many other early childhood feeding disorders, completely satisfactory estimates of the prevalence of FTT in the United States are unavailable. NFTT has been estimated to have a prevalence of 10%–20% in ambulatory health care centers and to account for from 1% to 5% of pediatric hospital admissions (Bithoney & Rathbun, 1983). These oft-cited statistics, however, are derived from small studies of clinically identified children and may not be representative of the prevalence of FTT in the general child population. Variations in diagnostic criteria for FTT (discussed previously under Definition) also complicate the issue of prevalence. Much of what is known about FTT, unfortunately, is derived from studies of hospitalized or high-risk populations, and generalizing to more representative populations must be done with considerable caution.

A careful whole-population study of the prevalence of growth deficiency was conducted in the United Kingdom by Skuse, Reilly, and Wolke (1994). This prospective longitudinal study surveyed all infants born during 1 year (1986) in an ethnically diverse, severely economically depressed inner-city health district in London, England. The study included only healthy full-term infants, excluding preterm infants and infants with IUGR—groups known to have poor early growth. FTT was defined as a weight-for-age falling below the 3rd percentile, attained by age 12 months, and sustained for at least 3 months. In this population, 3.3% of all children evidenced growth faltering. The prevalence of FTT in this population is less than would be expected on the basis of other studies of populations with similar demographics and may be due to the exclusion of children with poor growth potential and to the use of temporal criteria for the emergence and persistence of poor weight gain.

ETIOLOGY

Prior to the 1980s, it was common to differentiate strictly between organic and nonorganic FTT, with the former attributed to identified organic factors (e.g., celiac disease, congenital heart disease) and the latter—most often diagnosed by the exclusion of specific organic causes—attributed to environmental factors (e.g., lack of stimulation, irregular feeding). A variation of this binary diagnostic model classifies some cases of FTT as "mixed" etiology rather than as exclusively organic or nonorganic etiology (Homer & Ludwig, 1981). The distinction between organic and nonorganic etiology, however, is plagued by many conceptual problems, most of which are not remedied by the addition of a "mixed" etiology category; and it is generally more useful to conceptualize FTT as the end result of multiple, interacting risk factors, which may be biological or environmental (Bithoney & Rathbun, 1983; Casey, 1992; Frank & Drotar, 1994).

The risk factors for FTT are many, but the proximal cause of poor weight gain is always suboptimal nutrition, which results from inadequate *access* to food, inadequate *intake*, inadequate *utilization* (retention and absorption) of calories consumed, or some combination of these factors (Bell & Woolston, 1985; Bithoney et al., 1989; Whitten, Pettit, & Fischoff, 1969). Evidence for the definitive importance of suboptimal nutrition comes from several sources. For example, children who have NFTT that is thought to be caused by maternal deprivation will gain weight normally when they consume adequate calories, even in the absence of other environmental changes (Whitten et al., 1969). Likewise, weight gain in children with FTT is related directly to caloric intake, whether FTT is organic or nonorganic (Bell & Woolston, 1985).

The practical task of assessing children diagnosed with FTT is therefore one of identifying the origin(s) of suboptimal nutrition. The classification of etiological variables proposed in Chapter 1 (i.e., physical competence, appetite, diet, illness, interaction, child constitution, caregiver competence, systemic variables) can be used to organize and integrate the initial assessment. The following etiological factors—biological, environmental, and psychosocial—are among those that should be taken into consideration.

Biological Factors

Some biological factors (e.g., prematurity, IUGR) affect a child's growth potential and must be considered in the differential diagnosis of FTT. More pertinent to a workup of weight gain deceleration is an understanding of how an acute or chronic illness can affect a child's nutritional status. Underlying disease can affect the *absorption* of nutrients (e.g., celiac disease), can *increase metabolic requirements* (e.g., heart disease), can undermine the ability to *retain* nutrients (e.g., GER), or affect the *ability to consume* sufficient calories (e.g., neuromuscular disease). Malnutrition itself can cause important biochemical, endocrinological, immunological, gastrointestinal, and central nervous system alterations (Bithoney & Dubowitz, 1985). When FTT does result from disease or major organ dysfunction, it is seldom the only presenting symptom, and the medical diagnosis is usually made on the basis of a thorough history and physical examination. Laboratory tests should be guided by the clinical evaluation and, by themselves, seldom contribute new information (Berwick, Levy, & Kleinerman, 1982; Sills, 1978). Finally, children diagnosed with FTT may have unremarkable medical evaluations but present with subtle, organic problems, such as oral-motor immaturity (Mathisen, Skuse, Wolke, & Reilly, 1989). The medical evaluation of growth problems is discussed more extensively in Chapter 2.

Although the number of potential biological causes for FTT is vast, the proportion of children presenting with growth deceleration of exclusively organic origin is less certain. Earlier studies of children admitted to the hospital for FTT tended to report a relatively high proportion of cases classified as organic (Bithoney & Rathbun, 1983), but organic etiology is much less frequently diagnosed in children seen as outpatients. For example, 93% of children with growth deficiency presenting to a statewide network of outpatient growth and nutrition clinics were classified as having psychosocial or mixed etiology (Massachusetts Department of Public Health, 1991).

Psychosocial and Environmental Factors

Numerous child, family, and social factors have been cited as potential contributors to FTT (Bithoney & Rathbun, 1983; Drotar, 1995; Frank & Zeisel, 1988). The range of possible nonorganic determinants is extensive because any factor that might cause a child to undereat is a potential suspect. Poverty, family dysfunction, parent psychopathology, problematic parent–child interaction, child temperament, feeding disorder, and maladaptive nutritional practices all have been correlated with FTT in studies with varying degrees of rigor. Although these factors, considered separately, may not be necessary or sufficient causes of growth deceleration, each needs to be considered in a thorough evaluation of FTT and, when identified, linked to the proximal cause of FTT: suboptimal nutrition. In short, when identified, these factors must be shown either to reduce the child's *access* to an adequate diet or to operate to reduce the likelihood that the child will *accept* adequate nutrition.

Inadequate Access to Food   Many circumstances can affect the likelihood that a child will be offered sufficient calories for growth. Family income directly affects the child's potential access to adequate nutrition. *Poverty* can reduce both the quantity and the quality of food offered to the child. Adults and older children may compete with a young child for food, and the distribution of food resources may not favor the young child most in need of calories for growth. Of course, the relationship between poverty and growth deficiency is not a simple matter of food availability. Poor prenatal care, contributing to an increased prevalence of low birth weight infants, and poor postnatal health care also affect the growth potential of children from impoverished families. As Frank, Allen, and Brown (1985) observed, poverty is a complex variable that affects all aspects of family functioning, including the emotional availability of the parent and the child's capacity to respond positively to the parent.

Although children with FTT are thought to be found disproportionately among families with low incomes (Frank et al., 1985), not all children in low-income families grow poorly, and FTT occurs at all income levels. A child's access to appropriate foods also can be constrained by *maladaptive parental health beliefs and eating practices*, even in families with adequate income and an abundant food supply. Growth deficiency has been documented in children whose parents placed restrictions on the children's diets in the mistaken belief that the children would become obese, develop atherosclerosis, or develop "unhealthy" eating habits (Pugliese, Weyman-Daum, Moses, & Lifshitz, 1987). These parents may have family histories of heart disease, have personal problems with weight control, and/or may practice high levels of personal dietary restraint (McCann, Stein, Fairburn, & Dunger, 1994). Mistaken parental beliefs about childhood food allergies also can lead to dietary restrictions severe enough to cause FTT in their children (Roesler, Barry, & Bock, 1994). Growth retardation also has been documented in children from families practicing alternative diets such as macrobiotic diets (chiefly comprising whole grains and beans) (Dagnelie, Van Stavern, & Hautvast, 1991).

Finally, inattentive, preoccupied, or otherwise neglectful parents may fail to feed their children sufficiently, even when food is not scarce. For example, sleeping through feeds has been found to characterize a substantial proportion of children with growth faltering in the first year of life (Skuse et al., 1994), and this factor also was correlated significantly with lower weight-for-age in this group. Children in the care of multiple caregivers may be fed in several different locations throughout the day and week, and consequently, they may not receive enough to eat if communication about mealtimes is not optimal. In very rare cases, parents may restrict the child's access to food as a form of punishment (Krieger, 1964).

Inadequate Acceptance of Food   Poor weight gain can occur in otherwise healthy children who are offered nutritious diets but who fail to eat enough to grow adequately. It is a common clinical experience to find FTT associated with persistent *food refusal* or with extremely selective eating that significantly limits caloric intake. Parents of children with FTT frequently report early histories of feeding difficulty in their children as well as contemporaneous feeding problems (McCann et al., 1994; Politt & Eichler, 1976). Feeding disturbance also figures prominently in classification schema for FTT (Chatoor & Egan, 1983; Linscheid & Rasnake, 1985); likewise, a diagnosis of Feeding Disorder of Infancy or Early Childhood (characterized by persistent failure to eat adequately, resulting in poor weight gain that is not attributable to medical causes or to lack of access to food) is recognized in the *Diagnostic and Statistical Manual of Mental Disorders–Fourth Edition* (American Psychiatric Association, 1994).

Despite widespread agreement about its importance, the relationship between food refusal and poor weight gain has received little systematic research attention, and the proportion of children diagnosed with FTT who also exhibit selective eating or food refusal is entirely unknown. Furthermore, the presence of feeding resistance in a child with poor weight gain raises additional questions. How do children come to resist feeding to the extent that they do not grow adequately? Does the child feed poorly because of constitutional factors (e.g., difficult temperament), parental mismanagement of feeding, undetected oral-motor dysfunction (Ramsay, Gisel, & Boutry, 1993), or some combination of these factors? Is feeding difficulty the cause or the consequence of malnutrition? Satisfactory answers to these questions await further research. Some plausible causal pathways are discussed in the following paragraphs.

The quality of *parent–child interaction* in children with FTT often is observed to be problematic. This may be reflected primarily in feeding interactions but may also be observed in other spheres of interaction. Several studies in which interaction between parents and their children with FTT are compared with matched normally growing controls have identified problems that could affect caloric intake. For example, Drotar, Eckerle, Satotola, Pallotta, and Wyatt (1990) found that mothers of children with NFTT demonstrated generalized problems in social interactional behavior and, to a lesser extent, problems in feeding interaction (e.g., more arbitrary termination of feeding) in comparison with matched controls. Black, Hutcheson, Dubowitz, and Berenson-Howard (1994), in another case control study, found that parents of children with NFTT were less nurturant and more neglecting than parents of comparison children and found that children of nurturant parents demonstrated better social-cognitive development.

The relative contribution of child and parent to disordered interaction is often difficult to determine in individual cases. *Child temperament* and related child behavioral characteristics have been found to differentiate children with FTT from typically growing children. Parents of children with FTT often describe their children as more difficult (Bithoney, Van Sciver, Foster, Corso, & Tentindo, 1995), and behavioral differences frequently are recorded by objective observers. For example, Wolke et al. (1989), in a case control study, found children with NFTT to be more fussy, demanding, and unsociable, as well as less task oriented and less persistent. Polan et al. (1991) found that children with FTT, observed in both feeding and nonfeeding situations, expressed less positive affect and more negative affect, compared with children with normal growth.

Traditional accounts of NFTT assigned almost exclusive responsibility for disordered parent–child interaction to *diminished caregiver competence*. These early accounts relied heavily on the concept of "maternal deprivation," derived from the research of Spitz (1945), who studied the effects of mother–child separation in infants who were institutionalized. When similar effects (including growth failure and developmental delay) were found in children not separated from their mothers, it was assumed that a severe degree of maternal inadequacy functionally equivalent to "deprivation" must account for growth deficiency (Patton & Gardner, 1962).

Although diminished maternal competence is no longer assumed to be the sole or chief cause of FTT, some studies continue to show a correlation between FTT and maternal psychological status (Drotar, 1995). Maternal depression is the most frequently measured correlate of FTT (e.g., Polan et al., 1991; Skuse et al., 1994), but virtually any acute or ongoing psychological disturbance can potentially desynchronize the feeding relationship and contribute to clinically significant food refusal.

Child feeding resistance also may be related to broader, organizational aspects of meal management. Some forms of meal mismanagement (e.g., infrequent feeding, poor coordination of feeding and sleep) may result in inadequate access to food, but *meal mismanagement* also can affect the child's motivation to eat. Poor meal spacing (e.g., snacking before dinner), grazing, and feeding in distracting or inappropriate environments can increase the likelihood of food refusal. Some controlled studies have found the feeding environments of children with FTT to be less organized and meal schedules to be less predictable, but these environmental differences were not correlated with higher rates of food refusal (Heptinstall et al., 1987; Mathisen et al., 1989).

Finally, feeding resistance with significant nutritional implications may be acquired secondary to *aversive or traumatic events* associated with eating. Acute trauma (e.g., choking on a hot dog), recurrent pain associated with swallowing (e.g., esophagitis), or forced feeding can lead to suboptimal oral intake and significant weight loss. Food refusal secondary to aversive conditioning, sometimes described as a feeding phobia, is covered in more detail in Chapter 5, under the heading of Extreme Selectivity.

Because the number of potential biological and environmental factors contributing to poor growth is large and the complexity of potential interactions daunting, the idea of defining subtypes of FTT (Drotar, 1995) is appealing. Several subtype classifications have been proposed, some of which are summarized in Table 6.1. All of these FTT subtype classifications are clinically derived and await empirical validation.

In reality, the assessment of children with FTT is more straightforward than the above discussion may suggest. Considerable simplification is achieved by defining FTT as a disorder of undernutrition and identifying specific barriers to optimal nutrition for the individual child. Table 6.2 summarizes some elements of a clinical assessment of children with FTT. This assessment incorporates medical, anthropometric, nutritional, historical, interactional, developmental, and familial factors within a multidisciplinary context.

Table 6.1. Subtypes of failure to thrive

Reference	Subtypes	Characteristics (selected)
Casey (1992)	Neurodevelopmental	• Onset: less than 10 months • Child likely to have overt organic problems and have developmental delays
	Socioemotional	• Onset: after 10 months • Child likely to be healthy and developmentally normal but have "poor appetite," selective eating, and behavior problems
Chatoor, Dickson, Schaeffer, & Egan (1985)	Disorders of homeostasis	• Onset: 0–2 months • Child often has organic problems and/or self-regulatory problems; may be irritable or passive during feeding • Mother often anxious, depressed, narcissistic; misreads infant's feeding cues
	Disorders of attachment	• Onset: 2–6 months • Child may have organic problems and/or self-regulatory problems; poor interaction • Mother may appear detached, unresponsive, mechanical, or unaware of child's nutritional needs
	Disorders of separation	• Onset: 6–36 months • Child usually healthy, achieves normal milestones; often angry, defiant, stubborn, concerned with autonomy; selective food refusal • Mother may be anxious or insecure; may have history of unresolved eating problems; fails to set limits, multiple maladaptive feeding techniques
Linscheid & Rasnake (1985)	Type I Reactive Attachment Disorder of Infancy	• Early age of onset (before 8 months) • Caregiver–infant relationship is generally dysfunctional, characterized by noncontingency
	Type II	• Later age of onset (after 8 months) • Specific feeding interaction problems; multiple maladaptive feeding techniques

(*continued*)

Table 6.1. *(continued)*

Reference	Subtypes	Characteristics (selected)
Schmitt & Mauro (1989)	Neglectful FTT	• Caregiver competence issues (overwhelmed, preoccupied, mental health problems)
	Accidental FTT	• Nutrition knowledge deficits; maladaptive health beliefs; maladaptive feeding practices
	Poverty-related FTT	• Insufficient food available
	Deliberate starvation	• Food withheld to punish child
Woolston (1983)	Type I Reactive Attachment Disorder of Infancy	• Onset before 8 months • Infants often delayed; poor social responsivity; apathetic during feeding • Mother may be depressed, socially isolated
	Type II Simple calorie-protein malnutrition	• Onset before 12 months • Healthy, normal child • Mother perceives child as sick; parent–child interactions pleasurable; no feeding problems
	Type III Pathological food refusal	• Onset between 6 and 16 months • Child healthy, normal development; shows angry withdrawal and active avoidance during feeding • Mother depressed and hostile; few pleasurable social interactions

INTERVENTION

Interventions for children with poor growth often are guided as much by clinical lore as by empirically validated techniques. Controlled intervention studies with children with FTT are difficult to conduct—for both ethical and practical reasons—and many published reports are anecdotal or are based on single case studies. Larger studies often are limited by sampling errors, absent or inappropriate control groups, and nonrandom assignment to intervention groups (Drotar, 1990).

Even well-designed studies do not always share the same treatment goals or measure the same outcome variables. For example, one important implication of defining FTT as a disorder of undernutrition expressed in anthropometric terms is the use of growth changes to assess treatment efficacy. But some intervention studies have been exclusively concerned with psychological, behavioral, or

Table 6.2. Failure to thrive: Clinical guidelines for evaluation

Medical evaluation
- Identify prenatal factors affecting child's growth potential:
  - IUGR
  - Prematurity
  - Growth-retarding syndromes
- Identify chronic illness with implications for nutrition:
  - Malabsorption (e.g., cystic fibrosis)
  - Increased metabolic requirements (e.g., congenital heart disease)
  - Decreased ability to retain calories (e.g., vomiting secondary to GER)
  - Diminished ability to consume calories (e.g., neuromuscular disease)
- Identify frequent recurrent illness (e.g., otitis media).
- Identify sequelae of malnutrition (e.g., iron deficiency).
- Conduct basic screening lab tests and other testing as indicated by clinical evaluation (see Chapter 2).

Anthropometric measures
- Determine weight-for-age.
- Determine height-for-age.
- Determine weight-for-height.
- Determine head circumference.
- Review growth history for changes in rate of growth.

Nutrition assessment (3-day diet record and parent interview)
- Calculate estimated caloric/protein intake.
- Calculate energy requirements for catch-up growth.
- Assess dietary variety.
- Assess for over-reliance on liquids.
- Assess parent nutrition knowledge.
- Assess family health beliefs/unusual dietary practices.
- Assess food availability.
- Characterize mealtime structure:
  - Frequency of meals and snacks
  - Spacing of meals and snacks
  - Duration of meals

Feeding history (parent interview)
- Identify events associated with onset of growth deceleration.
- Identify events associated with onset of feeding problems.
- Identify acquisition of feeding milestones.
- Identify problems associated with feeding milestones.
- Identify current feeding problems.

Feeding behavior (observe at least one meal in home or at clinic)
- Identify oral-motor problems.
- Assess independent feeding skills/utensil use.
- Identify selective eating/feeding resistance.
- Identify feeding interaction/meal management problems.

(continued)

Table 6.2. *(continued)*

Developmental screening
- Complete developmental checklists (see Chapter 3).
- Perform or refer for individual testing, if indicated.

Family assessment
- Assess material resources.
- Identify other agency resources (e.g., WIC).
- Identify other social supports.
- Determine level of family support/marital accord.
- Determine need for additional mental health evaluation.

developmental outcome and have not reported changes in growth (e.g., Larson, Ayllon, & Barrett, 1987). When changes in growth *are* reported, variations in the measures used may complicate interpretation and foil attempts to compare studies. Finally, many interventions employ multiple treatment and intervention components, thus making it difficult to determine which element, or combination of elements, is responsible for outcome.

The following section reviews representative interventions for children with FTT. Controlled intervention studies that report changes in child growth status are emphasized, but common components of clinical intervention that have received less empirical evaluation also are discussed.

Multidisciplinary Outpatient Interventions

Multidisciplinary assessment and intervention have become the standard of care for children with FTT (Casey, 1992; Drotar, 1995; Frank & Drotar, 1994). Medical centers in major urban areas often have pediatric specialty clinics that are staffed by teams comprising some combination of physicians, nutritionists, and mental health professionals who specialize in the evaluation of children with FTT. Two studies have evaluated the efficacy of these multidisciplinary clinics.

Bithoney et al. (1991) assessed the effects of an outpatient multidisciplinary intervention on weight gain in children treated for NFTT. Multidisciplinary intervention was compared with treatment of a similar group of children with FTT followed in the primary care clinic of the same hospital. Children receiving multidisciplinary treatment were cared for by a team including members from several disciplines (pediatrics, nutrition, nursing, child development, gastroenterology, social work) and were provided comprehensive interdisciplinary assessment and individualized interven-

tions incorporating hypercaloric diets and behavioral feeding protocols. Children seen in the multidisciplinary clinic also were seen
more frequently and kept more appointments than the children
seen in primary care. Access to community resources, such
as visiting nurses and early intervention, also was emphasized for
children seen in the multidisciplinary clinic.

This study assessed weight gain using growth quotient (GQ)
analysis, in which observed weight gain over a period of time is compared with the expected weight gain (on the NCHS growth charts)
over the same period of time. When observed growth (the numera-
tor) equals expected growth (the denominator), the GQ is 1.0. When
the observed growth is twice the expected growth, the GQ equals
2.0, and so forth. Children with a GQ greater than 1.0 are achieving
some degree of "catch-up" growth over that period of time.

Children treated by the multidisciplinary team achieved better
weight gain than children treated in primary care. Because children
treated in both groups received a very high quality of medical care,
Bithoney et al. (1991) attributed superior outcome in the multidisciplinary group to individualized high-calorie diets, comprehensive behavioral intervention strategies, and the provision of other
psychosocial and community based services.

In another study of children receiving services from a multidisciplinary clinic, Black, Hutcheson, Dubowitz, and Berenson-
Howard (1994) assessed the effects of a randomized clinical trial of
home intervention on both the physical growth and the development of infants and young children with NFTT. Children receiving
home intervention services were matched with a group of children
not receiving these services. Children in both groups were followed
by a multidisciplinary outpatient growth and nutrition clinic similar to that described by Bithoney et al. (1991). Children in the home
intervention group also were scheduled to receive weekly home visits for 1 year by lay home visitors who provided maternal support,
developmental stimulation, and parent advocacy. At the end of 1
year, children in the home intervention group had better receptive
language skills and cognitive development, and their homes were
judged to be more child oriented. Both groups showed improved
weight-for-age, height-for-age, and weight-for-height; but there was
no difference between groups on these variables. Thus, the addition
of home intervention services did not enhance the positive effects
of multidisciplinary outpatient intervention on growth in children
with FTT.

A case study of a child treated in a multidisciplinary growth
and nutrition clinic is described next.

■ ■ ■

CASE 6.1. A CHILD WITH GROWTH DEFICIENCY
NAME: Tanya
AGE AT INTERVENTION: 22 months

BACKGROUND

A 22-month-old girl was referred to an interdisciplinary growth and nutrition clinic for the evaluation of precipitous weight loss and rumination. Tanya weighed 6 pounds, 3 ounces at birth, following a full-term pregnancy, which was complicated by maternal cocaine addiction. After an 8-day hospitalization for cocaine withdrawal, she was found to gain weight poorly in the care of her teenage mother, and the Department of Social Services assumed custody. She was placed in the first of three foster homes at 1 month of age. At the foster home, her weight-for-age increased from the 5th percentile to the 50th percentile by 2 months of age. She was subsequently placed in a second foster home at 12 months of age, after her original foster parents expressed concerns that she "ate incessantly." Tanya's second foster mother decided to wean her from the bottle and to normalize her meal schedule, offering three meals and three snacks per day. Tanya lost nearly 2 kilograms over the next 8 months, falling from the 50th percentile to well below the 1st percentile. Linear growth velocity also was affected, falling from the 25th percentile at 12 months of age to below the 5th percentile by 19 months. Rumination, the voluntary production and reconsumption of vomitus, also began during this period.

On examination, Tanya was found to have a weight-for-age and height-for-age below the 1st percentile. Her head circumference was at about the 5th percentile, having fallen from near the 50th percentile during the previous 10 months. Her physical exam was remarkable for significantly decreased subcutaneous tissue and wasted appearance. Otherwise, the physical exam was unremarkable and the neurological exam was grossly within normal limits. Nothing was known about the stature or weight of Tanya's biological parents, making it difficult to estimate her genetic growth potential.

Growth deficiency was accompanied by multiple behavioral disturbances. Tanya's appetite was described as insatiable. Rumination occurred both after and between meals. Much but not all of the vomitus was reconsumed. Vomiting without rumination was rare. She reportedly drank frequently and with great urgency but did not urinate excessively. Bowel movements were described as large but normal; there was no diarrhea. She was reported to be chronically irritable and prone to tantrums. She often banged her head and pulled out her hair during tantrums. She was reported to have poor sleep, arising four to five times per night, but she did not snore. In evaluation, she appeared withdrawn and lethargic, often blinking and closing her eyes when interaction was initiated by the examiners. During a brief feeding observation, she was noted to refuse some foods but to drink avidly.

Tanya's caloric intake, by 24-hour recall provided by her foster mother, far exceeded both the Recommended Dietary Allowance (RDA) and requirements for catch-up growth. Studies to rule out malabsorption were ordered. Tanya's remarkably precipitous weight loss, significant wasting, and severe behavioral disturbance were suggestive of diencephalic syndrome; and a magnetic resonance imaging study was ordered to look for evidence of hypothalamic glioma.

As an initial intervention, the foster mother was instructed to provide six cans of Pediasure (a high-calorie liquid supplement) per day on a regular schedule, and a follow-up appointment was scheduled for 2 weeks. All lab studies were found to be within normal limits. Of greater diagnostic value at follow-up was a 97-grams-per-day weight gain (the typical 22-month-old girl gains about 5 grams per day), which occurred in response to a simple nutrition intervention: provision of Pediasure. As a result, the foster mother's previous reports of caloric intake were discounted, and the social situation was reevaluated. Further assessment of the foster home subsequently revealed the presence of seven other foster children with whom Tanya had difficulty competing for parental attention. The assessment also raised concerns about the foster parents' ability to follow through with professional recommendations.

FORMULATION

A diagnosis of growth deficiency secondary to suboptimal caloric intake subsequently guided intervention. Inadequate access to food was assumed to be the chief determinant of poor weight gain and nutritional dwarfing the cause of poor linear growth. The onset of rumination appeared to coincide with an abrupt change in feeding practices: weaning from the bottle and "normalization" of meal schedule. Rumination is a relatively rare feeding disorder of infancy and early childhood (see Chapter 9), which may, in a hungry, malnourished child, be motivated by the desire to "prolong" ingestion. Even when rumination is relatively efficient, calories tend to be lost, and this can establish a "vicious cycle" in which increases in rumination lead to increases in hunger, which, in turn, motivate more rumination. Tanya's other behavioral disturbances also were believed to be secondary to chronic hunger and malnutrition, as well as to relative emotional neglect.

INTERVENTION

Subsequent intervention was interdisciplinary, incorporating frequent growth monitoring, medical surveillance, nutrition rehabilitation, behavioral counseling, and service coordination. The chief components of nutrition rehabilitation were the continued provision of Pediasure and ongoing nutrition counseling to increase caloric density of the diet. Behavioral recommendations included scheduling six to eight predictable meals and snacks per day, scheduled holding ("cuddling") for rumination, as well as behavior management guidelines for managing tantrums and head-banging. Case management included coordinating services with early intervention and advocating for placement in a less crowded foster home.

OUTCOME

As Tanya's weight increased, she became more interactive and less irritable, and her sleep improved. Her appetite continued to be described as "insatiable" and rumination continued, but at a significantly decreased rate. Her rate of weight gain at subsequent visits was less spectacular, but weight gain was accompanied by some modest catch-up of linear growth, as well as improvement in head circumference. During this period the frequency of rumination decreased, sleep improved, and head-banging ceased entirely.

Two months after Tanya's initial evaluation in the growth and nutrition clinic, Tanya was placed in a new foster home in which she again evidenced a remarkable spurt of catch-up growth (81 grams per day in 3 weeks), suggesting that she would indeed thrive in a home that provided more individual attention. In subsequent follow-up visits, Tanya's reliance on Pediasure was gradually decreased and finally discontinued. Her rate of weight gain moderated somewhat in subsequent visits but remained in the catch-up range, which brought an increase in linear growth to well above the 50th percentile by her 33rd month of age. Her head circumference was at the 90th percentile. Her weight-for-height, at this point, began to track above the 95th percentile, raising concerns about obesity! The decision was made not to place significant limits on her caloric intake until it was clear that she had met her potential for linear growth. At a 3-year visit, she was described as still somewhat preoccupied with food but no longer was described as insatiable. Indeed, she had become a little "picky." She was changed to 1% milk, and her foster mother was counseled to reduce dietary fat.

■ ■ ■

Children treated in multidisciplinary outpatient clinics receive intervention composed of a variety of medical, nutritional, and psychosocial therapies. Not all children seen in FTT clinics receive the same combination of interventions. Medical therapies may predominate in the management of some cases, whereas nutritional counseling or case management may predominate in others. The following section describes some of these treatment components in more detail, citing supporting studies, when these are available. These interventions also may be provided as discipline-specific services to children with FTT.

Medical Treatments

When organic disease is the sole or partial cause of poor growth, it must be treated before, or concurrent with, other interventions. Sometimes the treatment of the underlying disease is sufficient to correct the growth problem. For example, poor weight gain is frequently seen in children with upper airway obstruction (enlarged tonsils and adenoids) and tonsillectomy/adenoidectomy can, by itself, result in a pronounced recovery of weight gain (Everett, Koch, & Saulsbury, 1987). Often relatively minor changes in medical management can make a big difference in growth status. For example, recurrent infections are commonly associated with poor appetite and weight loss. Children with chronic otitis media and poor weight gain will often benefit from antimicrobial prophylaxis (Frank, 1995). Because children who are malnourished are at increased risk of illness, close medical follow-up is warranted even when illness is not the original cause of poor growth (Frank, 1985).

Medical therapies also may be employed when the origins of FTT remain obscure and are not clearly organic. Nasogastric or gastrostomy feedings are sometimes used with children who are unable or unwilling to eat (Tolia, 1995). Zinc supplementation has been found useful in some studies of children with poor growth (Castillo-Duran, Rodriguez, Venegas, Alvarez, & Icaza, 1995; Walravens, Hambridge, & Koepfer, 1989). Finally, medications are sometimes prescribed to enhance appetite in children with poor weight gain (see Chapter 2).

Dietary Intervention

The primary objective of intervention for children with FTT is the achievement of accelerated or catch-up growth (i.e., a sustained growth rate greater than the average expected for a child of a certain age). There is considerable variation in the degree to which children with FTT achieve catch-up growth (Sturm & Drotar, 1989). To achieve catch-up growth, children must consume calories and protein in excess of the RDA. Exact catch-up needs can be easily calculated (Peterson, 1993), and these calculations help establish reasonable dietary goals for intervention. If a child has not previously been offered adequate amounts of food, or if a child is to be fed via nasogastric tube or gastrostomy, catch-up growth can be rapid, and growth recovery often can be achieved within a matter of weeks. More often, removing the obstacles to adequate intake requires more than knowing the exact number of calories required for catch-up growth.

Increases in energy intake can be achieved by 1) increasing the number of meals, 2) increasing the volume of meals, and 3) increasing the caloric density of meals. In some cases, parents may have inappropriate expectations regarding meal frequency, and recommendations to add nutritious snacks at a regular time between meals and before bedtime can be helpful. Some infants and young children may not clearly communicate hunger, and meals may be terminated before adequate volume has been consumed. For these children, educating parents about developmentally appropriate portion sizes and increasing parents' sensitivities with regard to hunger and satiety cues are useful. Sometimes both meal frequency and volume are adequate, but caloric density is not. Suggestions for increasing the caloric density of the child's diet can take several forms. For formula-fed infants, the concentration of formula can be increased gradually, from 20 kilocalories per ounce to 24 kilocalories per ounce, in consultation with the child's pediatrician (Peterson, 1993). The child's tolerance of increased concentrations of formula should be monitored carefully. Infant cereal and dietary fat (e.g., butter, margarine) can be added to commercial infant foods.

Parents of older children can be counseled about the caloric density of age-appropriate foods and can be given lists of high-calorie foods. Dietary fat (e.g., butter, margarine, oil) can be added as appropriate. Drinking whole milk is encouraged, and parents also are advised to limit the child's intake of juices and soft drinks. High-calorie liquid supplements designed for children (Morales, Craig, & MacLean, 1991) are available, and high-calorie drinks and shakes can be prepared using instant breakfast products. When parents understand and are receptive to dietary advice, when the family has adequate access to food, and when child feeding resistance is not an issue, catch-up growth can sometimes be achieved with nutritional counseling alone (Pugliese et al., 1987).

Psychosocial Intervention

Psychosocial interventions are often useful or necessary in removing barriers to adequate caloric intake. These interventions can take many forms, operating at different levels of the presenting problem. Some interventions focus on reducing child feeding resistance, improving parent feeding skills, or enhancing the quality of more general aspects of parent–child interaction. Other interventions support the emotional adjustment and mental health of individual parents or address aspects of family functioning such as communication among family members. Finally, a broad spectrum of advocacy and service coordination interventions focus primarily on increasing the family's access to supportive services in the community.

Reducing Feeding Resistance/Food Refusal The use of behavioral techniques such as differential attention, stimulus control, contingent access to preferred foods or other reinforcers, and negative reinforcement procedures such as escape extinction in the intervention for selective eating and food refusal has been well documented with several child populations (see Chapters 4, 5, 7, and 8). Behavioral interventions also are frequently recommended as an important component of the multidisciplinary intervention for children with FTT (Bithoney et al., 1991; Frank & Drotar, 1994; Linscheid & Rasnake, 1985). There is, however, surprisingly little research that directly evaluates the use of these techniques for interventions with children with suboptimal weight gain. Behavior studies in which poor growth is a stated concern are briefly reviewed in the following paragraphs.

A single-case study by Hatcher (1979) describes the use of behavioral contingencies in the intervention with a 26-month-old girl hospitalized for poor eating and weight loss. A complex medical history, including multiple hospitalizations and maternal–child feeding conflicts, preceded inpatient behavioral intervention for feeding problems, which were characterized by subsistence on liquids and strained foods and a refusal to eat solid foods. Intervention included reinforcing acceptance of solid foods with liquids, her preferred food. When solid foods were refused, liquids were withheld, and attention was directed to other children sitting at her table. Both increased acceptance of solid foods as well as significant weight gain—during and after hospitalization—are reported in this case study.

Larson et al. (1987) described an intervention used to treat three infants, ranging in age from 4 to 21 months, who were hospitalized with FTT. Organic factors contributed to growth deficiency in each of these cases, and two of the three children also presented with vomiting. Two of three children received nasogastric feeds to sustain weight. The parent-mediated intervention consisted of differential reinforcement of eating and time-out for food refusal. Stimulus control was maximized by playing music during the feeding intervention that precedes each feeding session. Music was terminated during time-out periods. This combination of procedures resulted in increased rates of food acceptance, decreased vomiting and gagging, maintenance of weight, and decreased reliance on nasogastric feeding. Although weight gain is reported, the primary focus of this study was treatment of food refusal.

Systematic desensitization also has been studied as an intervention component in treating feeding resistance in children with FTT. Ramsay and Zelazo (1988) reported on the treatment of five hospitalized infants with FTT, using a combination of nasogastric feeding and interactive-behavioral therapy. In addition to poor weight gain, all five infants displayed feeding resistance and frequent vomiting. Intervention began with therapist-mediated desensitization of feeding avoidant behavior using tactile stimulation, interactive social stimulation, and music scheduled during nasogastric feeding. Oral desensitization proceeded, in this context, from distal areas to locations more proximal to the oral area, ending with milk drops introduced to the lips, first by finger and then by nipple. The therapeutic desensitization procedure then was modeled for the child's mother, and when infants began to respond positively to oral stimulation, nasogastric feeding was decreased.

An intervention that combines the use of differential reinforcement with observational learning has been described by Greer, Dorow, Williams, McCorkle, and Asnes (1991). This intervention, discussed in Chapters 4 and 5, has been used for children with food refusal and swallowing problems who also may have poor weight gain.

All of the studies that the previous paragraphs discuss describe intensive behavioral interventions that were initially implemented by trained staff in highly structured settings. Most of the children had complex medical histories and significant developmental delays. Although all of the children in these studies were diagnosed with FTT, their growth histories and anthropometric assessment before and after intervention are not described sufficiently to determine how many would meet accepted anthropometric criteria for FTT. When weight gain outcome is reported, it is not clear whether catch-up growth or recovery of normal growth velocity is achieved. Therefore, whether behavioral interventions, by themselves, are sufficient to induce catch-up growth has not been established.

Less formal behavioral interventions, in the form of behavioral feeding guidelines similar to those used in the treatment of selective eating (see Chapter 5), are often provided to parents of children with FTT. For example, Chatoor, Dickson, Schaeffer, and Egan (1985) included a list of "food rules" as a part of a multi-element psychosocial intervention for children with FTT. These rules include eating at regular times; not offering food between meals and scheduled snacks; offering solid foods before liquids; limiting meals to 30 minutes or less; encouraging self-feeding; cleaning up after (not during) meals; not approving, disapproving, or force feeding; not using foods as presents or rewards; not playing games at mealtimes; removing food after 10–15 minutes if the child stops eating; and terminating meals if the child throws food in anger. These, and similar mealtime guidelines, usually are offered to parents of children between 1 and 3 years of age, when feeding autonomy struggles are especially evident. Feeding guidelines are intended to reduce feeding conflicts and, in some theoretical formulations, to help the child distinguish physiological hunger from emotional hunger for attention (Chatoor, 1989). As described by Chatoor, food rules are provided in the context of parent psychotherapy, but similar guidelines may be offered to parents of children with FTT during the course of primary care or multidisciplinary clinic visits (Frank, 1995). Mealtime guidelines are also a component of interventions for more common feeding problems such as selective eating (see Chapter 5). The extent to which all or each of these guidelines is effective, or the degree of support parents may require to implement them, is unknown.

Enhancing Parent–Child Interactions Interactional intervention, sometimes also known as interactional coaching or interaction guidance (McDonough, 1995), targets and seeks to modify aspects of parent–child interaction. These interventions are linked to the practice of traditional infant–parent psychotherapy and tend to conceptualize feeding problems and FTT as specific manifestations of broader mental health issues (Shapiro, Fraiberg, & Adelson, 1975). The focus of intervention is the parent–child relationship, rather than the individual participants or specific feeding behaviors. In the typical case, parents and children are seen together—often in the context of play—while the therapist makes nonjudgmental comments on and suggestions for alternative interpretations of the child's affect and behavior. Parent–child play sessions often are videotaped so that the tapes can provide a basis for therapist commentary. Although the rationale for the use of interaction guidance in the intervention for children with FTT is sound, support for the use of this technique is based entirely on case studies (Chatoor, 1989; McDonough, 1995).

Parent- and Family-Focused Interventions Although maternal psychopathology is no longer considered the primary cause of FTT, some parents of children with FTT may indeed have untreated mental health problems that interfere with dietary or mealtime management recommendations. In such cases, intervention may be required at the level of the individual parent. For example, some studies (Polan et al., 1991) have found a higher incidence of major depression in mothers of children with FTT. Untreated depressive disorder would potentially undermine the parent's ability to provide optimal nutrition in several ways. Organizing regular meal schedules, dealing with child feeding resistance, and attending to the child's feeding cues could present challenges for a parent who is depressed. In such cases, psychotherapy and antidepressant medications can serve to ameliorate depression and to make the parent's emotional resources more available to the child.

Daly and Fritch (1995) described an interesting example of FTT effectively managed by diagnosing and treating the parent. This case involved a 2-month-old boy hospitalized on two occasions for FTT. An extensive medical workup during the first admission failed to identify organic contributions to poor weight gain. Neither parent nutrition education nor visiting nursing in the home sufficed to avert a second admission. A feeding observation during the second hospitalization revealed a healthy, affectively typical child with a vigorous and effective suck. The mother, however, was observed to be extremely inattentive, easily distracted, and fidgety. She was subsequently diagnosed with residual adult attention-deficit/hyperactivity disorder and was treated with methylphenidate. Feeding observation after pharmacological treatment revealed a more attentive mother with significantly increased ability to feed her child. The child subsequently gained weight at an appropriate rate and did not require rehospitalization.

In some cases, significant family dysfunction interferes with the child's treatment (Drotar, Wilson, & Sturm, 1989), and intervening at the level of the child, the parent–child relationship, or the individual parent is insufficient. These cases may respond to intensive service coordination coupled with family-focused, often home-based, educational and therapeutic efforts. As a last resort, child protective services may need to intervene by placing the child with chronically poor growth in foster care.

Advocacy/Service Coordination Children with FTT are frequently identified in families with multiple and complex needs that require comprehensive, long-term service coordination. Service coordination is a component of the multidisciplinary approach to FTT intervention but is not usually studied in its own right. Community agencies and programs that may play an important role in serving the families of children with FTT include Women, Infants, and Children (WIC), early intervention programs, state departments of public health, and child protective services. Even families that have access to these services may benefit from more active coordination of services.

Developmental Stimulation   A variety of child stimulation and developmental therapy modalities often is incorporated into interventions for infants with FTT, especially those with developmental delays or those from disadvantaged home environments (e.g., Black et al., 1995; Casey et al., 1994). The opportunity to gain access to developmental services is critical given the increased risk of cognitive and behavior difficulties in undernourished children. The effects of infant stimulation and early intervention programs on developmental attainment are generally conceded, but effects on weight gain are less well established (Black et al., 1995).

One particular infant intervention, tactile and kinesthetic stimulation, *has* been found to enhance the growth of preterm infants, in some studies (Field, Schanberg, & Scafidi, 1986; Scafidi et al., 1990); but comparable, controlled studies with children with FTT have not been conducted. It is interesting to note that there is some evidence that mothers of children with FTT provide less frequent touch stimulation during feeding and play as compared with mothers of normally growing children (Polan & Ward, 1994).

Hospitalization

In previous decades, it was not uncommon to hospitalize children with FTT. This treatment reflected the then-more-prevalent belief that FTT often was caused by occult organic factors requiring elaborate medical workups. In addition, by removing children from the home, hospitalization was used to confirm a diagnosis of maternal psychopathology: Children who gained weight in the hospital were presumed to have been deprived at home. These beliefs are no longer widely held, and health care utilization practices in the late 1990s discourage hospital admissions in general. Nevertheless, hospitalization remains an important treatment option for children with one or more of the following characteristics: 1) severe malnutrition, 2) evidence of or risk of nonaccidental trauma, 3) serious neglect, 4) significant concurrent illness, 5) conspicuous parental incompetence, or 6) failure of outpatient intervention (Frank, 1995; Schmitt & Mauro, 1989).

Subgroups/Tailoring Interventions

Each of the intervention modalities discussed in the previous sections plays a potentially important role in the amelioration of growth deficiency. The degree to which each intervention component should be utilized with individual children and families is a matter of clinical judgment. Different subgroups of FTT may well benefit from different combinations of intervention (Drotar, 1995; Drotar et al., 1989), but the validity of specific FTT subgroups has yet to be established. In the meantime, most children with poor weight gain will benefit from a multidisciplinary team assessment and comprehensive intervention and treatment including close medical follow-up, individualized nutritional and psychosocial counseling, and service coordination.

Clinical guidelines for intervention with children with FTT are summarized in Table 6.3. Intervention planning begins with consideration of general issues regarding treatment priorities, the schedule of growth monitoring, and ways to involve the child's parents in intervention. Specific treatments or interventions may be directed at increasing caloric intake, improving mealtime structure, enhancing feeding interactions, and providing or coordinating additional child or family services.

NUTRITIONAL DWARFING

Short stature (significantly reduced height-for-age) in children and young adolescents may occur as a result of suboptimal caloric intake unaccompanied by poverty, psychiatric disorder, or organic illness. This type of growth stunting is called nutritional dwarfing (Lifshitz & Tarim, 1993) or benign nutritional dwarfing (Woolston, 1991). Nutritional dwarfing is described as usually originating in middle childhood; being associated with weight gain deceleration (without loss of weight); and occurring as the result of maladaptive or mistaken nutritional beliefs in the absence of body image distortion, family dysfunction, or other psychopathology (Sandberg, Smith, Fornari, Goldstein, & Lifshitz, 1991; Woolston, 1991). It is not clear why nutritional dwarfing should be classified differently from other disorders of growth secondary to undereating. Weight gain deceleration often precedes or accompanies nutritional dwarfing (Lifshitz & Tarim, 1993), as does the stunting characteristic of younger children with chronic FTT.

Interventions for children with nutritional dwarfing have not been described in detail. Nutritional counseling and rehabilitation are most often mentioned (Lifshitz & Moses, 1989); family counsel-

Table 6.3. Failure to thrive: Clinical guidelines for intervention

GENERAL CONSIDERATIONS

- Treat any identified illness or refer for medical treatment.
- Determine optimal intervention site:
    - Primary care?
    - Outpatient specialty clinic?
    - Hospital admission?
    - Other inpatient admission?
    - Regular home visits?
- Determine frequency of growth monitoring:
    - Monthly visits (at a minimum)
    - Weekly visits (for infants and children who are severely malnourished)
- Establish parent–professional partnership:
    - Assess parent attributions/fears/concerns.
    - Work with all family members.

SPECIFIC INTERVENTIONS

Suboptimal caloric intake

- Increase meal frequency (three meals, three snacks is often optimal).
- Provide a list of calorically dense foods.
- Increase dietary fat:
    - Add butter/margarine/mayonnaise, when appropriate.
    - Use whole milk.
    - Add cheese to pasta, vegetables, and so forth.
    - Increase milk intake.
    - Decrease intake of juice and water.
- Increase formula density, when appropriate.
- Add supplements, when appropriate:
    - Pediasure
    - Instant breakfast, added to whole milk
    - Supermilk (1 cup of powdered milk added to 4 cups whole milk)
- Increase food variety.
- Offer child's favorite (high-calorie) foods more frequently.
- Change food texture:
    - Advance gradually to more developmentally appropriate foods.
    - Reduce texture to compensate for oral-motor difficulties.
- Change liquid/solid ratio.

Suboptimal mealtime schedule or food presentation

- Limit meal duration (20–30 minutes is usually sufficient).
- Space meals/snacks (try for even spacing between meals, no nibbling/drinking/nursing in the hour before a meal or snack).
- Change sleep schedule to maximize meal frequency.
- Order presentation of foods/liquids:
    - Offer solids before liquids for children who favor liquids.
    - Offer higher-calorie foods first.
- Limit portion size (smaller portions often are less intimidating).

Suboptimal feeding environment

- Change to more supportive seating.
- Feed in less distractive environment.
- Use one-to-one feeding.

(continued)

Table 6.3.   *(continued)*

Suboptimal feeding interaction
- Provide brief cue-sensitivity counseling.
- Discontinue forced or coercive feeding.
- Use differential attention (ignore food refusal/attend to food acceptance).
- Use specific rewards (e.g., favored foods).
- Encourage feeding independence (e.g., finger-feeding).
- Reduce play and other distractions during meals.
- Use modeling (provide appropriate adult or peer models).
- Modify feeding rate.
- Use contingency management for disruptive mealtime behavior.
- Provide interaction guidance sessions.
- Provide individual parent/family therapy sessions.
  COMPREHENSIVE SERVICE COORDINATION
- Refer children with possible developmental problems for
  - More specialized testing or consultation (e.g., occupational therapy, speech evaluation)
  - Early intervention programs (for children under 3 years of age)
  - Head Start or special needs preschool
- Refer children with complex medical needs for visiting nurse or for home health aide services.
- Refer eligible children to WIC.
- Inform parents about food pantries and other resources.
- Recommend child protective services for neglected or abused children and/or massively overwhelmed parents.

ing also is reported (Pugliese et al., 1987). In short, children with nutritional dwarfing do not eat enough, and the recommendations for assessment and intervention appropriate to children with FTT should apply to this disorder as well.

PSYCHOSOCIAL DWARFISM

Psychosocial dwarfism (PD) is a very rare growth disorder of young children characterized by linear growth deceleration, growth hormone insufficiency, and characteristic behavior disturbances, which occurs in children raised in unusually impoverished and abusive environments by parents with significant psychopathology (Woolston, 1991). Unlike FTT and nutritional dwarfing, psychosocial dwarfism is *not* a disorder of undereating and is discussed here only because there is still some tendency to confuse PD with FTT. Children with PD tend to be short and plump because linear growth deceleration occurs in the absence of weight gain deceleration. Bizarre eating behaviors are commonly associated with psychosocial dwarfism, and include polydipsia, hyperphagia, food hoarding, and eating marginal foods (e.g., cat food, garbage). Skuse, Albanese, Stanhope, Gilmour, and Voss (1996) suggested that hyperphagic symptoms are diagnostic criteria for a syndrome of "hyperphagic short stature." Hyperphagia also is discussed in Chapter 10.

There have been no systematic evaluations of treatment for psychosocial dwarfism, in part because the disorder is so rare. But with a change in psychosocial environment, normal linear growth usually resumes, growth hormone insufficiency is reversed, and behavior problems are ameliorated (Skuse et al., 1996).

PREPUBERTAL ANOREXIA NERVOSA

A thorough consideration of anorexia nervosa, an eating disorder primarily of late adolescence and early adulthood, is beyond the scope of this chapter. It should be noted, however, that in very rare cases this disorder presents in preadolescent children. The cardinal features of prepubertal anorexia nervosa are the same as those for anorexia nervosa in adolescents and adults: an intense fear of becoming fat, body image distortion, significant weight loss, and a refusal to gain weight (Woolston, 1991). Assessment of body image distortion, fear of weight gain, and intentional dieting are central to making the diagnosis and differentiating prepubertal anorexia nervosa from other childhood disorders of undereating. Prepubertal anorexia nervosa may co-occur with other mental disorders such as depression (Alessi, Krahn, Brehm, & Wittekindt, 1989). There is at least limited evidence that behavioral intervention can play an important role in the multidisciplinary, usually inpatient, treatment of prepubertal anorexia nervosa (Alessi et al., 1989; Lask & Bryant-Waugh, 1993; Linscheid & Fleming, 1995). It is important, however, to note that treatment and intervention considerations relevant to anorexia nervosa often go well beyond those relevant to FTT and nutritional dwarfing.

SUMMARY

Children with FTT show poor weight gain relative to age and/or height. The proximal cause of FTT is suboptimal nutrition, secondary to inadequate acceptance, offering, utilization, or retention of calories. Many factors, both organic and nonorganic, play a potential role in causing growth deficiency, with several interacting factors often responsible for growth failure in an individual child. Treatment of FTT consequently requires the expertise of several professional disciplines, and multidisciplinary assessment and treatment have become the standard of care for these children. Effective intervention requires the close coordination of medical, nutritional, and psychosocial therapies. Behavioral interventions can play an important role in children with FTT, especially those children demonstrating food refusal, extreme selectivity, or significant mealtime management problems. Other psychosocial interventions, at the level of the parent, family, and community, are often helpful. Comprehensive service coordination usually is required to address the complex needs of children with FTT and their families.

Psychosocial dwarfism is a rare growth disorder of early childhood sometimes confused with FTT. It is characterized by primary linear growth deceleration and behavior disturbance. Unlike FTT, psychosocial dwarfism is not a disorder of undereating. Benign nutritional dwarfism and prepubertal anorexia nervosa are growth disorders that may emerge, albeit infrequently, in early childhood, both of which *do* result from undereating.

REFERENCES

Alessi, N.E., Krahn, D., Brehm, D., & Wittekindt, J. (1989). Prepubertal anorexia nervosa and major depressive disorder. *Journal of the American Academy of Child and Adolescent Psychiatry, 28,* 380–384.

American Psychiatric Association. (1994). *Diagnostic and statistical manual of mental disorders* (4th ed.). Washington, DC: Author.

Bell, L.S., & Woolston, J.L. (1985). The relationship of weight gain and caloric intake in infants with organic and nonorganic failure to thrive syndrome. *Journal of the American Academy of Child Psychiatry, 24,* 447–452.

Berwick, D.M., Levy, J.C., & Kleinerman, R. (1982). Failure to thrive: Diagnostic yield of hospitalization. *Archives of Disease in Childhood, 57,* 347–351.

Bithoney, W.G., & Dubowitz, H. (1985). Organic concomitants of nonorganic failure to thrive: Implications for research. In D. Drotar (Ed.), *New directions in failure to thrive: Implications for research and practice* (pp. 47–68). New York: Plenum.

Bithoney, W.G., & Rathbun, J.M. (1983). Failure to thrive. In M. Levine, W. Carey, A. Crocker, & R. Gross (Eds.), *Developmental-behavioral pediatrics* (pp. 557–572). Philadelphia: W.B. Saunders.

Bithoney, W.G., McJunkin, J., Michalek, J., Snyder, J., Egan, H., & Epstein, D. (1991). The effect of a multidisciplinary team approach on weight gain in nonorganic failure-to-thrive children. *Journal of Developmental and Behavioral Pediatrics, 12,* 254–258.

Bithoney, W.G., Van Sciver, M.M., Foster, S., Corso, S., & Tentindo, C. (1995). Parental stress and growth outcome in growth-deficient children. *Pediatrics, 96,* 707–711.

Black, M., Dubowitz, H., Hutcheson, J., Berenson-Howard, J., & Starr, R.H. (1995). A randomized clinical trial of home intervention for children with failure to thrive. *Pediatrics, 95,* 807–814.

228 ■ ■ ■ Childhood Feeding Disorders

Black, M., Hutcheson, J.J., Dubowitz, H., & Berenson-Howard, J. (1994). Parenting style and developmental status among children with non-organic failure to thrive. *Journal of Pediatric Psychology, 19,* 689–707.

Casey, P.H. (1992). Failure to thrive. In M.D. Levine, W.B. Carey, & A.C. Crocker (Eds.), *Developmental and behavioral pediatrics* (2nd ed., pp. 375–383). Philadelphia: W.B. Saunders.

Casey, P.H., Kelleher, K.J., Bradley, R.H., Kellogg, K.W., Kirby, R.S., & Whiteside, L. (1994). A multifaceted intervention for infants with failure to thrive. *Archives of Pediatric and Adolescent Medicine, 148,* 1071–1077.

Castillo-Duran, C., Rodriguez, A., Venegas, G., Alvarez, P., & Icaza, G. (1995). Zinc supplementation and growth of infants born small for gestational age. *Journal of Pediatrics, 127,* 206–211.

Chatoor, I. (1989). Infantile anorexia nervosa: A developmental disorder of separation and individuation. *Journal of the American Academy of Psychoanalysis, 17,* 43–64.

Chatoor, I., Dickson, L., Schaeffer, S., & Egan, J. (1985). A developmental classification of feeding disorders associated with failure to thrive: Diagnosis and treatment. In D. Drotar (Ed.), *New directions in failure to thrive: Implications for research and practice* (pp. 235–258). New York: Plenum.

Chatoor, I., & Egan, J. (1983). Nonorganic failure to thrive and dwarfism due to food refusal: A separation disorder. *Journal of the American Academy of Child Psychiatry, 22,* 294–301.

Dagnelie, P.C., Van Stavern, W.A., & Hautvast, J.G.J.A. (1991). Stunting and nutrient deficiencies in children on alternative diets. *Acta Paediatrica Scandinavia Supplement, 374,* 111–118.

Daly, J.M., & Fritch, S.A. (1995). Case study: Maternal residual attention deficit disorder associated with failure to thrive in a two-month-old infant. *Journal of the American Academy of Child and Adolescent Psychiatry, 34,* 55–57.

Drotar, D. (1989). Behavioral diagnosis in nonorganic failure to thrive: A critique and suggested approach to behavioral assessment. *Journal of Developmental and Behavioral Pediatrics, 10,* 48–57.

Drotar, D. (1990). Sampling issues in research with nonorganic failure-to-thrive children. *Journal of Pediatric Psychology, 15,* 255–272.

Drotar, D. (1995). Failure to thrive (growth deficiency). In M.C. Roberts (Ed.), *Handbook of pediatric psychology* (2nd ed., pp. 516–536). New York: Guilford Press.

Drotar, D., Eckerle, D., Satotola, J., Pallotta, J., & Wyatt, B. (1990). Maternal interactional behavior with nonorganic failure-to-thrive infants: A case comparison study. *Child Abuse & Neglect, 14,* 41–51.

Drotar, D., & Sturm, L. (1988). Prediction of intellectual development in young children with early histories of failure to thrive. *Journal of Pediatric Psychology, 13,* 281–295.

Drotar, D., Wilson, F., & Sturm, L. (1989). Parent intervention in failure to thrive. In C.E. Schaefer & J.M. Briesmeister (Eds.), *Handbook of parent training* (pp. 364–391). New York: John Wiley & Sons.

Everett, A.D., Koch, W.C., & Saulsbury, F.T. (1987). Failure to thrive due to obstructive sleep apnea. *Clinical Pediatrics, 26,* 90–92.

Field, T.M., Schanberg, S.M., & Scafidi, F. (1986). Tactile/kinesthetic stimulation effects on preterm neonates. *Pediatrics, 77,* 654–658.

Frank, D.A. (1985). Biologic risks in "nonorganic" failure to thrive: Diagnostic and therapeutic implications. In D. Drotar (Ed.), *New directions in failure to thrive: Implications for research and practice* (pp. 17–26). New York: Plenum.

Frank, D.A. (1995). Failure to thrive. In S. Parker & B. Zuckerman (Eds.), *Behavioral and developmental pediatrics: A handbook for primary care* (pp. 134–139). Boston: Little, Brown.

Frank, D.A., Allen, D., & Brown, J.L. (1985). Primary prevention of failure to thrive: Social policy implications. In D. Drotar (Ed.), *New directions in failure to thrive: Implications for research and practice* (pp. 337–357). New York: Plenum.

Frank, D.A., & Drotar, D. (1994). Failure to thrive. In R.M. Reece (Ed.), *Child abuse: Medical diagnosis and management* (pp. 298–324). Philadelphia: Lea & Febiger.

Frank, D.A., & Zeisel, S.H. (1988). Failure to thrive. *Pediatric Clinics of North America, 35,* 1187–1206.

Galler, J.R., Ramsey, F., Solimano, G., Lowell, W.E., & Mason, E. (1983). The influence of early malnutrition on subsequent behavioral development: I. Degree of impairment in intellectual performance. *Journal of the American Academy of Child Psychiatry, 22,* 8–15.

Greer, R.D., Dorow, L., Williams, G., McCorkle, N., & Asnes, R. (1991). Peer-mediated procedures to induce swallowing and food acceptance in young children. *Journal of Applied Behavior Analysis, 24,* 783–790.

Hamill, P.V., Drizd, T.A., Johnson, C.L., Reed, R.B., Roche, A.F., & Moore, W.M. (1979). Physical growth: National Center for Health Statistics percentiles. *American Journal of Clinical Nutrition, 32,* 607–629.

Hatcher, R.P. (1979). Treatment of food refusal in a two-year old child. *Journal of Behavior Therapy and Experimental Psychiatry, 10,* 363–367.

Heptinstall, E., Puckering, C., Skuse, D., Start, K., Zur-Szpiro, S., & Downey, L. (1987). Nutrition and mealtime behaviour in families of growth-retarded children. *Human Nutrition: Applied Nutrition, 41A,* 390–402.

Homer, C., & Ludwig, S. (1981). Categorization of etiology of failure to thrive. *American Journal of Diseases of Children, 135,* 848–851.

Krieger, J. (1964). Food restriction as a form of child abuse in ten cases of psychosocial dwarfism. *Clinical Pediatrics, 13,* 127–130.

Larson, K.L., Ayllon, T., & Barrett, D.H. (1987). A behavioral feeding program for failure-to-thrive infants. *Behaviour Research and Therapy, 25,* 39–47.

Lask, B., & Bryant-Waugh, R. (1993). *Childhood onset anorexia nervosa and related eating disorders.* Hillsdale, NJ: Lawrence Erlbaum Associates.

Lifshitz, F., & Moses, N. (1989). Growth failure: A complication of dietary treatment of hypercholesterolemia. *American Journal of Diseases of Children, 143,* 537–542.

Lifshitz, F., & Tarim, O. (1993). Nutritional dwarfing. *Current Problems in Pediatrics, 23,* 322–336.

Linscheid, T.R., & Fleming, C.H. (1995). Anorexia nervosa, bulimia nervosa, and obesity. In M.C. Roberts (Ed.), *Handbook of pediatric psychology* (pp. 676–700). New York: Guilford Press.

Linscheid, T.R., & Rasnake, L.K. (1985). Behavioral approaches to the treatment of failure to thrive. In D. Drotar (Ed.), *New directions in failure to thrive: Implications for research and practice* (pp. 279–294). New York: Plenum.

Maggioni, A., & Lifshitz, F. (1995). Nutritional management of failure to thrive. *Pediatric Clinics of North America, 42,* 791–810.

Massachusetts Department of Public Health. (1991). *Catching up: Report of the Massachusetts Growth and Nutrition Clinics, FY 1985–1989.* Boston: Author.

Mathisen, B., Skuse, D., Wolke, D., & Reilly, S. (1989). Oral-motor dysfunction and failure to thrive among inner city infants. *Developmental Medicine and Child Neurology, 31,* 293–302.

McCann, J.B., Stein, A., Fairburn, C.G., & Dunger, D.B. (1994). Eating habits and attitudes of mothers of children with non-organic failure to thrive. *Archives of Disease in Childhood, 70,* 234–236.

McDonough, S.C. (1995). Promoting positive early parent–infant relationships through interaction guidance. *Child and Adolescent Psychiatric Clinics of North America, 4,* 661–671.

Morales, E., Craig, L.D., & MacLean, W.C. (1991). Dietary management of malnourished children with a new enteral feeding. *Journal of the American Dietetic Association, 91,* 1233–1238.

Patton, R.G., & Gardner, L.I. (1962). Influence of family environment on growth: The syndrome of "maternal deprivation." *Pediatrics, 30,* 957–962.

Pelletier, D.L. (1994). The potentiating effects of malnutrition on child mortality: Epidemiologic evidence and policy implications. *Nutrition Reviews, 52,* 409–415.

Peterson, K.E. (1993). Failure to thrive. In P.M. Queen & C.E. Lang (Eds.), *Handbook of pediatric nutrition* (pp. 366–383). Rockville, MD: Aspen Publishers.

Peterson, K.E., Rathbun, J.M., & Herrera, M.G. (1985). Growth analysis in FTT treatment and research. In D. Drotar (Ed.), *New directions in failure to thrive: Implications for research and practice* (pp. 157–176). New York: Plenum.

Polan, H.J., Kaplan, M.D., Kessler, D.B., Shindeldecker, R., Newmark, M., Stern, D.N., & Ward, M.J. (1991). Psychopathology in mothers of children with failure to thrive. *Infant Mental Health Journal, 12,* 55–64.

Polan, H.J., Leon, A., Kaplan, M.D., Kessler, D.B., Stern, D.N., & Ward, M.J. (1990). Disturbances of affect expression in failure-to-thrive. *Journal of the American Academy of Child and Adolescent Psychiatry, 30,* 897–903.

Polan, H.J., & Ward, M.J. (1994). Role of the mother's touch in failure to thrive: A preliminary investigation. *Journal of the American Academy of Child and Adolescent Psychiatry, 33,* 1098–1105.

Pollitt, E., & Eichler, A. (1976). Behavioral disturbances among failure-to-thrive children. *American Journal of Diseases of Children, 130,* 24–29.

Powell, G.F., Low, J., & Speers, M.A. (1987). Behavior as a diagnostic aid in failure-to-thrive. *Journal of Developmental and Behavioral Pediatrics, 8,* 8–18.

Pugliese, M.T., Weyman-Daum, M., Moses, N., & Lifshitz, F. (1987). Parental health beliefs as a cause of nonorganic failure to thrive. *Pediatrics, 80*, 175–182.

Ramsay, M., Gisel, E.G., & Boutry, M. (1993). Nonorganic failure to thrive: Growth failure secondary to feeding skills disorder. *Developmental Medicine and Child Neurology, 35*, 285–297.

Ramsay, M., & Zelazo, P.R. (1988). Food refusal in failure-to-thrive infants: Nasogastric feeding combined with interactive behavioral treatment. *Journal of Pediatric Psychology, 13*, 329–347.

Roesler, T.A., Barry, P.C., & Bock, S.A. (1994). Factitious food allergy and failure to thrive. *Archives of Pediatric and Adolescent Medicine, 148*, 1150–1155.

Rosenn, D.W., Loeb, L.S., & Jura, M.D. (1980). Differentiation of organic from nonorganic failure to thrive in infancy. *Pediatrics, 66*, 698–704.

Sandberg, D.E., Smith, M.M., Fornari, V., Goldstein, M., & Lifshitz, F. (1991). Nutritional dwarfing: Is it a consequence of disturbed psychosocial functioning? *Pediatrics, 88*, 926–933.

Scafidi, F.A., Field, T.M., Schanberg, S.M., Bauer, C.R., Tucci, K., Roberts, J., Morrow, C., & Kuhn, C.M. (1990). Massage stimulates growth in preterm infants: A replication. *Infant Behavior and Development, 13*, 167–188.

Schmitt, B.D., & Mauro, R.D. (1989). Nonorganic failure to thrive: An outpatient approach. *Child Abuse & Neglect, 13*, 235–248.

Shapiro, V., Fraiberg, S., & Adelson, E. (1975). Infant–parent psychotherapy on behalf of a child in a critical nutritional state. *Psychoanalytic Study of the Child, 31*, 461–491.

Sills, R.H. (1978). Failure to thrive: The role of clinical and laboratory evaluations. *American Journal of Diseases of Children, 32*, 967–969.

Skuse, D., Albanese, A., Stanhope, R., Gilmour, J., & Voss, L. (1996). A new stress-related syndrome of growth failure and hyperphagia in children, associated with reversibility of growth-hormone insufficiency. *Lancet, 348*, 353–358.

Skuse, D., Reilly, S., & Wolke, D. (1994). Psychosocial adversity and growth during infancy. *European Journal of Clinical Nutrition, 48*, S113–S130.

Spitz, R.A. (1945). Hospitalism: An inquiry into the genesis of psychiatric conditions in early childhood. *Psychoanalytic Study of the Child, 1*, 53–74.

Sturm, L., & Drotar, D. (1989). Prediction of weight for height following intervention in three-year old children with early histories of nonorganic failure to thrive. *Child Abuse & Neglect, 13*, 19–28.

Tolia, V. (1995). Very early onset nonorganic failure to thrive in infants. *Journal of Pediatric Gastroenterology and Nutrition, 20*, 73–80.

Villee, D.B. (1989). Endocrinology. In M.E. Avery & L.R. First (Eds.), *Pediatric medicine* (p. 808). Baltimore: Williams & Wilkins.

Walravens, P.A., Hambridge, M., & Koepfer, D.M. (1989). Zinc supplementation in infants with a nutritional pattern of failure to thrive: A double-blind, controlled study. *Pediatrics, 83*, 532–538.

Whitten, C.F., Pettit, M.G., & Fischoff, J. (1969). Evidence that growth failure from maternal deprivation is secondary to undereating. *Journal of the American Medical Association, 209*, 1675–1682.

Wilcox, W.D., Nieburg, P., & Miller, D.S. (1989). Failure to thrive: A continuing problem of definition. *Clinical Pediatrics, 28,* 391–394.

Wolke, D., Skuse, D., & Mathisen, B. (1989). Behavioral style in failure-to-thrive infants: A preliminary communication. *Journal of Pediatric Psychology, 15,* 237–254.

Woolston, J.L. (1983). Eating disorders in infancy and early childhood. *Journal of the American Academy of Child Psychiatry, 22,* 114–121.

Woolston, J.L. (1991). *Eating and growth disorders in infants and children.* Beverly Hills, CA: Sage Publications.

Wright, J.A., Ashenburg, C.A., & Whitaker, R.C. (1994). Comparison of methods to categorize undernutrition in children. *Journal of Pediatrics, 124,* 944–966.

7 Children with Chronic Illness

Illness is a causal variable with potential implications across the complete spectrum of early childhood feeding disorders (see Chapter 1). The onset of many childhood feeding problems often can be traced to common, acute childhood illnesses; and more severe or protracted illnesses frequently play a prominent role in shaping extreme selectivity and food phobia (see Chapter 5). This chapter focuses on feeding disorders in children with specific chronic health conditions. Most of the feeding problems covered in this chapter can be classified as disorders of extreme selectivity; but the emphasis in the following discussion is on the unique contribution of specific illnesses to disordered feeding and how the medical management of illness affects feeding. The discussion also explores how illness interacts with other causal variables (e.g., appetite, diet, parent–child interaction) in the genesis and maintenance of childhood feeding disorders.

Illness can influence feeding in multiple and complex ways. The immediate effects of an acute illness frequently include decreased appetite; fatigue; nausea; and various discomforts, such as mouth sores and abdominal pain. These symptoms can create temporary disinterest in eating and may result in reduced caloric intake. Coupled with the increased energy expenditure often associated with illness, reduced oral intake can result in poor weight gain. The effects of acute illness on feeding usually dissipate when the illness runs its course; however, when illness is recurrent or chronic, poor appetite, discomfort, reduced intake, and weight loss can have more lasting and serious consequences. Feeding problems severe enough to result in malnutrition can further weaken the child with chronic illness and can exacerbate effects of the original illness (see Chapter 6). With each succeeding illness, or with prolonged symptoms, the child becomes more malnourished and more vulnerable to infection—an effect known as the infection–malnutrition cycle (Scrimshaw, 1981). Reduced food intake and weight loss also set the occasion for increased parental anxiety, and this may contribute to maladaptive learning and dysfunctional feeding interaction, which may, in turn, result in further reduction of food intake.

Chronic illness also functions as a potent family stressor, independent of its effects on feeding. A chronic health condition can place a significant burden on family finances, challenge marital relationships, and undermine the emotional adjustment of parents and siblings. Children with chronic illness, especially those with life-threatening diseases, also may be perceived as "vulnerable" by their parents, who then may feel that they are unable to set limits on their children's behavior (Thomasgard & Metz, 1995). The sum of these effects may further diminish parental competence in the feeding arena. Finally, chronic illness is often associated with medical treatments—including medication, restricted diets, and technology dependence—that have the potential to further compromise oral feeding. Figure 7.1 illustrates the potential synergistic interaction of some of the factors that can produce serious feeding problems in children with chronic illness.

The next section examines feeding disorders in high-risk infants for multiple ongoing health conditions. The section also discusses iatrogenic and environmental factors that contribute to difficult feeding. This is followed by a discussion that covers feeding problems associated with specific respiratory, gastrointestinal (GI), cardiac, neurological, and metabolic diseases and includes two case studies of behavioral feeding interventions for children with chronic illness.

HIGH-RISK INFANTS

Nowhere is the complex interrelationship between chronic illness and feeding more apparent than in high-risk infants—those children born preterm and/or with very low birth weights (VLBW). Nearly one quarter of a million infants are born prematurely each year in the United States. In 1983, 9.2% of all births in the United States were premature (less than 37 weeks' gestation); the rate of low birth weight (2,500 grams or less) infants was 6.4%; and the rate of VLBW (1,500 grams or less) was 1.1% (Kotelchuck & Wise, 1987). Advances in neonatology have resulted in increasing survival rates for infants in each of the preceding categories. Hack et al. reported in 1991 that 90% of infants with birth weights in the 1,000- to 1,500-gram range, nearly 70% of infants in the 750- to 1,000-gram range, and about

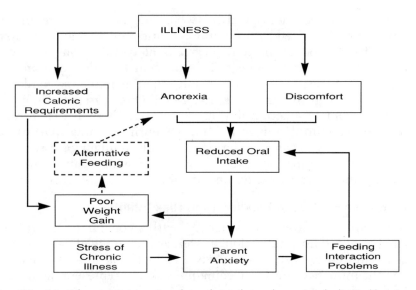

Figure 7.1. Potential synergistic interaction of some factors that produce serious feeding problems in children with chronic illnesses.

33% of infants with birth weights between 500 and 750 grams survive (Hack et al., 1991).

Although survival rates continue to improve, premature and VLBW infants are at increased risk for multiple health and developmental problems, which reflect their reduced capacity to adapt to the extrauterine environment. Some of the immediate complications of prematurity include respiratory distress syndrome (which may lead to bronchopulmonary dysplasia [BPD]), patent ductus arteriosus, apnea, intraventricular hemorrhage (IVH), retinopathy of prematurity, and necrotizing enterocolitis (Batshaw, 1997). In the longer term, high-risk infants are also at significantly greater risk for mental retardation, learning disabilities, and academic problems (Brandt, Magyary, Hammond, & Barnard, 1992).

The prevalence of feeding problems in high-risk infants is unknown, but many factors—including neurological immaturity, adverse nutritional sequelae of illness, and iatrogenic effects of medical treatment—combine to jeopardize the development of normal feeding. The infant's neurological immaturity is a primary risk factor for feeding, the direct effects of which are seen in a diminished ability to suck and swallow and more indirectly in behavioral immaturity, which can affect feeding. Sucking behavior in premature infants is inefficient and poorly coordinated with swallowing and breathing (Kramer & Eicher, 1993). The behavior of preterm infants is characterized by immature motoric processes and a relative difficulty in modulating state (degree of alertness). Compared with infants born at term, preterm infants seem less alert and are less behaviorally responsive; as a result, their parents try harder to stimulate them (Barnard & Kelly, 1990). Observational studies of infant–parent interaction during feeding have shown that parents tend to overstimulate high-risk infants during feedings (DiVitto & Goldberg, 1979). Overstimulation can result in infant gaze aversion, increased irritability, or even sleep—all of which can complicate feeding and set the stage for ongoing interaction problems.

Iatrogenic Factors in Feeding High-Risk Infants

Environmental stressors associated with neonatal intensive care and prolonged hospitalization, as well as specific medical technologies required to ensure the survival of high-risk infants, have important influences on the feeding process and represent significant feeding risk factors.

Neonatal Intensive Care Unit Environment   High-risk infants are born in or transferred to neonatal intensive care units (NICUs). The NICU is designed to maximize an infant's fragile respiratory and metabolic condition. Therapies typically include heating and fluorescent light therapy, vigorous ventilation and oxygenation, multiple medications, and high-calorie intravenous feeding. The infant's vital signs are constantly monitored in noisy, brightly lit rooms, and infants are frequently subjected to invasive and painful procedures such as intravenous (IV) line placement, suctioning, and spinal taps. There is often a very high level of staff activity and many scheduled interactions with the infant that occur independent of the infant's behavior, social–affective needs, or sleep–wake state. Although this therapeutic environment maximizes the likelihood of survival, it is also highly stressful to the immature nervous system; and it is thought to contribute to a compromised ability to regulate sleep, modulate movement, and interact attentively (Als, 1986). These self-regulatory competencies all are critical to effective feeding. The NICU is also a difficult environment for the infant's parents, who are still struggling with the crisis of prematurity. Parents also may experience medical technology as distancing and may find it difficult to relate to the ever-changing stream of busy professionals (O'Brien, Soliday, & McCluskey-Fawcett, 1995).

Although the NICU environment may seem singularly iatrogenic and its stresses blessedly temporary, it should be noted that some features of this environment are characteristic of hospital life in general and that for many high-risk infants, the hospital is "home" for months or sometimes years. The hospital environment is a "systems" factor that must be taken into consideration when diagnosing and treating early childhood feeding disorders in any child with chronic illness.

Alternative Feeding Because sucking and swallowing may not be fully developed in high-risk infants (Hack & Estabrook, 1985), alternative feeding methods are routinely used to provide optimal nutrition for premature and low birth weight infants. Alternative methods of feeding include nasogastric, gastrostomy, or jejunostomy tubes and IV (parenteral) nutrition. Nasogastric tubes are passed through the nares and the esophagus, whereas gastrostomy tubes are surgically implanted through the abdominal wall. Nasogastric tubes are considered a short-term solution to meeting a child's nutritional needs and are generally replaced by gastrostomy after 2–3 months if supplemental feeding continues to be required (Moore & Greene, 1985). Percutaneous gastrostomy placement can eliminate the need for an open abdominal procedure (Gauderer, 1992). Jejunostomy tubes are surgically implanted in the small bowel and may be indicated when there is risk of aspiration (Moore & Greene, 1985). Total parenteral nutrition (TPN) initially may be required for VLBW infants because the GI tract is not sufficiently mature to tolerate tube feeding. These infants have extremely limited nutritional reserves and a very rapid growth rate and are especially vulnerable to acquired brain injury secondary to malnutrition (Zlotkin, Stallings, & Pencharz, 1985).

Prolonged Dependence on Alternative Feeding Prolonged dependence on alternative feeding methods often is associated with resistance to oral feeding (Blackman & Nelson, 1985, 1987; Geertsma, Hyams, Pelletier, & Reiter, 1985; Handen, Mandell, & Russo, 1986; Schauster & Dwyer, 1996). Factors thought to contribute to feeding resistance in children who are maintained on nasogastric feeding include nasal and pharyngeal irritation, altered breathing patterns, suppressed swallow (conditioned dysphagia), and habituation to sensory input (Bazyk, 1990; Tuchman, 1994). An increased risk of gastroesophageal reflux (GER) after gastrostomy tube placement also can contribute to oral feeding resistance (Tuchman, 1994). Interference with the development of normal hunger–satiety cycles and generalized appetite suppression secondary to any method of alternative feeding also contribute to oral feeding resistance. Finally, deprivation of oral feeding experiences during "critical periods," especially the transition from reflexive to voluntary feeding, is often cited as a cause of oral feeding resistance (Blackman & Nelson, 1985; Tuchman, 1994).

At what point dependence on non-oral feeding should be considered "prolonged" has not been established and depends on several factors in addition to the duration of alternative feeding, including whether there has been a prior history of oral feeding, the child's developmental status, and the presence of other medical problems. Bazyk (1990) reviewed 100 infants who had been fed by nasogastric tubes sometime during the first 6 months of life. Of these, 6 infants were "poor feeders" and had extremely lengthy (14–16 months) transitions or never progressed to oral feeding. All of the poor feeders had multiple medical conditions (from 6 to 14 different conditions) and poor sucking abilities at the onset of the nasogastric feeding. The remaining 94 infants ("good feeders") made the transition in an average of 17.5 days. The total number of medical complications in this group of good feeders was significantly correlated with the length of transition. Digestive, respiratory, and cardiac conditions were the strongest predictors of long transitions to oral feeding. It is not unusual for high-risk infants to be started on alternative feeding at birth and to be maintained on tube feeding for many months—or even years—before weaning is successful or even attempted. Studies of feeding resistance secondary to prolonged alternative feeding, unfortunately, do not always describe the alternative feeding history in detail.

Tracheostomy   A tracheostomy is an operation in which a surgical incision is made in the trachea and a tracheostomy tube or cannula is inserted to provide for a free airway. Congenital airway obstruction, cardiopulmonary problems, and ventilator dependence are among the conditions requiring tracheostomy. Both the incidence and the duration of pediatric tracheostomy have increased (Singer, Wood, & Lambert, 1985; Wetmore, Handler, & Potsic, 1982), and children with tracheostomies are thought to be at risk for growth and feeding problems (Fowler, Simon, & Handler, 1985; Singer et al., 1985). Because the presence of tracheostomy is often superimposed on a variety of other associated medical conditions— both concurrent and historical—the specific contribution of this procedure to feeding disorders may be difficult to determine. Indeed, as of this writing, there are no studies demonstrating the unique impact of tracheostomy on feeding. Fowler et al. (1985) speculated that swallowing problems secondary to tracheostomy may be related to the following: 1) limitations on head flexion, 2) discomfort as the larynx is elevated during swallowing, 3) possible aspiration due to prevention of complete glottic closure, and 4) increased risk of aspiration due to a less effective cough. Wolf and Glass (1992) suggested that the coordination of sucking, swallowing, and breathing is impaired in children with tracheostomies. There also may be discomfort associated with frequent suctioning due to increased tracheal secretions (Simon & McGowan, 1989). If suctioning is aversive then a conditioned aversion may generalize to any procedure performed around the oral area, including feeding. Behavioral interventions for children with tracheostomies and feeding problems, therefore, often begin with a desensitization phase (see Chapter 4).

Ventilator Dependence Children with prolonged ventilator dependence constitute a small but growing population (Schreiner, Downes, Kettrick, Ise, & Voit, 1987) at risk for feeding problems. An early study by Fitzhardinge et al. (1976) found that infants who weighed less than 1,501 grams at birth and who were mechanically ventilated had inadequate caloric intake during and after the period of ventilation and had poor growth relative to premature infants who were unventilated. Children on ventilators are subject to all of the feeding risk factors associated with tracheostomy and tube feeding. Furthermore, the degree of technology dependence, including the need for ongoing monitoring, is often socially distancing and disruptive of typical social interaction. Feeding interventions with infants on ventilators also are subject to multiple systems obstacles. These obstacles include busy schedules of developmental intervention, chest physiotherapy, and aerosol therapy, as well as more difficulty in creating a comforting, low-distraction environment for feeding.

Clinical experience also suggests that the high level of medical risk associated with children on ventilators contributes enormously to family stress with the predicted secondary consequence of exacerbated feeding interaction dysfunction. Preoccupation with the child's very survival can overshadow interest in promoting greater feeding independence, even when the child seems to be a good candidate. Finally, mechanical ventilation may have direct effects on the sensory aspects of appetite. It is not uncommon for children without prior history of feeding problems who become ventilator dependent secondary to trauma (e.g., spinal cord transection) to show a striking disinterest in eating during the initial phase of ventilator dependency. Some of these children report that food now tastes "funny" or different, and it is possible that reduced olfactory input contributes to gustatory disinterest in children who are dependent on ventilators.

INTERVENTIONS WITH HIGH-RISK INFANTS

Interventions for feeding problems in high-risk infants often include many of the techniques used to treat selectivity and food refusal described in previous chapters. The next section summarizes interventions that tend to be more specific to this population: the amelioration of environmental stress in the NICU, the use of nonnutritive sucking (NNS), and systematic approaches to weaning children from nonoral feeding.

NICU Stress Reduction

Als (1986) proposed a number of environmental and caregiver modifications to reduce NICU stress. Environmental modifications include relocation of the infant's crib or incubator to reduce auditory and visual stimulation and use of soothing bedding, swaddling blankets, and specially designed hammocks and bunting. Placing infants in flexed positions to promote restfulness, holding them supportively during and after stressful procedures, and instituting dark and quiet times are other recommended interventions. Caregiver modifications relevant to feeding include providing the opportunity for NNS during gavage feeding (discussed further in the next section); conducting feeding in quiet, shielded locations, without simultaneous talking or looking at the infant; and timing of feeding in coordination with the infant's sleep cycle. Instituting these interventions requires close monitoring of the infant's neurobehavioral status, with special attention given to behavioral indicators of stress, including variations in autonomic activity, levels of arousal, and regulatory motor movements.

A randomized controlled trial of the intervention package described in the previous paragraph, referred to as "individualized developmentally focused care," provided by specially trained nurses in consultation with a developmental psychologist, has been shown to significantly affect medical and developmental outcome of VLBW preterm infants (Als et al., 1994). Infants who received this intervention developed less severe BPD and pneumothorax and had a lower incidence of IVH. Treated infants also stayed in the hospital for fewer days and spent fewer days on mechanical ventilation or oxygen. Especially relevant is the finding that infants receiving individualized developmental intervention showed increased weight gain and began bottle feeding significantly earlier than infants receiving standard care.

Effects of Nonnutritive Sucking

Measel and Anderson (1979) reported that providing preterm infants the opportunity to suck on a pacifier during tube feeding facilitated earlier transition to bottle feeding as well as earlier discharge from the hospital. In a replication of this study, Field et al. (1982) found that treated infants were ready for bottle feeding 3 days earlier and required fewer tube feedings, gained more weight, and were discharged sooner than control infants who were not offered NNS during tube feeding. The infants' behavior during bottle feeding, as well as neurobehavioral maturity, also were measured in this study, but these measures failed to distinguish treated and control children. Bernbaum, Pereira, Watkins, and Peckham (1983) replicated the findings of these previous studies, finding that NNS resulted in increased weight gain and earlier hospital discharge as well as in easier and more effective transition to total oral feeds (measured by time required for oral feeding and days required before total oral feeding was achieved). Bernbaum et al. (1983) also found that NNS infants showed accelerated maturation of sucking and decreased GI transit times. Ernst et al. (1989), in a study that controlled for type and amount of nutrient intake, however, found that NNS during gavage feeding did not affect weight gain, nutritional outcome, or GI transit time nor did treated infants show improved energy absorption or decreased energy expenditure, which have been hypothesized to be responsible for increased weight gain in NNS infants. The effects of NNS on duration of hospitalization, maturity of suck, or oral feeding behavior were not examined in the study by Ernst et al. (1989).

The inconsistent findings of these four studies—Bernbaum et al. (1983), Ernst et al. (1989), Field et al. (1982), and Measel and Anderson (1979)—are summarized in Table 7.1. Although at the time of this writing, NNS during gavage feeding cannot be recommended on the basis of growth enhancement, it does seem reasonable to ex-

Table 7.1. Effects of nonnutritive sucking during gavage feeding

	Measel & Anderson (1979)	Field et al. (1982)	Bernbaum et al. (1983)	Ernst et al. (1989)
Increased bottle readiness	Yes	Yes	Yes	NM
Increased weight gain	Yes	Yes	Yes	No
Earlier discharge	Yes	Yes	Yes	NM
Increased suck maturity	NM	NM	Yes	NM
Decreased energy expenditure	NM	NM	NM	No
Decreased GI transit	NM	NM	Yes	No
Improved feeding	No	No	NM	NM
Other behavior improved	NM	No	NM	NM

NM = not measured in this study

pect that NNS will ease and perhaps hasten the transition to oral feeding. Additional well-controlled studies are needed to further assess the effects of NNS on subsequent feeding behavior. It also should be noted that all of the premature infants in these studies did make a successful transition to oral feeding regardless of whether they were offered NNS experiences during gavage feeding. It is unlikely, therefore, that the absence of NNS experience, by itself, could account for the degree of feeding resistance often reported in high-risk infants.

Although the effects of NNS on feeding and growth remain unclear, several studies support the value of NNS in modulating iatrogenic stress in preterm infants (DiPietro, Cusson, Caughy, & Fox, 1994; McCain, 1993; Miller & Anderson, 1993). NNS appears to have a generally soothing effect, which reduces behavioral distress and facilitates inactive waking states and also the infant's return to sleep after a waking state.

Review of Tube-Weaning Studies   A number of clinical studies describe procedures for weaning feeding-resistant children from reliance on tube feeding. Geertsma et al. (1985) reported on a behavioral intervention used to treat feeding resistance in a 7.5-month-old child with a history of 30-week gestation, bowel resection, necrotizing enterocolitis, and dependence on alternative feeding methods (including parenteral hyperalimentation and gastrostomy feeding) since birth. Feeding resistance in this child was characterized by head aversion to presentation of rubber nipples, extrusion of the inserted nipple by tongue movement and thrusting, and pushing the nipple away with her hands. Geertsma et al. (1985) attributed feeding resistance in this child to "the association of noxious procedures such as nasogastric tube placement, endotracheal intubation, and oropharyngeal suctioning with oral stimulation" (p. 256). The inpatient feeding intervention consisted of the following elements: 1) The number of feeders was kept to a minimum (most feedings were conducted by a single nurse); 2) feeding sessions were scheduled frequently (at least 3 sessions per day); 3) therapy began with oral desensitization (gentle stroking of oral area during positive interaction); 4) after oral desensitization had been accomplished, objects (e.g., finger, rubber objects) were gradually inserted into the child's mouth; 5) invasive oral procedures were kept to a minimum and clearly distinguished in time and setting from feeding intervention periods; and 6) after the child began to accept the nipple, tube feeds were given concurrently with oral feeding opportunities. Successful weaning from both the central line and the gastrostomy feeding was accomplished, and the gastrostomy tube removed at 13.5 months of age.

Similar interventions were described by Blackman and Nelson (1985), who reported on 17 children with gastrostomies (placed at a mean age of 6.7 months) who were considered for oral feeding programs. Of these, 10 children were considered suitable for an oral feeding program and, of these 10, 9 were successfully weaned using the following procedures: 1) normalizing the gastrostomy feeding schedule (gastrostomy feeds were provided as bolus feeds, with durations approximating typical meals [30 minutes] and snacks [15 minutes] at typical mealtimes); 2) providing gentle but firm and consistent handling (including forced feeding); 3) rewarding acceptance of food; 4) ignoring refusal of food; 5) tube feeding scheduled after each oral meal; and 6) removing the gastronomy tube 6 weeks after all nutrition needs were met with oral feeding. The duration of intervention varied from 2–3 weeks to 2.5 years with inpatient treatment resulting in a mean treatment time of 1 month and outpatient treatment requiring a mean of 16.6 months to discontinuation of all gastrostomy feeding.

In another series of children, 14–29 months of age, seen on an inpatient basis using the interventions listed in the previous paragraph, Blackman and Nelson (1987) reported rapid introduction of oral feeding in a period of 2–3 weeks. Blackman and Nelson (1987) also recommended multidisciplinary evaluation, careful selection of children, and the graded introduction and training of parents by feeding specialists.

Handen et al. (1986) used a feeding induction protocol with a series of seven children with a variety of chronic illnesses, ranging in age from 10 to 66 months, all of whom exhibited food aversions and were dependent on central intravenous feeding or enteral feeding as the primary source of nutrition. A feeding protocol, using the following procedures, was observed for all children: 1) limiting the number of people assigned to feed the child; 2) using preferred, or easy to digest, foods; 3) feeding in a low-distraction environment; 4) developing a hierarchy of feeding steps with specified criteria for success; 5) providing frequent meals of short duration; 6) limiting the child's access to reinforcers at nonmealtimes to increase reinforcer potency during meals; and 7) using immediate consequences for food acceptance and refusal. All seven children established consistent oral intake subsequent to initiation of the feeding intervention, and three were discontinued on supplemental feeding prior to discharge. Neither the scheduling of supplemental feeds nor the protocol for reduced supplemental feeds was described in this study.

These interventions have several common elements (see Table 7.2). Contingency management, limiting the number of feeders, using frequent feeding sessions, and scheduling postprandial tube feeds are common features of two of the three studies and thus may warrant special consideration when treating children with feeding resistance secondary to prolonged tube feeding. Because these studies involved multifactorial interventions, however, further study is required to identify which combination of elements would be expected to have the most potency.

Two of these studies explicitly scheduled bolus tube-feeding after oral feeding sessions, and this practice, sometimes referred to as "normalizing" the tube-feeding schedule, is routinely recommended (Blackman & Nelson, 1987; Davis, 1994; Pipes & Glass, 1989; Schauster & Dwyer, 1996). The rationale often provided for this practice is that it helps to establish normal hunger and satiety cycles and that the association between oral sensations (during feeding therapy) and postprandial satiety (from bolus tube feeds) serves to facilitate the transition to oral feeding. Although this rationale is entirely plausible, there are no studies that show this temporal schedule of tube feeding to be necessary or sufficient for supporting oral feeding, and there are some studies (e.g., Linscheid, Tarnowski, Rasnake, & Brams, 1987, discussed in the next section) that employ an alternative strategy of scheduling all tube feedings at night. A rationale for this practice is establishing a gradient of increasing appetite throughout the day, with the child becoming progressively hungrier and more likely to accept oral feeding. It also could be argued that the complete absence of tube feeding during the day promotes greater social normalization than intermittent bolus feeds. Clearly this is an issue that warrants further study.

Table 7.2. Components of selected tube-weaning programs

	Geertsma et al. (1985)	Blackman & Nelson (1985)	Handen et al. (1986)
Limited number of feeders	X		X
Frequent feeding sessions	X		X
Oral desensitization	X		
Postprandial tube feeding	X	X	
Minimized invasive oral procedures	X		
Forced feeding		X	
Contingency management		X	X
Dietary modification			X
Specified feeding environment			X
Reinforcer restriction			X

When to initiate a reduction in the caloric content of alternative feedings and at what rate has received little study. Blackman and Nelson (1987) described caloric reductions in successive 25% increments, with tube feeding discontinued entirely when the child is taking 75% of his or her caloric needs by mouth. This protocol was used for carefully selected children who could tolerate an initial weight loss and were being treated in an intensive inpatient feeding program. Reduction of tube feeds to as little as 30% of the child's daily needs, in selected children who were treated as inpatients, also has been suggested (Linscheid, Budd, & Rasnake, 1995).

Screening for Oral-Feeding Programs   What criteria should be used to screen tube-dependent children for oral-feeding programs? Glass and Lucas (1990) proposed that resolution of the original medical difficulty, quality of oral-motor skills, documentation of swallowing abilities, and parental readiness be considered before making the transition from tube to oral feeding. Although these are reasonable criteria, the following qualifications and elaborations are in order. First, children often are ready for oral-feeding programs well before the original medical problem has resolved. Medical *stability* and the absence of acute illness are, therefore, more pertinent considerations. Second, the type of feeding program needs to be considered. Children often are ready for oral stimulation or desensitization well before they would be considered candidates for weaning from supplemental feeding. The degree to which food ingestion should be a part of oral stimulation depends on the risk of aspiration, as determined by medical history and swallowing studies. Oral-motor competence contributes to the success of weaning, but many children with substantial oral-motor impairment can be partially or wholly weaned from supplemental feeding.

Although parental readiness is clearly crucial for outpatient intervention, systems readiness (e.g., availability of a sufficient number of trained feeders, distraction-free environments) is an equally important criterion for inpatient intervention. It is also important to note that therapist-mediated interventions may be warranted even when parental readiness is in doubt and that a successful therapist-mediated feeding intervention can remove an important obstacle to the ultimate re-integration of the child with chronic illness into his or her family. These issues are discussed in more detail in Chapter 4.

An example of an outpatient intervention with a child with oral-feeding resistance subsequent to prolonged gastrostomy feeding is described in the following case study.

▪ ▪ ▪

CASE 7.1. OUTPATIENT INTERVENTION
FOR TUBE DEPENDENCE
NAME: Zoe
AGE AT INTERVENTION: 4 years, 4 months

BACKGROUND

Zoe was the 33-week product of a pregnancy complicated by gestational diabetes. She sustained a bilateral, Grade IV intraventricular hemorrhage; spent 9 weeks in the NICU; and was later rehospitalized for 3 months for failure to thrive (FTT). Hydrocephalus was diagnosed at 9 months of age, and multiple shunt revisions were subsequently required. She had been fed entirely by gastronomy tube since the age of 5 months, being unable to take sufficient calories by mouth. She also had been treated for GER, chronic vomiting, and delayed gastric emptying. Zoe had mild cerebral palsy, and at the time of intervention she ambulated with the assistance of a walker. Zoe's weight and height both were between the 10th and 25th percentile for age. She received all of her nutrition via gastrostomy feeds of 1,300–1,400 kilocalories per day.

In an interdisciplinary feeding evaluation conducted immediately prior to this intervention, Zoe was found to have a high, narrow, arched palate; oral-facial hypersensitivity; hyperactive gag; and mild decreased oral-facial tone. Her tongue and jaw movements were within normal limits; biting, chewing, sucking, and swallowing were believed to be functional, although biting and chewing were not observed. Zoe was capable of self-feeding (somewhat inefficiently) with a spoon and able to drink with a cup held bilaterally. Although capable of independent feeding, in this evaluation she merely mimicked eating (by bringing an empty spoon to within an inch of her mouth), and no actual self-motivated oral intake occurred.

Zoe presented as a socially engaging, talkative, young girl. When food was initially brought into view, she promptly became extremely anxious, hyperverbal, and red in the face. With much encouragement, she was able to touch, smell, and lick a french fry; but she could not be encouraged to eat it. When she was subsequently offered puréed apples and bananas by her mother, her distress increased, and she coughed and gagged as each spoonful was brought to her mouth. Her distress seemed to decrease significantly after several spoonfuls of food were actually consumed.

Zoe had received several prior feeding evaluations and interventions during previous hospitalizations, at home by visiting nurses, through an early intervention program, and by therapists in her special-needs preschool. Zoe previously had taken "tastes" of Popsicles, infant fruits, infant mixed cereal, and apple juice. But she would often gag and always become extremely distressed when feeding efforts were persistent. Feeding usually was discontinued when Zoe began to gag. Zoe's mother would occasionally continue past the point of gagging, but she expressed guilt and uncertainty about this practice. Zoe's mother also expressed considerable discouragement about Zoe's lack of progress in oral feeding and about the conflicting advice she had received regarding approaches to feeding Zoe. For example, she had been advised to encourage self-feeding as a way for Zoe to assume more control over eating. This practice led to Zoe playing with utensils and with food but did not result in her eating. Normalization and reduction of tube feeding to promote appetite also had been attempted without success. She also had been advised to discontinue puréed foods and to "insist" that Zoe eat "age-appropriate" table foods.

FORMULATION

Zoe's extreme feeding resistance had the characteristic of a feeding phobia, acquired secondary to a long history of aversive oral experiences. Diminished appetite secondary to gastronomy feeding, diminished oral-motor competence, and inconsistent feeding practices contributed to her feeding resistance. Distress and food avoidance during oral feeding attempts at home and in feeding therapies were typically reinforced by the cessation of feeding attempts. Feeding therapy sessions in early intervention and preschool largely had been devoted to increasing self-feeding skills, with little time having been spent on reducing feeding aversion. Thus, previous interventions had served to maintain rather than ameliorate Zoe's feeding phobia.

INTERVENTION

Zoe's mother agreed to work closely with a behavioral psychologist and a nutritionist to overcome Zoe's resistance to oral feeding. To promote consistency and therapeutic focus, all other feeding therapies were suspended during this intervention. This included postponing therapeutic goals for improved self-feeding. The behavioral feeding intervention had three phases. The first phase was designed to reduce aversion to feeding, the second was to stimulate appetite and meaningfully increase oral intake by decreasing the volume of tube feeds, and the third was to increase self-feeding skills.

Phase 1

1. All feeding sessions were conducted in the home by Zoe's mother.
2. One feeding session per day, scheduled at the same time each day, was conducted during the first week. This was increased to two sessions per day during the second week and to three sessions after the fourth week. Sessions were scheduled prior to tube feeds.
3. The goal of each session was to provide systematic, invariant exposure to and intake of food. To accomplish this, Zoe was fed puréed food by her mother. Puréed rather than age-appropriate foods were chosen because they elicited less distress and gagging. The initial intake goal was set at 2 ounces of puréed fruit per feeding session. The intake goal was adjusted each week.
4. Each session was conceptualized as a series of trials beginning with a specific verbal prompt ("Take a bite") and the presentation of a teaspoon of puréed fruit. The spoon was not withdrawn until Zoe took it into her mouth—a procedure similar to "escape extinction" (see Chapter 4). Zoe's mother was instructed to strictly ignore coughing, gagging, and negative verbal behavior. She was advised to praise acceptance and intake, to remain calm and reassuring, to end each meal on a pleasant note, and to plan a pleasant activity after each feeding session.
5. Feeding progress, weight gain, and diet were monitored in biweekly sessions with the psychologist and the nutritionist.

Phase 2

1. Tube feeds were reduced by 250 kilocalories after the fifth week of Phase 1, by another 250 kilocalories after the seventh week, and by another 250 kilocalories at the end of 14 weeks. At the end of 36 weeks, Zoe was taking all but 250 calories per day by mouth.
2. Both increased oral intake and weight gain were used as criteria for progressive reductions in tube feeding.

Phase 3

1. After the 16th week, feeding-related therapies were reinstated in school, with emphasis focused on refining self-feeding skills and promoting oral-motor skills, especially those relevant to drinking, which was identified as an area of special difficulty during the course of this intervention.
2. Special rewards for drinking small amounts of juice at home also were incorporated into the parent-mediated program.

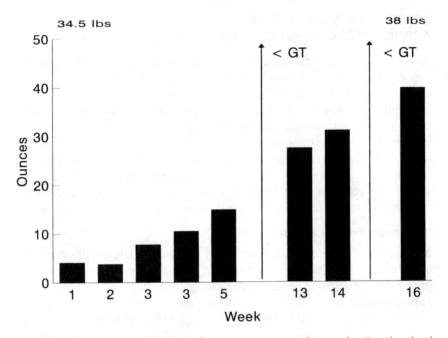

Figure 7.2. Zoe's average oral intake per day in mean ounces per day, as a function of weeks of intervention, for the first 16 weeks of intervention. Vertical lines indicate points at which GT feeds were reduced. Zoe's weight gain (from 34.5 pounds to 38 pounds) was satisfactory.

OUTCOME

Outcome was measured by parent report of daily oral intake, expressed in ounces of food consumed. Figure 7.2 shows Zoe's average oral intake per day, as a function of weeks of intervention, for the first 16 weeks of intervention. Intake over the first 2 weeks averaged about 4 ounces per day and then began to increase with each subsequent week. At the end of the fifth week of intervention, intake was judged to be sufficient to begin reduction of tube feeds. At this point, appetite manipulation supported increased oral intake. Zoe accepted an increased variety of foods as intervention progressed. Initially accepting only puréed fruits, she gradually was offered and accepted a wide variety of puréed and "chunky" vegetables and meats, as well as cereals, yogurt, and puddings. As each novel food was introduced, Zoe's distress re-emerged but soon abated with increased exposure to the new food. Zoe also became more interested in finger-feeding as intervention proceeded, and this was vigorously encouraged. It was not possible to wean Zoe from gastrostomy feeds entirely during the course of this intervention because of her very limited intake of liquids.

OTHER CHRONIC ILLNESSES
ASSOCIATED WITH FEEDING PROBLEMS

As is seen in the case of high-risk infants, many biological, iatrogenic, and behavioral factors can converge and interact to increase the likelihood of feeding disorders in children with chronic illness. The following examples of pediatric illness are grouped according to three major factors that potentially increase feeding difficulty: the increased energy needs associated with some illnesses, restrictive diets required in treating some illnesses, and illnesses that may directly decrease appetite or increase the aversiveness of feeding. These are certainly not mutually exclusive categories, and many chronic illnesses could be multiply classified.

Increased Energy Requirements

Many illnesses complicate feeding by increasing the child's need for calories. Because the child's appetite may not be sufficient to support his or her metabolic needs, caregivers may force feed and/or supplemental non-oral feeding may become necessary. Many pulmonary and cardiac diseases provide examples of increased energy needs.

Bronchopulmonary Dysplasia   BPD is a chronic pulmonary disease common in premature infants when respiratory distress syndrome is treated with supplemental oxygen and with mechanically assisted ventilation (Bancalari & Gerhardt, 1986). The disease is characterized by damage to lung tissue, edema, abnormal surfactant production, atelectasis, and emphysema. Children with BPD are at elevated risk for malnutrition and growth retardation because respiratory disease is associated with increased energy needs and both the treatment and the complications of the disease make oral feeding and nutrition therapy difficult. At the same time, satisfactory nutritional status is of crucial importance in supporting optimal treatment of the respiratory disease (Adams, 1991).

Several factors—including fatigue, breathlessness, fluid restriction, and appetite suppression caused by illness or medication—work directly or indirectly to complicate oral intake in children with BPD. Infants with BPD are prone to episodes of low oxygen saturation during feeding (Garg, Kurzner, Bautista, & Keens, 1988). Episodes of hypoxia can last from 15 to 20 seconds and are unassociated with apnea, bradycardia, or cyanosis; hypoxia is therefore difficult to detect by routine clinical assessment. Singer et al. (1992) found that infants with BPD who had been weaned from oxygen and discharged from the hospital showed more hypoxia before, during, and after feeding than same-age controls who were VLBW or healthy. Singer and her colleagues (1992) also found that increased volume of formula consumed and faster feeding were related to severe desaturation and speculated that the slower feeding often observed in infants with BPD may be related to the infant's attempts to minimize desaturation.

The energy expenditure of infants with BPD can be 25%–50% above that of same-age infants without lung disease (Yeh, McClenan, Ajay, & Pildes, 1989). It is not surprising, therefore, that the combination of high-energy needs and multiple oral intake risk factors often results in partial or complete reliance on supplemental non-oral feeding. As already noted, this can introduce additional problems for oral feeding. Those infants with BPD who are maintained on ventilators for prolonged periods are, of course, subject to additional feeding problem risk factors. Children with BPD are also at increased risk for cerebral palsy and compromised cognitive outcome, factors with additional implications for feeding (see Chapter 8).

Medications commonly used in the treatment of BPD include corticosteroids, diuretics, bronchodilators, and antibiotics. Some of these medications have potential adverse effects on the GI system and may cause anorexia, nausea, vomiting, or diarrhea (see Chapter 2).

Table 7.3 summarizes several recommendations for feeding children with BPD. Some of these recommended techniques (e.g., use of small, frequently scheduled meals; reinforcement of positive eating behaviors) are common to the interventions for feeding problems in other populations, whereas other techniques (e.g., providing additional oxygen during feeding, administering prescribed bronchodilator prior to feeding) are specific to feeding children with BPD. The clinical utility of most of these techniques requires additional study. An example of the systematic assessment of positioning and support techniques with a 10-month-old boy with BPD was described by Kerwin, Osborne, and Eicher (1994). This inpatient study assessed the effects of an upright (90°) versus angled (45°) feeding position and the effects of chair-seating versus held support on several feeding variables, including bites accepted, swallowed, and expelled. An angled feeding position initially facilitated feeding and quickly generalized to upright feeding. Type of support did not affect feeding.

Case 7.2 illustrates many of the factors that impede oral feeding of children with BPD. A multicomponent, behavioral inpatient intervention was used to establish oral feeding in this child.

Table 7.3. Feeding interventions for children with BPD

Adams (1991)
  1. High-calorie diet
  2. Small, frequent meals
  3. Feeding in "protected zones" (i.e., areas in which no aversive procedures are administered)

Singer et al. (1992)
  1. Teach caregivers to "slow down" feeding through frequent pauses or alteration of nipple size
  2. Provide home oxygen for infants who do not gain satisfactory weight and are difficult feeders secondary to suspected hypoxia

Wolf & Glass (1992)
  1. Administering prescribed bronchodilator prior to feeding
  2. Providing additional oxygen during oral feeding
  3. Postponing or eliminating feeding if the infant's respiratory rate remains high
  4. Encouraging a short sucking burst pattern
  5. Attending carefully to body posture and alignment during feeding
  6. Minimizing aversive oral input by attending to the timing, sequencing, and frequency of procedures
  7. Maximizing pleasurable oral-tactile input
  8. Building trust between therapists and the child by respecting the infant's control over the feeding process
  9. Using behavioral management techniques, focusing on reinforcement of positive eating behaviors

■ ■ ■

CASE 7.2. INPATIENT INTERVENTION FOR A CHILD WITH BPD
NAME: Mark
AGE AT INTERVENTION: 1 year, 3 months

BACKGROUND

Mark was the product of a 26-week pregnancy complicated by pre-eclampsia, which required an emergency cesarean section. Mark required assisted ventilation for the first 66 days of life, was extubated, and then re-intubated on Day 78. Other neonatal complications included intraventricular hemorrhage, patent ductus arteriosus, renal calcification, retinopathy of prematurity, strabismus, and a fractured femur. Tracheostomy and gastrostomy tubes were placed at 6 months of age. He was cared for in a NICU for the first 5 months of his life, transferred to another acute care hospital for 2 months, and then transferred to a pediatric rehabilitation hospital for developmental intervention, respiratory care, and further treatment of BPD.

At the time of behavioral feeding intervention, he presented with mild cerebral palsy and significant delays in all developmental domains. Mark's language skills were especially delayed, and he also presented with significant oral-motor problems. Initial feeding attempts, conducted in his hospital room, had found him to be very easily distracted by both visual and auditory stimulation. His oral intake prior to intervention was highly variable: He would occasionally have what was described as a "good" meal, taking a few ounces of formula or puréed food, but would subsequently become extremely resistant, refusing any feeds for days at a time, as well as vomiting most meals that were accepted.

Family involvement at the onset of feeding intervention was minimal. Mark's 16-year-old mother gradually became more involved as discharge grew imminent and was ultimately included in the feeding protocol, becoming one of Mark's designated feeders. Weekly outpatient sessions were scheduled after discharge to help his mother capitalize on gains that had been made during the inpatient intervention.

FORMULATION

The following factors were thought to contribute to Mark's feeding resistance:

1. History of oral intake prior to behavioral intervention was highly variable and was marked by inconsistent feeding practices. For example, during 1 week, Mark was fed by 11 different individuals; some offered only formula, some attempted solid foods; many meals were missed because of a variety of staffing- and patient-related factors.
2. Behavior observation indicated extreme liability to distraction. Mark would stop feeding each time a monitor sounded or people entered his room, even when the bedside curtain was drawn.
3. Mark's oral-motor skills were judged to be mildly impaired but functional for bottle feeding and puréed foods. Oral-motor dysfunction contributed to feeding inefficiency and fatigue.
4. Mark was necessarily subjected to multiple and recurrent aversive events in the oral area, including suctioning and treatment of recurrent keloid formation around the tracheostomy. All of these aversive procedures were implemented in the same room that feeding typically was attempted.
5. Prolonged dependence on alternative feeding had served to dissociate feeding behavior from its natural consequence: satiety. Bolus gastrostomy feeds were distributed evenly throughout the day.

INTERVENTION

A feeding protocol was developed to establish consistent oral intake. The essential features of the protocol included using a limited number of designated feeders, feeding in a distraction-free environment, initially feeding only formula (both to promote consistency and to ensure high caloric density), using differential attention to strengthen acceptance of eating, scheduling gastronomy feeds at night to promote increased appetite during the day, followed by tapering of gastronomy feeds when this was justified by reliable intake. The complete treatment protocol, with detailed instructions for staff, is reproduced in the next section.

Mark's Feeding Program

1. Feeding will be conducted by a minimum number of staff to foster consistency in implementation.
2. Feedings will be conducted in a distraction-free setting. Because Mark's room is seldom free of distractions, even with the curtains drawn, we will use the shower room. The light should be *off* during feeding, and the door open about 6 inches to provide dim illumination. Mark should face away from the partially open door to minimize visual distraction associated with staff activity in the hallway.
3. Three oral feeding sessions will be scheduled at the following times: 9 A.M., 12 noon, and 4 P.M. Tube feeds will be scheduled during the evenings at 8 P.M., 12 midnight, and 4 A.M. Mark will not be fed at any other time.
4. Offer only formula during this phase of the intervention and record the amount consumed at the end of each meal. Use the red "preemie" nipple to minimize oral fatigue.
5. Mark is very often "fussy" and irritable when he first begins a meal. Wait him out: Ignore his fussing, hold him quietly, do not speak to him, and do not offer the bottle until he settles down. This may take a few minutes. When he has calmed down, he will usually accept the bottle and will guide it into his mouth with his hands, often holding it there by himself.
6. Follow each successful meal with a period of pleasant social interaction (e.g., 15 minutes of play). Any meal in which Mark consumes 80 millimeters or more of formula is a successful meal during this phase of the intervention.
7. Implement consistent consequences for refusing to eat and for inappropriate eating. Ignore food refusal by turning away from Mark for 15 seconds; at the end of this period, re-present food. When Mark becomes very fussy or overly active, it often helps to place him in a stroller for about 1 minute before resuming the meal. Ter-

minate the meal after five refusals. No social or other reinforcers should be available for 15 minutes after an unsuccessful meal. Place Mark in his crib, without toys, for 15 minutes after unsuccessful meals. If he spits up or vomits during a meal, clean him quickly, with minimal social attention, and resume feeding.

8. If Mark requires suctioning during the beginning of a meal (before refusals begin), then have him suctioned, and restart the meal. If he requires suctioning toward the end of a meal (after several refusals), then terminate the meal.

OUTCOME

The results of the first phase of the behavioral intervention are shown in Figure 7.3. Notable is an immediate improvement in the consistency of oral intake, with reliable intake on each day of the intervention. Second, there is a gradual increase in intake, presumably due to environmental modification and behavioral contingencies. Finally, there is a pronounced increase in the rate of oral intake when alternative feeding is discontinued, showing the direct effect of appetite enhancement. Small amounts of puréed foods were subsequently introduced during each meal, and other caregivers—including his mother—were trained and added to the list of designated feeders. Mark's respiratory status improved gradually and, after many months, he was discharged home.

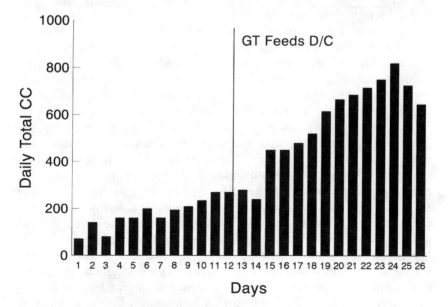

Figure 7.3. Graphic representation of the first phase of behavioral intervention showing rate of oral intake in cubic centimeters (CC). After Day 12, GT feeds were discontinued (D/C).

At discharge, he was taking 100% of his required calories by mouth, in the form of both formula and puréed foods. The gastrostomy tube was not removed prior to discharge, but its use at home was limited to periods of acute illness.

■ ■ ■

Cystic Fibrosis   Cystic fibrosis (CF) is a lethal genetic disease of the exocrine system that affects 1 in every 2,000 newborns (Batshaw & Rose, 1997; Wood, Boat, & Doershuk, 1976). Malnutrition is a common problem in children with CF. It has been recommended that children with CF consume 120%–200% of the calories recommended for children who are healthy, but a 1991 review (Bowen & Stark) concluded that most children with CF do not meet this caloric standard, and many do not meet the Recommended Dietary Allowance for healthy children. Short-term supplemental feeding (via oral supplement or nasogastric feeding) often is used to treat malnutrition in children with CF, but weight gains may not persist following treatment termination. The following two studies illustrate the utility of behavioral interventions for poor intake and food refusal in children with CF.

Singer, Nofer, Benson-Szekely, and Brooks (1991) described four children with CF, malnutrition, and feeding problems who were treated on an inpatient unit. The children ranged in age from 10 to 42 months. All were below the 5th percentile weight-for-age despite appropriate treatment of CF, nutritional counseling, and prior hospitalizations. All children were treated with a basic feeding protocol that included the following components: 1) using a hierarchy of steps and providing clearly specified criteria for success, 2) allowing the child access to food and drink only at mealtime, 3) reinforcing food acceptance, 4) ignoring food refusal or using time-out, and 5) training parents prior to discharge. Additional procedures were used for individual children. These included the following techniques: 1) feeding in a nondistracting environment, 2) modifying medication and aerosol schedules, 3) enlarging bottle nipples or using a Tippy cup to reduce feeding fatigue, 4) slowing the pace of the meal to allow for rest and breathing between bites, and 5) using a sharp verbal "no" contingent on gagging. Children in this study increased their daily caloric intake from a mean of 54% of requirements at treatment initiation to a mean of 92% at discharge. Three of the four children demonstrated continued catch-up growth postdischarge with percentiles of weight-for-height at follow-up ranging from the 10th to the 50th percentile.

Stark, Bowen, Tyc, Evans, and Passero (1990) reported on an outpatient, interdisciplinary behavioral intervention for five children with CF (ages 5–12) whose weights-for-age ranged from the 35th percentile to below the 5th percentile. Children and parents met weekly in separate groups to receive nutrition education and parent behavior management training to deal with food refusal. Children received rewards for achieving clearly specified dietary intake goals in a systematic stepwise intervention across snacks, breakfasts, lunches, and dinners. The children in this study increased oral intake by an average of 900 calories per day during the course of the intervention. Increased caloric intake was maintained at 1- and 9-month follow-up observations.

Feeding disorders in children with CF are paradigmatic of the genesis of feeding disorders in chronic illness. The combination of increased caloric requirements and decreased appetite due to disease process, as well as heightened parental anxiety due to malnutrition and the mortal implications of this disease, are typical of the issues involved in treating feeding problems in children with chronic health conditions.

Congenital Heart Disease   Congenital heart disease (CHD) can be associated with growth deficiency, which is generally thought to result from inadequate caloric intake (Huse, Feldt, Nelson, & Novak, 1975). Factors contributing to reduced oral intake include fatigue during feeding, competition between breathing and swallowing, medication intoxication, restricted diets, intestinal dysfunction, and weakness from diuretic-induced loss of electrolytes (Greecher, 1990). (Diuretics frequently are used to control fluid balance in children with CHD.) Breast feeding children with CHD is usually discouraged, and recommendations for bottle feeding have focused on using a soft nipple, enlarging the nipple hole, and altering the pattern of feeding to reduce fatigue (Wolf & Glass, 1992). Tube feeding often is used to maintain weight gain and nutritional balance in children with CHD.

The multitude of pathophysiological contributions to feeding problems in children with CHD can cause, or can be accompanied by, interactional feeding problems. Lobo (1992), in a study that compared feeding interaction in CHD dyads with matched healthy infants, found that children with CHD evidenced more ambiguous feeding cues and were less responsive to parents during feeding than healthy controls (Barnard & Kelly, 1990). Mothers of children with CHD demonstrated less emotional growth fostering. Whether these feeding problems are inherent to CHD or emerge over the course of months or years of difficult feeding is unclear.

Aversion and/or Anorexia

Many illnesses can directly affect the desire to eat by reducing appetite or by making ingestion painful. Cancer and several GI diseases provide specific examples of this process.

Cancer Anorexia, feeding aversion, and malnutrition are common in children (and adults) with cancer. In their most extreme expression, these can culminate in cancer cachexia, severe emaciation, and death by starvation (Fearon & Carter, 1988). The evidence suggests that most children newly diagnosed with cancer are no more malnourished than healthy controls; thus, the growth of the tumor and complications of antitumor therapy appear to be responsible for eating and nutrition problems (Bernstein, 1986).

Tumor growth can affect appetite and intake in several ways. Effects on the GI system include maldigestion, malabsorption, and anatomical obstruction. There is also evidence that learned food aversions may be more specifically induced by physiological changes related to the growth of the tumor (Bernstein, 1986). Significant anorectic effects also are associated with radiotherapy and chemotherapy. These include nausea, vomiting, altered taste sensitivity, and oral ulceration, as well as depression and anxiety. Bernstein (1978) has shown that children develop learned aversions to novel foods consumed prior to GI-toxic chemotherapy and that a single pairing of food and chemotherapy was sufficient to induce food aversion.

The treatment of cancer-related feeding problems in children has received little systematic study, but clinical recommendations are available. Kelly (1986) summarized multiple practical suggestions for dealing with specific "dietary dilemmas" and obstacles to oral intake. These include many techniques validated in the treatment of feeding problems in other populations (e.g., small, frequent meals; avoiding noncaloric drinks; behavior modification techniques; cognitive behavior pain management), as well as more disease-specific recommendations to address alterations in taste sensitivity (e.g., using herbs and spices, varying color and texture) and nausea (e.g., avoiding foods with strong odors, avoiding very sweet foods). Bernstein (1986) also recommended some specific techniques, derived from clinical research with children with cancer, for managing learned food aversions. These include the following: 1) consuming novel foods prior to chemotherapy to "block" the formation of learned aversions to familiar foods, 2) eating lightly before drug treatment, and 3) avoiding protein foods before chemotherapy because protein sources are more likely to become the target of learned food aversions than are foods that are high in carbohydrates.

Hypnosis, guided imagery, and other variants of relaxation therapy have been used with some success in managing anticipatory nausea and vomiting (Culbert, Kajander, Kohen, & Reaney, 1996; Zeltzer, LeBaron, & Zeltzer, 1984). Cognitive-behavioral and relaxation therapies have proved useful in treating feeding phobias in children with secondary extreme selectivity (see Chapter 5) and show promise in treating feeding aversion, cancer anorexia, and secondary malnutrition in children with cancer.

Gastroesophageal Reflux GER refers to the reflux (reverse flow) of gastric acid into the esophagus. Occasional reflux is common and benign in children and adults. GER can be associated with regurgitation but also can occur without manifest symptoms. GER is especially prevalent in infants younger than 12 months of age and is assumed to result from developmental variations in the maturation of the GI tract (Glassman, George, & Grill, 1995). About 40% of healthy infants younger than 12 months of age regurgitate at least once per day (Orenstein, 1994). Individuals with clinically significant GER have more frequent and longer episodes of reflux, which can lead to serious pathological consequences. Severe GER can result in esophagitis, with consequent chronic blood loss, and possible esophageal strictures due to permanent tissue damage. GER with regurgitation also may be associated with caloric loss and undernutrition. Recurrent pneumonia secondary to aspiration is also a risk, especially in children with neurological impairments (Sondheimer, 1988). There is an increased incidence of GER in children with severe disabilities (Orenstein & Orenstein, 1988) and in children following placement of GTs (Tuchman, 1994). Although the etiology of GER is not completely understood, it is generally considered to be an involuntary process and, as such, should be clearly distinguished from rumination and voluntary vomiting (see Chapter 9) with which it may co-exist.

GER affects feeding in a number of important ways. First, reflux is perceived as chest pain and is therefore an aversive stimulus around which maladaptive learning can occur. In preverbal children, postprandial chest pain may be expressed as crying or irritability, during or after feeding. Feeding resistance and poor weight gain can develop when an infant with recurrent postprandial pain learns to avoid pain by limiting meal size (Hyman, 1994). Esophagitis secondary to chronic reflux may make swallowing uncomfortable and contribute to feeding resistance. GER with regurgitation can be especially disruptive to feeding, affecting the child's nutritional status and the quality of feeding interaction. Impaired feeding interaction resulting from GER-induced vomiting can establish a vicious cycle in which ongoing maternal and infant distress results in increased vomiting as a visceral response to stress (Fleisher, 1995).

Conservative interventions for GER include dietary modifications and recommendations for mealtime positioning. Foods that may be contraindicated for children with GER include chocolate, citrus juices, fatty foods, carbonated beverages, and caffeine. These foods can have the effect of decreasing tone in the lower esophageal sphincter, increasing gastric acidity, or increasing intragastric pressure, which all are mechanisms that have been implicated in the etiology of GER. Other dietary interventions include thickening infant feeds; providing small, frequent meals; and fasting before bedtime. Upright positioning during and after meals is also frequently recommended. Pharmacological treatment includes medications to reduce gastric acidity and prokinetic agents, which are medications that improve gastric motility. When conservative measures and pharmacological treatments fail and when there is risk of severe esophagitis or aspiration pneumonia, surgery often is considered. The most common surgical procedure, the Nissen fundoplication, serves to reduce reflux by tightening the passage between the esophagus and the stomach.

Short-Gut Syndrome   Short-gut syndrome (SGS) is a disorder in which loss of intestinal length, as a result of resection, significantly compromises the ability to absorb and digest nutrients. Children with SGS initially are managed with TPN and are only gradually advanced to enteral feeding; the transition to oral feeding may take weeks to months (Biller, 1987). Lengthy hospitalizations, prolonged dependence on parenteral and enteral feeding, and some of the clinical manifestations of SGS, including anorexia, impaired taste, and ongoing risk of malnutrition and dehydration (Biller, 1987), contribute to feeding problems in these children.

Linscheid et al. (1987) described a behavioral intervention for a 6-year-old boy with SGS who had been born with jejunal atresia and malrotation, had numerous surgeries related to SGS, and had life-long dependence on alternative feeding, including TPN and a gastrostomy tube. At the beginning of intervention, this child's oral intake was limited to small amounts of a liquid food supplement, and attempts to encourage consumption of other liquids or solids elicited reactions of fear and distress (i.e., crying, trembling). The child was admitted for an inpatient behavioral feeding intervention, which included the following features: 1) three time-limited meals daily; 2) contingent access to ward privileges; 3) token reinforcement for meeting oral intake requirements during a meal; 4) contingent attention during the meal; 5) all gastrostomy feeds scheduled at night; 6) all meals provided in a distraction-free environment; 7) a limited number of designated feeders; 8) gradually increasing intake requirements; and 9) parent training, planned implementation of the protocol at home, and outpatient follow-up. At discharge after a 60-day hospitalization, the child was accepting milk, chocolate milk, orange juice, pudding, mashed potatoes, bananas, spaghetti, and turkey. At a 1-month follow-up visit, 75% of his calories were taken orally, and eight new foods had been added to his diet; 2 months after discharge, all foods were taken orally. This case illustrates the value of behavioral intervention for feeding disorders with a complex medical etiology in which there had been minimal oral intake over a period of years.

Restrictive Diets

Ongoing health conditions that require restrictive diets as a part of medical treatments may raise feeding issues as well. When the diet is unappetizing, is socially unconventional, or requires careful calibration, mealtime struggles and adherence can become issues. Diabetes and phenylketonuria (PKU) are illnesses that raise these issues, as do specific food allergies.

Diabetes   Diabetes mellitus is a chronic disease of insufficient insulin production. Insulin-dependent diabetes (IDDM) results from pancreatic beta cell failure and requires that the individual replace insulin by injection. IDDM is the most common childhood metabolic disease, affecting 1.7 per 1,000 individuals younger than the age of 20 years (American Diabetes Association, 1996). Potential health complications of diabetes include retinopathy, neuropathy, renal disease, hypertension, vascular problems, and, ultimately, a shortened life expectancy (Johnson, 1995). Management of diabetes requires mastery of a complex regimen including two to four daily insulin injections, blood glucose testing several times per day, dietary modifications, and careful timing and insulin dose adjustments to compensate for variations in diet and exercise.

Although dietary prescriptions for children with IDDM are based on foods essential to any healthy diet, consistent meal schedules, portion control, and careful attention to the energy and nutrient content of foods are required to achieve optimal metabolic control and to reduce the risk of complications. These requirements challenge the abilities of children and parents alike. Eating appropriate foods and sticking to meal plans are, in fact, often found to be the elements of the diabetes treatment regimen that children find most difficult (LaGreca, 1988). Children often are asked to adhere to a meal structure of three meals and three snacks per day, at regular and fixed intervals, and to moderate their intake of foods with concentrated sweets. Thus, they are often in the position of eating when peers are not or of being unable to consume the same foods (especially sweets) as peers. Common mealtime struggles can be intensified because insulin injections are typically scheduled prior to meals, and a child who refuses to eat after an insulin injection is at risk for severe hypoglycemia.

Understanding and attending to the energy and nutrient content of foods on a daily basis is also challenging. Many newly diagnosed children and their parents receive nutrition education and individualized meal planning, but the efficacy of these interventions is uncertain. Delamater, Smith, Kurtz, and White (1988) found that a sample of mostly middle-class parents and children who had been given 4 hours of intensive dietary instruction at the time of diagnosis were able to recall only about 50% of their dietary prescriptions. They also performed poorly on a test of dietary skills that assessed judgments of food quantity and exchange equivalence values. Child-acknowledged adherence with diet also was poor, with 24% reporting rarely adhering to their afternoon snack, 18% rarely adhering to diet in school, and 12% rarely adhering while dining in restaurants or with friends. Mean glycosylated hemoglobin (a reliable measure of diabetic control) was significantly correlated with child adherence but not with child dietary skills. Another study of dietary compliance in 69 children (40 in hospitals and 29 in outpatient treatment) with IDDM, ages 4–18 years, found a mean daily deviation from prescribed diet of 23.8% (Schmidt, Klover, Arfken, Delamater, & Hobson, 1992). Children in this study consumed significantly more calories than prescribed, with the majority of excess energy intake coming from fat sources.

Although a review of issues associated with medical adherence is beyond the scope of this chapter, it has been suggested (Varni & Wallander, 1984) that noncompliance with medical regimen should be *expected* in children, and it would appear that children with IDDM are no exception. Children with complex medical regimens often require special incentives to improve health care compliance. Although there are no studies that specifically target dietary compliance in children with diabetes, several studies (e.g., LaGreca, 1988) demonstrate the value of systematic use of rewards and incentives to improve children's diabetes care. Delamater et al. (1988) also recommended that dietary knowledge and skills be enhanced by the use of behavior rehearsal, role-playing, and actual practice at diet implementation.

Phenylketonuria PKU is an inborn error of metabolism in which phenylalanine, an essential amino acid, is not metabolized, accumulates in the blood, and causes injury to the brain. Newborn screening programs for PKU are well established, and, with early and appropriate dietary intervention, mental retardation can be prevented in most children with PKU. Intervention involves limiting dietary phenylalanine. Unfortunately, it is impossible to devise a diet of natural foods sufficiently low in phenylalanine and a synthetic diet is required. Most PKU clinics in the United States recommend indefinite continuation of the low phenylalanine diet (Schuett & Brown, 1984). The issue of dietary compliance is therefore one that persists throughout childhood and into adulthood. For women with PKU, continuing the low phenylalanine diet can reduce the risk of giving birth to a child with mental retardation (Batshaw, 1997; Lowitzer, 1987).

The PKU diet has been described as drab, monotonous, and unappetizing, resulting in dietary compliance problems for some children (Finney & Friman, 1988). MacDonald et al. (1994) found that feeding problems were significantly more common in children with PKU (ages 1–5 years) than in a matched control group. Parents of children with PKU rated them as having poorer appetites, as consuming a more limited range of foods, and as having more difficulty in feeding. Significantly more children with PKU had GI symptoms such as constipation and abdominal pain, and eating in isolation also was significantly more common in children with PKU.

Archer, Cunningham, and Whelan (1988) reported on the treatment of a 7-year-old child with PKU who had a phobic-like response to eating characterized by frequent gagging and vomiting for no apparent reason and who had many other eating-avoidant behaviors. Family meals were marked by tension, anxiety, and coercive feeding practices. Treatment involved family systems therapy and child behavior management counseling and resulted in a significant reduction of mealtime problems.

The routine use of behavioral techniques, including use of preferred (nonsynthetic foods) to reward consumption of synthetic foods and the use of observational learning (e.g., having parents and siblings eat portions of the synthetic foods) have been recommended to increase dietary compliance in children with PKU (Finney & Friman, 1988).

Other Metabolic Disorders Anorexia and food refusal often are associated with urea cycle and organic acid disorders, with both biological and behavioral mechanisms contributing to feeding disturbance (Hyman et al., 1987). Diminished appetite is thought to result from neurotransmitter alterations associated with these metabolic disorders. Ongoing feeding problems in these children often result in nasogastric tube or GT feedings. Hyman et al. (1987) reported on a series of six children, three with urea cycle disorders and three with acidemia, who were treated in hospitals for feeding disturbance with behavior management protocols. All children had functional oral-motor skills but exhibited inappropriate mealtime behaviors including food selectivity and avoidance, food refusal, expulsion, vomiting, and disruptive behaviors. These children required nasogastric and gastrostomy feedings to maintain adequate nutrition. Five of the six children responded to behavioral intervention, with food acceptance improving from 0%–41% to 69%–99% during hospital intervention and with all five children taking all food orally at follow-up. Three of the five children responding to behavioral intervention also had improved metabolic control measured by fewer short-term hospitalizations due to hyperammonemic episodes. Metabolites of serotonin and dopamine also were measured in this study and were found to be elevated in the children with feeding disorders. This study is notable for the successful behavioral intervention of feeding disorders in children with metabolic disorders even when anorexia appears to be induced by objectively identified neurochemical alterations.

Seizure Disorders   Children with seizure disorders are usually treated with anticonvulsant medication regimens. These medications can have side effects that have an impact on feeding. Gastric irritation, decreased appetite, lethargy, mild incoordination, and vomiting are among the observed side effects of anticonvulsant therapy (see Chapter 2). Dilantin therapy also may have the side effect of gum hypertrophy, which can make eating painful. Some anticonvulsant medications are unpleasant to taste and—when it is necessary to administer them in liquid form—may produce resistance. In some cases, resistance to medication administration can generalize to feeding or can lead to generalized noncompliance.

Some cases of intractable epilepsy are treated with a ketogenic diet. This diet, consisting largely of high-fat foods, is generally considered to be unappetizing and must be observed strictly to be effective. Compliance is therefore a significant issue, especially with children. Amari, Grace, and Fisher (1995) described a case in which a 15-year-old girl's compliance with a ketogenic diet was maintained using behavioral interventions. First, a stimulus choice procedure was used to assess the child's preference for a list of 33 ketogenic foods. The stimulus choice procedure involves the pair-wise presentation of all foods, with the child choosing and consuming the preferred choice on each trial. This resulted in the rank ordering of preference for the complete list of foods. Second, preferred foods were used to reinforce consumption of less-preferred foods, a procedure common to interventions for extreme selectivity (see Chapter 5). Compliance with the ketogenic diet improved from 60% in the pre-intervention baseline to 99% following intervention, with a 40% reduction in seizures relative to baseline.

Adverse Food Reactions   Adverse reactions to specific foods are frequent presenting complaints in pediatric practice. Bock (1987) found that 43% of a group of 480 children who were followed from birth to 3 years of age had some negative reactions attributed to food, but only 8% had reactions that were probably truly caused by food. Not all confirmed adverse reactions to food represent true allergies (i.e., reactions with an immunological basis). Enzyme deficiency (e.g., lactase deficiency), pharmacological effects (e.g., arrhythmia resulting from caffeine), and toxic reactions (e.g., to pollutants carried in breast milk) are examples of organic nonallergic adverse food reactions (Bock & Sampson, 1994; Ferguson, 1992). Psychogenic food aversions also may be mistaken for allergies. Bock and Sampson (1994) estimated that the incidence of true food allergies in infancy is 1%–2% and decreases as children get older. Cow's milk, eggs, nuts, wheat, soy products, fish, and crustacea are foods that are often suspected of eliciting allergic reactions.

The diagnosis of specific food intolerance is difficult because the most frequent symptoms (e.g., diarrhea, vomiting, abdominal pain, dermatitis, coughing) are usually nonspecific and may mimic symptoms of other health conditions. In very rare cases, food allergies can result in severe anaphylactic reactions requiring emergency treatment. Elimination diets with double-blind food challenges are the most reliable way to identify a true food allergy (Bock & Sampson, 1994). The presumed offending food is deleted from the diet, symptoms are observed, and then the food is reintroduced, with symptoms again closely observed. Elimination diets are, themselves, a considerable source of stress for children and their families. Thus, these diets should not be undertaken without strong presumptive evidence that food intolerance is the problem. If a food allergy is objectively identified, then offending foods are eliminated from the diet. These foods then should be reintroduced, under medical supervision, after a period of several months, to reassess for clinical sensitivity. When allergies to several foods or to a large class of foods is identified, children often perceive the resulting acceptable diet as rigid or monotonous. The child's intake may be reduced as a result of limited gustatory interest, parents may consequently become anxious about dietary adequacy, and mealtime struggles then may ensue (Pipes, 1989). Finally, unidentified allergens, or allergens consumed as a result of dietary noncompliance, can produce aversive symptoms and a more generalized disinterest in eating. Fortunately, most children outgrow food hypersensitivity (Bock & Sampson, 1994), and prolonged elimination diets are usually not necessary.

It is important for the feeding therapist to consider the possibility that behavioral difficulty around feeding may have a basis in an adverse reaction to specific foods and to refer the child back to his or her pediatrician for further consideration of this possibility. It is equally important to remember that interactional feeding difficulties may be mistakenly attributed to food allergies (Satter, 1986). Indeed, parental attribution of feeding problems to food sensitivity far exceeds the incidence of true food allergies. Factitious food allergies (a parent's mistaken attribution of feeding problems to food sensitivity) can result in severely restricted diets and consequently lead to FTT (Roesler, Barry, & Bock, 1994).

SUMMARY

Chronic illness can negatively affect feeding in many ways. The effects of illness can be direct and immediate (e.g., loss of appetite, increased caloric needs) or indirect and cumulative (e.g., poor weight gain, increased parental stress leading to mealtime problems). Significant feeding problems are frequently associated with a number of different chronic health conditions. Premature birth, LBW, respiratory disease, GI disease, inborn errors of metabolism, diabetes, heart disease, cystic fibrosis, cancer, seizure disorder, and adverse reactions to specific foods all place children at risk for feeding problems. Although the etiology of feeding problems in children with chronic illness is often specifically related to the biologic disease process, illness typically potentiates and interacts with other causal variables (e.g., physical competence for feeding, interaction/management, caregiver competence, systemic factors). Behavioral interventions have been demonstrated to be useful primary or adjunctive therapies for many children with feeding problems secondary to chronic illness.

REFERENCES

Adams, E. (1991). Nutrition for the young child with bronchopulmonary dysplasia (BPD). *Nutrition Focus, 6,* 1–6.
Als, H. (1986). A synactive model of neonatal behavioral organization: Framework for the assessment of neurobehavioral development in the premature infant and for support of infants and parents in the neonatal

intensive care environment. *Physical and Occupational Therapy in Pediatrics, 6,* 3–55.

Als, H., Lawhon, G., Duffy, F., McAnulty, G.B., Gibes-Grossman, R., & Blickman, J.G. (1994). Individualized developmental care for the very low-birth-weight preterm infant. *Journal of the American Medical Association, 272,* 853–858.

Amari, A., Grace, N.C., & Fisher, W. (1995). Achieving and maintaining compliance with the ketogenic diet. *Journal of Applied Behavior Analysis, 28,* 341–342.

American Diabetes Association. (1996). *Vital statistics.* Alexandria, VA: Author.

Archer, L.A., Cunningham, C.E., & Whelan, D. (1988). Coping with dietary therapy in phenylketonuria: A case report. *Canadian Journal of Behavioural Science, 20,* 461–466.

Bancalari, E., & Gerhardt, T. (1986). Bronchopulmonary dysplasia. *Pediatric Clinics of North America, 33,* 1–23.

Barnard, K.E., & Kelly, J.F. (1990). Assessment of parent–child interaction. In S.J. Meisels & J.P. Shonkoff (Eds.), *Handbook of early childhood intervention* (pp. 278–302). Cambridge, MA: Cambridge University Press.

Batshaw, M.L. (Ed.). (1997). *Children with disabilities* (4th ed.). Baltimore: Paul H. Brookes Publishing Co.

Batshaw, M.L., & Rose, N.C. (1997). Birth defects, prenatal diagnosis, and fetal therapy. In M.L. Batshaw (Ed.), *Children with disabilities* (4th ed., pp. 35–52). Baltimore: Paul H. Brookes Publishing Co.

Bazyk, S. (1990). Factors associated with the transition to oral feeding in infants fed by nasogastric tubes. *American Journal of Occupational Therapy, 44,* 1070–1077.

Bernbaum, J.C., Pereira, G.R., Watkins, J.B., & Peckham, G.J. (1983). Nonnutritive sucking during gavage feeding enhances growth and maturation in premature infants. *Pediatrics, 71,* 41–45.

Bernstein, I.L. (1978). Learned taste aversions in children receiving chemotherapy. *Science, 200,* 1302–1303.

Bernstein, I.L. (1986). Etiology of anorexia in cancer. *Cancer, 58,* 1881–1886.

Biller, J.A. (1987). Short small-bowel syndrome. In R.J. Grand, J.L. Sutphen, & W.H. Dietz (Eds.), *Pediatric nutrition: Theory and practice* (pp. 481–487). Boston: Butterworths.

Blackman, J.A., & Nelson, C.L.A. (1985). Reinstituting oral feedings in children fed by gastrostomy tube. *Clinical Pediatrics, 24,* 434–438.

Blackman, J.A., & Nelson, C.L.A. (1987). Rapid introduction of oral feedings to tube-fed patients. *Journal of Developmental and Behavioral Pediatrics, 8,* 63–67.

Bock, S.A. (1987). Prospective appraisal of complaints of adverse reactions to foods in children during the first 3 years of life. *Pedatrics, 79,* 683–688.

Bock, S.A., & Sampson, H.A. (1994). Food allergy in infancy. *Pediatric Clinics of North America, 41,* 1047–1067.

Bowen, A.M., & Stark, L.J. (1991). Malnutrition in cystic fibrosis: A behavioral conceptualization of cause and treatment. *Clinical Psychology Review, 11,* 315–331.

Brandt, P., Magyary, D., Hammond, M., & Barnard, K. (1992). Learning and behavioral–emotional problems of children born preterm at second grade. *Journal of Pediatric Psychology, 17,* 291–311.

Culbert, T.P., Kajander, R.L., Kohen, D.P., & Reaney, J.B. (1996). Hypno-behavioral approaches for school-age children with dysphagia and food aversion: A case series. *Journal of Developmental and Behavioral Pediatrics, 17*, 335–341.

Davis, A. (1994). Transitional and combination feeds. In S.B. Baker, R.D. Baker, & A. Davis (Eds.), *Pediatric enteral nutrition* (pp. 139–156). New York: Chapman & Hall.

Delamater, A.M., Smith, J.A., Kurtz, S.M., & White, N.H. (1988). Dietary skills and adherence in children with Type I Diabetes Mellitus. *The Diabetes Educator, 14*, 33–36.

DiPietro, J.A., Cusson, R.M., Caughy, M.O., & Fox, N.A. (1994). Behavioral and physiological effects of nonnutritive sucking during gavage feeding in preterm infants. *Pediatric Research, 36*, 207–214.

DiVitto, B., & Goldberg, S. (1979). The effects of newborn medical status on early parent–child interaction. In T.M. Field, A.M. Sostek, S. Goldberg, & H.H. Shuman (Eds.), *Infants born at risk* (pp. 311–322). New York: Spectrum Publications.

Ernst, J.A., Rickar, K.A., Neal, P.R., Yu, P., Oei, T.O., & Leamons, J.A. (1989). Lack of improved growth outcome related to nonnutritive sucking in very low birth weight premature infants fed a controlled nutrient intake: A randomized prospective study. *Pediatrics, 83*, 706–716.

Fearon, K.C.H., & Carter, D.C. (1988). Cancer cachexia. *Annals of Surgery, 208*, 1–5.

Ferguson, A. (1992). Definitions and diagnosis of food intolerance and food allergy: Consensus and controversy. *Journal of Pediatrics, 121*, S7–S11.

Field, T., Ignatoff, E., Stringer, S., Brennan, J., Greenberg, R., Widmayer, S., & Anderson, G.C. (1982). Nonnutritive sucking during tube feedings: Effects on preterm neonates in an intensive care unit. *Pediatrics, 70*, 381–384.

Finney, J.W., & Friman, P.C. (1988). Behavioral medicine approaches to the prevention of mental retardation. In D.C. Russo & J.H. Kedesdy (Eds.), *Behavioral medicine with the developmentally disabled* (pp. 173–200). New York: Plenum.

Fitzhardinge, P.M., Pape, K., Arstikaitis, M., Boyle, M., Ashby, S., Rowley, A., Netley, C., & Swyer, P.R. (1976). Mechanical ventilation of infants of less than 1,501 gm birth weight: Health, growth, and neurologic sequelae. *Journal of Pediatrics, 88*, 531–541.

Fleisher, D.R. (1995). Comprehensive management of infants with gastro-esophageal reflux and failure to thrive. *Current Problems in Pediatrics, 25*, 247–253.

Fowler, S.M., Simon, B.M., & Handler, S.D. (1985). Communication development in children. In E.N. Meyers, S.E. Stool, & J.T. Johnson (Eds.), *Tracheotomy* (pp. 156–163). New York: Churchill Livingstone.

Garg, M., Kurzner, S.I., Bautista, D.B, & Keens, T.G. (1988). Clinically unsuspected hypoxia during sleep and feeding in infants with bronchopulmonary dysplasia. *Pediatrics, 81*, 635–642.

Gauderer, M.W. (1992). Gastrostomy techniques and devices. *Surgical Clinics of North America, 76*, 1285–1298.

Geertsma, M.A., Hyams, J.S., Pelletier, J.M., & Reiter, S. (1985). Feeding resistance after parenteral hyperalimentation. *American Journal of Diseases of Children, 139*, 255–256.

Glass, R.P., & Lucas, B. (1990). Making the transition from tube feeding to oral feeding. *Nutrition Focus, 5,* 1–6.

Glassman, M., George, D., & Grill, B. (1995). Gastroesophageal reflux in children. *Gastroenterology Clinics of North America, 24,* 71–98.

Greecher, C. (1990). Congenital heart disease: A nutrition challenge. *Nutrition Focus, 5,* 1–6.

Hack, M., & Estabrook, M.M. (1985). Development of sucking rhythm in preterm infants. *Early Human Development, 11,* 133–140.

Hack, M., Horbar, J.D., Malloy, M.H., Tyson, J.E., Wright, E., & Wright, L. (1991). Very low birth weight outcomes of the National Institute of Child Health and Human Development Neonatal Network. *Pediatrics, 87,* 587–597.

Handen, B.L., Mandell, F., & Russo, D.C. (1986). Feeding induction in children who refuse to eat. *American Journal of Diseases of Children, 140,* 52–54.

Huse, D.M., Feldt, R.H., Nelson, R.A., & Novak, L.P. (1975). Infants with congenital heart disease. *American Journal of Diseases of Children, 129,* 65–69.

Hyman, P.E. (1994). Gastroesophageal reflux: One reason why baby won't eat. *Journal of Pediatrics, 125,* S103–S109.

Hyman, S.L., Porter, C.A., Page, T.J., Iwata, B.A., Kissel, R., & Batshaw, M.L. (1987). Behavior management of feeding disturbances in urea cycle and organic acid disorders. *Journal of Pediatrics, 111,* 558–562.

Johnson, S.B. (1995). Insulin-dependent diabetes mellitus in childhood. In M.C. Roberts (Ed.), *Handbook of pediatric psychology* (2nd ed., pp. 263–285). New York: Guilford Press.

Kelly, K. (1986). An overview of how to nourish the cancer patient by mouth. *Cancer, 58,* 1897–1901.

Kerwin, M.E., Osborne, M., & Eicher, P.S. (1994). Effect of position and support on oral-motor skills of a child with broncho-pulmonary dysplasia. *Clinical Pediatrics, 33,* 8–13.

Kotelchuck, M.C., & Wise, P.H. (1987). Epidemiology of prematurity and goals for prevention. In H.W. Taeusch & M.W. Yogman (Eds.), *Follow-up management of the high-risk infant* (pp. 3–14). Boston: Little, Brown.

Kramer, S.S., & Eicher, P.M. (1993). The evaluation of pediatric feeding abnormalities. *Dysphagia, 8,* 215–224.

LaGreca, A.M. (1988). Adherence to prescribed medical regimens. In D.K. Routh (Ed.), *Handbook of pediatric psychology* (pp. 299–320). New York: Guilford Press.

Linscheid, T.R., Budd, K.S., & Rasnake, L.K. (1995). Pediatric feeding disorders. In M.C. Roberts (Ed.), *Handbook of pediatric psychology* (2nd ed., pp. 501–515). New York: Guilford Press.

Linscheid, T.R., Tarnowski, K.J., Rasnake, L.K., & Brams, J.S. (1987). Behavioral treatment of food refusal in a child with short-gut syndrome. *Journal of Pediatric Psychology, 12,* 451–459.

Lobo, M.L. (1992). Parent–infant interaction during feeding when the infant has congenital heart disease. *Journal of Pediatric Nursing, 7,* 97–105.

Lowitzer, A. (1987). Maternal phenylketonuria: Cause for concern among women with PKU. *Research in Developmental Disabilities, 8,* 1–14.

MacDonald, A., Rylance, G.W., Asplin, D.A., Hall, K., Harris, G., & Booth, I.W. (1994). Feeding problems in young PKU children. *Acta Paediatrica Supplement, 407,* 73–74.

McCain, G.C. (1993). Facilitating inactive awake states in preterm infants: A study of three interventions. *Nursing Research, 41,* 157–160.

Measel, C.P., & Anderson, G.C. (1979). Nonnutritive sucking during tube feedings: Effect on clinical course in premature infants. *Journal of Obstetrical and Gynecological Neonatal Nursing, 8,* 265–272.

Miller, H.D., & Anderson, G.C. (1993). Nonnutritive sucking: Effects on crying and heart rate in intubated infants requiring assisted mechanical ventilation. *Nursing Research, 42,* 305–307.

Moore, M.C., & Greene, H.L. (1985). Tube feeding in infants and children. *Pediatric Clinics of North America, 32,* 401–417.

O'Brien, M., Soliday, E., & McCluskey-Fawcett, K. (1995). Prematurity and the neonatal intensive care unit. In M.C. Roberts (Ed.), *Handbook of pediatric psychology* (2nd ed., pp. 463–478). New York: Guilford Press.

Orenstein, S.R. (1994). Gastroesophageal reflux disease. *Seminars in Gastrointestinal Disease, 5,* 2–14.

Orenstein, S.R., & Orenstein, D.M. (1988). Gastroesophageal reflux and respiratory disease in children. *Journal of Pediatrics, 112,* 847–858.

Pipes, P.L. (1989). *Nutrition in infancy and childhood.* St. Louis: C.V. Mosby.

Pipes, P.L., & Glass, R.P. (1989). Nutrition and feeding of children with developmental delay and related problems. In P.L. Pipes (Ed.), *Nutrition in infancy and childhood* (pp. 361–386). St. Louis: C.V. Mosby.

Roesler, T.A., Barry, P.C., & Bock, S.A. (1994). Factitious food allergy and failure to thrive. *Archives of Pediatrics and Adolescent Medicine, 148,* 1150–1155.

Satter, E. (1986). *Child of mine: Feeding with love and good sense.* Palo Alto, CA: Bull.

Schauster, H., & Dwyer, H. (1996). Transition from tube feedings to feedings by mouth in children: Preventing eating dysfunction. *Journal of the American Dietetic Association, 96,* 277–281.

Schmidt, L.E., Klover, R.V., Arfken, C.L., Delamater, A.M., & Hobson, D. (1992). Compliance with dietary prescriptions in children and adolescents with insulin-dependent diabetes mellitus. *Journal of the American Dietetic Association, 92,* 567–570.

Schreiner, M.S., Downes, J.J., Kettrick, R.G., Ise, C., & Voit, R. (1987). Chronic respiratory failure in infants with prolonged ventilator dependency. *Journal of the American Medical Association, 258,* 3398–3404.

Schuett, V.E., & Brown, E.S. (1984). Diet policies of PKU clinics in the United States. *American Journal of Public Health, 74,* 501–503.

Scrimshaw, N.S. (1981). Significance of the interactions of nutrition and infection in children. In R.M. Suskind (Ed.), *Textbook of pediatric nutrition* (pp. 229–240). New York: Raven Press.

Simon, B.M., & McGowan, J.S. (1989). Tracheostomy in young children: Implications for assessment and treatment of communication and feeding disorders. *Infants and Young Children, 1,* 1–9.

Singer, L., Martin, R.J., Hawkins, S.W., Benson-Szekely, L.J., Yamashita, T.S., & Carlo, W.A. (1992). Oxygen desaturation complicates feeding in infants with bronchopulmonary dysplasia after discharge. *Pediatrics, 90,* 380–384.

Singer, L.T., Nofer, J.A., Benson-Szekely, L.J., & Brooks, L.J. (1991). Behavioral assessment and management of food refusal in children with cystic fibrosis. *Journal of Developmental and Behavioral Pediatrics, 12,* 115–120.

Singer, L.T., Wood, R., & Lambert, S. (1985). Developmental follow-up of long-term infant tracheostomy: A preliminary report. *Journal of Developmental and Behavioral Pediatrics, 6,* 132–136.

Sondheimer, J.M. (1988). Gastroesophageal reflux: Update on pathogenesis and diagnosis. *Pediatric Clinics of North America, 35,* 103–116.

Stark, L.J., Bowen, A.M., Tyc, V.L., Evans, S., & Passero, A. (1990). A behavioral approach to increasing calorie consumption in children with cystic fibrosis. *Journal of Pediatric Psychology, 15,* 309–326.

Thomasgard, M., & Metz, W.P. (1995). The vulnerable child syndrome revisited. *Journal of Developmental and Behavioral Pediatrics, 16,* 47–53.

Tuchman, D.N. (1994). Oropharyngeal and esophageal complications of enteral tube feeding. In S.B. Baker, R.D. Baker, & A. Davis (Eds.), *Pediatric enteral nutrition* (pp. 179–191). New York: Chapman & Hall.

Varni, J.W., & Wallander, J.L. (1984). Adherence to health-related regimens in pediatric chronic disorders. *Clinical Psychology Review, 4,* 585–596.

Wetmore, R.F., Handler, S.D., & Potsic, W.P. (1982). Pediatric tracheostomy: Experience during the past decade. *Annals of Otology, Rhinology and Laryngology, 91,* 628–632.

Wolf, L.S., & Glass, R.P. (1992). *Feeding and swallowing disorders in infancy.* Tucson, AZ: Therapy Skill Builders.

Wood, R.E., Boat, T.F., & Doershuk, C.F. (1976). State of the art of cystic fibrosis. *American Review of Respiratory Disease, 113,* 833–878.

Yeh, T.F., McClenan, D.A., Ajay, O.A., & Pildes, R.S. (1989). Metabolic rate and energy balance in infants with bronchopulmonary dysplasia. *Journal of Pediatrics, 114,* 448–451.

Zeltzer, L., LeBaron, S., & Zeltzer, P.M. (1984). The effectiveness of behavioral intervention for reduction of nausea and vomiting in children and adolescents receiving chemotherapy. *Journal of Clinical Oncology, 2,* 683–690.

Zlotkin, S.H., Stallings, V.A., & Pencharz, P.B. (1985). Total parenteral nutrition in children. *Pediatric Clinics of North America, 32,* 381–400.

8 Children with Delays in Feeding Skills

Children who have significant delays in developing and mastering feeding skills are the focus of this chapter. In contrast with factors such as illness or developmental transitions that produce mild or temporary disruptions in typical feeding patterns, a host of developmental disabilities can have pervasive impacts on children's acquisition and performance of feeding skills (Eicher, 1997; Luiselli, 1989; Stevenson, 1995). Developmental disabilities are structural, anatomical, and/or neurological impairments in one or more functions controlled by the brain that emerge prenatally, in infancy, or in childhood and that either preclude or significantly impede normal development (Accardo & Whitman, 1996).

Several types of developmental disabilities frequently are associated with delays in feeding skills, including congenital anomalies (e.g., Down syndrome), neuromuscular conditions (e.g., cerebral palsy, acquired brain injury), global developmental disorders (e.g., mental retardation, autism), and sensory impairments (e.g., visual, hearing). These impairments are not mutually exclusive in presentation or in etiology. For example, children may display a combination of cognitive, motor, and sensory impairments secondary to cerebral palsy or head trauma; and mental retardation frequently co-occurs with other developmental disabilities. Because of the overlap in feeding problems across different developmental disabilities, this chapter is organized by feeding skills domains rather than by specific etiological factors.

The next section provides a brief overview of the prevalence of feeding difficulties in children with various developmental disabilities. Subsequent sections describe feeding delays, environmental interventions, and clinical issues related to three basic areas of feeding skills: 1) oral-motor competence, 2) self-feeding capabilities, and 3) social skills and behavior skills at mealtimes. Consistent with the book's focus on behavioral approaches, interventions employing behavioral perspectives are emphasized; however, other treatment approaches also are described. Although this chapter focuses primarily on children with developmental disabilities, many of the interventions apply to children whose feeding skills are delayed for other reasons.

PREVALENCE OF FEEDING PROBLEMS IN CHILDREN WITH DEVELOPMENTAL DISABILITIES

Feeding problems reportedly are quite common among children with developmental disabilities (Brown, Davis, & Flemming, 1979). A frequently cited source is a database described by Palmer and colleagues (Palmer, 1978; Palmer & Horn, 1978; Palmer, Thompson, & Linscheid, 1975) monitoring 500 individuals with various forms of developmental disabilities who were served in the Nutrition Division of the Georgetown University Affiliated Program for Child Development over a 4-year period in the 1970s. This database, as well as other surveys cited by Palmer and Horn (1978), suggested that as many as one in three children with developmental disabilities has one or more types of feeding problems. Reported problems included having difficulties with food intake (e.g., sucking, swallowing, chewing), lacking independent feeding skills (e.g., using a spoon and fork), having bizarre food habits (e.g., eating nonfood items), refusing certain food types or textures, having disruptive or messy eating habits, eating too quickly or too slowly, eating too much or too little, and having nutrient deficiencies. Many of these problems are similar to those eating difficulties that are reported in normally developing children, although the level of skills often is lower and the severity of problems greater in children with developmental disabilities.

The prevalence of feeding problems appears to vary somewhat according to the type and overall severity of developmental disability. Palmer (1978) noted, for example, that obesity is more commonly reported in children with Down syndrome, myelomeningocele, spastic cerebral palsy, and Klinefelter syndrome, whereas being underweight is more frequent in children with athetoid cerebral palsy, attention-deficit/hyperactivity disorder (ADHD; termed "minimal brain dysfunction" by Palmer), autism, and congenital anomalies. Presumably because of the greater breadth and extent of functioning areas affected, feeding problems reportedly are more common in people with severe developmental disabilities than in those with mild to moderate conditions. Perske and his colleagues estimated that 80% or more of individuals with severe developmental disabilities evidence some type of feeding disorder (Perske, Clifton, McLean, & Stein, 1977). Specific types of feeding delays and potential intervention approaches are described next.

ORAL-MOTOR DELAYS

This section discusses delays in oral-motor skills, which can be attributed to numerous factors, including anatomical developmental disorders, neuromuscular diseases, and physiological impairments. The section then discusses various interventions and treatments found to be effective with children with oral-motor delays.

Problems and Etiologies

Attainment of oral-motor competency is essential to successful feeding. Oral-motor competency includes the ability to take food into the mouth, to form a bolus (i.e., small parcel of food), to propel the bolus into the pharynx from mid-tongue area, and to complete the swallowing process by moving food from the pharynx into the esophagus (Eicher, 1997; Tuchman & Walter, 1994). In addition, biting and chewing are integral skills for intake of solid foods. Oral-motor dysfunction can hinder any of these crucial steps.

A variety of developmental disorders are commonly associated with oral-motor dysfunction. These include anatomical causes such as cleft lip and/or cleft palate, a disorder in which structural abnormalities interfere with oral suction and swallowing. Likewise, Robin sequence is associated with facial malformations in the jaw and tongue as well as with a U-shaped cleft, resulting in obstruction of the airway by the tongue (Shprintzen, 1992). Co-existing physical conditions (e.g., cardiac problems, respiratory distress, prematurity) or required treatment regimens (e.g., gastrostomy feedings, surgical procedures) may further complicate oral-motor functioning and feeding in children with developmental disabilities (e.g., Kerwin, Osborne, & Eicher, 1994). Additional discussion of feeding issues related to these health conditions may be found in Chapter 7.

Another group of developmental disorders associated with oral-motor dysfunction involves neuromuscular conditions (e.g., myelodysplasia, cerebral palsy, muscular dystrophy) or damage caused by traumatic brain injury. Neuromuscular damage may be manifested by problems such as an inefficient suck; persistence of primitive reflexes (e.g., rooting, suck–swallow); presence of atypical reflexes (e.g., tonic bite); reduced range of motion of the jaw, tongue, and lips (e.g., drooling); tongue thrust; swallowing disorder; gagging; or vomiting (Lewis, 1982; Reilly & Skuse, 1992; Ylvisaker & Logemann, 1985). Oral-motor complications also may present as one aspect of chromosomal anomalies, such as Down syndrome or Prader-Willi syndrome (PWS) (Pipes & Glass, 1993). Children with Down syndrome usually do not have severe feeding difficulties; however, hypotonia, open mouth posture, poor tongue control, and global developmental delay associated with Down syndrome reduce oral-motor effectiveness (Gisel, Lange, & Niman, 1984; Zausmer & Pueschel, 1978). Infants with PWS often display hypotonia and weak suck and may be diagnosed as having failure to thrive (FTT), whereas problems with obesity begin to predominate in children with PWS by preschool age. Overeating problems related to PWS and other conditions are discussed in Chapter 10.

Regardless of etiology, children with severe to profound mental retardation typically have neuromotor coordination impairments that interfere with the acquisition of oral-motor feeding skills (Eicher, 1997; Sisson & Van Hasselt, 1989). These impairments are related to the persistence of primitive oral reflexes that interfere with mature feeding patterns, impairments in neuromotor structures and integration, difficulties with imitative and receptive language abilities involved in learning, or other factors concomitant with developmental disabilities. Problems specific to oral-motor functioning are discussed in this section, whereas problems in acquiring and performing self-feeding or social/behavioral feeding skills are covered in later sections.

INTERVENTIONS FOR ORAL-MOTOR DELAYS

Interventions for children with significant oral feeding delays consist of a variety of therapeutic techniques focused on compensating for specific anatomical or physiological limitations, teaching functional skills, and facilitating more typical feeding responses. These techniques often are described as being "neurodevelopmental" in approach and are generally implemented by rehabilitative specialists (e.g., speech-language pathologists, occupational therapists, physical therapists). Lewis (1982), Morris and Klein (1987), Schuberth (1994), and Wolf and Glass (1992), among others, provided clinical descriptions of these therapeutic approaches; the interested reader is referred to these sources for a more detailed description. With the exception of Gisel and colleagues (e.g., Gisel, 1996; Gisel, Applegate-Ferrante, Benson, & Bosma, 1996), limited research has been published on the effectiveness of these oral-motor interventions; therefore, much of the following information is based on clinical sources. Interventions derived from behavioral frameworks are less frequently used for oral-motor problems, but some examples of behavioral interventions also are described (cf. Babbitt, Hoch, & Coe, 1994).

By way of introduction, Table 8.1 summarizes the basic features of the neurodevelopmental and behavioral intervention approaches for children with significant feeding delays, and it describes general characteristics of feeding intervention regardless of conceptual approach. Neurodevelopmental programs emphasize the following: 1) achieving whole-body stability and integration during feeding, 2) normalizing muscle tone and movement patterns, 3) designing adaptive equipment or specialized seating systems to support feeding, and 4) modifying the child's sensory environment (e.g., via touch, sound, motion) to enhance responding. Behavioral intervention programs employ the following techniques: 1) using antecedent stimuli (e.g., prompts) to set the occasion for specific feeding responses; 2) designing consistent positive consequences to strengthen desired feeding responses and, correspondingly, using negative consequences to weaken maladaptive responses; 3) providing step-by-step modification of intervention via shaping or fading procedures in response to a child's progress; and 4) using systematic desensitization procedures to reduce avoidance responses and to increase desired feeding. Regardless of the conceptual approach, feeding intervention programs strive to 1) begin at the child's current skill level and proceed toward greater independence, 2) communicate about intervention techniques with regular caregivers, and 3) monitor the child's medical and nutritional status throughout treatment. Further reference is made to these characteristics in the sections that follow.

The application of oral-motor intervention techniques is illustrated in the next section for three target problems, which overlap in some children: low oral-muscle tone, swallowing disorders, and oral-sensory disorders.

Low Oral-Muscle Tone

Muscle weakness in the oral region may be manifested by motor fatigue across the course of feeding, slow-paced eating, difficulty manipulating food in the mouth, drooling, inefficient lip closure, and tongue protrusion (Schuberth, 1994; Zausmer & Pueschel, 1978). Intervention for low oral-muscle tone usually begins by ensuring that the child is seated in a stable, well-supported position for feeding. Concern for positioning is consistent with Point 1 of the

Table 8.1. Features of feeding treatment programs for children with significant feeding delays

Basic features	Examples of application
Neurodevelopmental aspects	
1. Intervention emphasizes whole-body approach in which steps of the feeding program proceed from proximal to distal parts of the body.	Position child for stable head and trunk support.
2. Intervention focuses on normalizing muscle tone and movement patterns in major areas of oral-motor functioning.	Provide jaw support to assist chewing; practice tongue lateralization by placing a drop of food on side of tongue.
3. Intervention involves use of adaptive equipment and altered textures/bite sizes to support feeding.	Use specialized cups, plates, food stimuli, and seating systems as needed.
4. Sensory experiences are incorporated into intervention.	Apply gentle pressure to gums and teeth for oral stimulation.
Behavioral aspects	
1. Antecedent stimuli are arranged to set the occasion for specific feeding responses.	Provide prompts to assist child with moving spoon to mouth.
2. Positive consequences are delivered for desired feeding behavior, and negative consequences are delivered for undesired behavior.	Praise child for desired feeding, and briefly ignore or interrupt disruptive feeding behavior.
3. Shaping and fading procedures are used to facilitate child's progress.	Reduce extent of prompts systematically as child improves.
4. Systematic desensitization procedures are used to reduce avoidance and to increase desired behavior.	Pair pleasurable stimuli (e.g., music, massage) with meals or food offers.
General aspects	
1. Techniques begin at child's present skill level and progress to greater independence.	Begin training at a response that the child can perform consistently.
2. Communicate about intervention with child's regular caregivers.	Have parents watch therapy sessions.
3. The child's medical and nutritional state is monitored carefully throughout intervention.	Record caloric intake during intervention.

neurodevelopmental intervention features listed in Table 8.1, which stress working from proximal to distal regions of the body in planning intervention (Morris & Klein, 1987). For infants, stable positioning usually consists of an upright or partially upright posture with the head well supported at the body's mid-line. For older children, a high chair or other upright chair that provides adequate back, hip, and feet support is recommended. Some children with structural anomalies or motor impairments, however, benefit from adapted seating systems with specialized feeding positions (e.g., prone, with chin tucked, with side-support head rests) (Kosowski & Sopczyk, 1985; Morris & Klein, 1987).

A variety of techniques related to the second, third, and fourth points (i.e., muscle tone, adaptive equipment and altered textures, and sensory experiences) of the basic features of neurodevelopmental intervention listed in Table 8.1 are used to improve functioning of the oral musculature. The specific techniques vary according to the child's developmental level, the source of oral-motor problems, and potential areas of strength in oral-motor functioning. With infants, techniques to compensate for low muscle tone include selecting a nipple with an appropriate flow rate (e.g., faster or slower than a conventional nipple), stabilizing the infant's jaw and cheeks with the feeder's fingers to facilitate lip closure, and introducing a pacifier outside mealtimes to strengthen oral muscles (Morris & Klein, 1987; Zausmer & Pueschel, 1978). When solid foods are introduced, low muscle tone can result in inefficient or counterproductive tongue movements. Potential intervention techniques at this developmental point include help in positioning the spoon in the child's mouth, stabilizing the jaw to maintain the tongue in the mouth, changing the consistency of the food (i.e., to a smoother or coarser texture depending on the case) to facilitate transport in the mouth, and altering the size or shape of the spoon (Kosowski & Sopczyk, 1985; Zausmer & Pueschel, 1978).

Tongue Thrust Tongue protrusion, or a more exaggerated tongue thrust, occurs in some children with low oral-muscle tone. The typical reflex pattern of pushing the tongue forward when contacting food or swallowing usually subsides with maturation; however, a continued high amount of force, degree of protrusion, or amount of tooth surface area contacted by the tongue during swallowing can severely compromise food intake (Lewis, 1982). Intervention techniques usually consist of one or more of the techniques noted above or involve neurophysiological stimulation to the oral area, which is described later in this chapter in the section on oral-sensory disorders.

In addition to the neurodevelopmental techniques noted in the previous section, Thompson, Iwata, and Poynter (1979) demonstrated that behavioral procedures could be used to extinguish pathological tongue thrust. They conducted a case study with a 10-year-old boy with profound mental retardation and spastic cerebral palsy for whom oral-motor stimulation therapy had been unsuccessful. Thompson and colleagues (1979) systematically used two techniques to facilitate eating: First, food was presented only when the boy's tongue was inside his mouth; and, second, the tongue was gently but promptly pushed back into the mouth ("contingent pushback") with the spoon each time thrusting occurred. These techniques illustrate the use of specific antecedent conditions and consequences within behavioral feeding intervention, as noted in Points 1 and 2 in Table 8.1 under "Behavioral aspects." By alternately introducing and withdrawing intervention in a single-subject reversal design, the study demonstrated that intervention resulted in substantially decreased tongue thrusting as well as in less food expulsion and in more chewing. Some of the procedures used by Thompson and colleagues (1979) were similar to those recommended clinically by oral-motor specialists; however, Thompson and colleagues' report is distinguished by its systematic application of techniques contingent on child behavior, along with repeated observation of behavior changes and use of experimental control procedures, which provide a behavior analysis of the effectiveness of intervention.

Repeated use of oral-motor techniques is integral to their effectiveness. Thus, as listed in Point 2 of the "General aspects" of intervention in Table 8.1, caregivers are encouraged to implement the techniques as part of everyday feeding routines. Feeding specialists often view parents as the primary recipients of their recommendations, and thus they provide informal suggestions and model techniques as part of the therapy process. Most research in which parents have participated in oral-motor intervention concerns children referred because of ongoing food refusal and disruptive behavior in addition to oral-motor delays. In these cases (e.g., Ahearn, Kerwin, Eicher, Shantz, & Swearingin, 1996; Butterfield & Parson, 1973; Thompson & Palmer, 1974), parents were trained to implement behavior management techniques (e.g., differential social attention, modeling of appropriate eating, reinforcement using preferred foods) to increase cooperative feeding behavior. Intervention reportedly led to concomitant improvements in independent chewing and intake of solid foods, although oral-motor skills were not specifically evaluated in these studies.

Oral-motor intervention presumably facilitates feeding skills; however, children with severe developmental disabilities are at risk for medical and nutritional deterioration if intervention is not effective or if it proceeds too slowly. Thus, it is essential that Point 3 noted in the "General aspects" of intervention in Table 8.1 be honored (i.e., that the child's health and growth status be carefully monitored as intervention proceeds). Gisel and Patrick (1988) studied children with severe cerebral palsy and growth failure who were not adequately maintained by oral feeding regimens. Cerebral palsy places children at heightened risk of growth failure due to motor difficulties with food intake, and the problem may be exacerbated by increased energy requirements secondary to atypical movements or seizures. Gisel and colleagues (e.g., Gisel, 1994, 1996; Gisel et al., 1996) evaluated the effects of 10–20 weeks of sensorimotor therapy focused on strengthening the oral-motor skills of tongue lateralization, lip closure, and chewing in children with cerebral palsy. For children with moderate oral-motor impairments, intervention resulted in limited but measurable improvements in eating skills but not in drinking skills or growth rates. Children with more severe impairments or with aspiration problems did not show improvements in eating skills from therapy. Gisel et al. (1996) advocated monitoring both feeding skills and growth parameters in children with cerebral palsy to determine those who can and do benefit from sensorimotor therapy versus those who require supplemental nutrition. Their work also highlighted the fact that some children with feeding delays require alternative treatment (e.g., nutritional supplements, non-oral feeding regimens) to meet their basic health needs, even as oral-motor intervention proceeds (cf. Camp & Kalscheur, 1994).

Swallowing Disorders

Swallowing involves a coordinated sequence of motor actions to transport fluids and nutrients from the oral cavity to the stomach without allowing the entry of material into the airway. (See Chapter 2 for a more detailed review of the biological aspects of swallowing and for diagnostic procedures to detect swallowing dysfunction.) Disorders in swallowing are referred to as dysphagia, which is derived from the Greek words meaning "with difficulty" and "to eat" (Tuchman & Walter, 1994).

In the pediatric population, clinicians have used the term dysphagia both to describe physiological impairments in swallowing due to atypical functioning of the swallowing apparatus and to refer more broadly to any difficulties with swallowing (Eicher, 1997;

Tuchman & Walter, 1994; Wolf & Glass, 1992). It is useful, however, to distinguish physiologically based swallowing disorders (referred to in this chapter as dysphagia) from functional swallowing problems in which biological explanations for the current problems have been ruled out. Whereas dysphagia may result from disease, accident, physiological malformation, or neurological system disorders, functional swallowing problems are presumed to result from learning experiences. In particular, negative conditioning—involving repeated pairing of swallowing with aversive events such as pain, disgusting tastes, or other unpleasant experiences—has been implicated in functional swallowing refusal (DiScipio & Kaslon, 1982; Riordan, Iwata, Finney, Wohl, & Stanley, 1984).

Interventions for swallowing disorders range from the use of physical stimuli, altered methods of food presentation, positioning techniques, and/or behavior management techniques designed to initiate and strengthen swallowing patterns. Except for the last example, these interventions fit with the neurodevelopmental perspective outlined in Table 8.1.

Physical Stimulation Techniques   The use of physical stimuli is exemplified by thermal stimulation, which involves applying a cold substance to the back of the mouth, thereby triggering a swallowing reflex more quickly. Drawing on Logemann's (1986) use of this technique with adults, Wolf and Glass (1992) reported substantial improvement in infants' swallowing as a result of feeding refrigerator-chilled formula or food. They also suggested using a frozen pacifier to enhance speed of swallowing during nonnutritive sucking. Morris and Klein (1987) recommended applying cold stimulation through frozen water in a straw, through small amounts of sherbet on a cotton swab, and by other therapeutic techniques. Despite their potential usefulness in the hands of experienced clinicians, physical stimulation techniques for swallowing have not been rigorously evaluated with children. Physical stimulation techniques have the potential to be frightening, intrusive, and therefore aversive experiences for children; thus, they merit careful examination and cautious use.

Food Delivery and Alteration Techniques   The second approach to swallowing intervention involves changing the texture, amount, placement, or method of food offered to facilitate the organization of a bolus prior to the swallow (Morris & Klein, 1987; Schuberth, 1994). Thickened liquids, smaller amounts of food, or bites offered slowly in a controlled fashion often facilitate bolus organization. During the rehabilitation process following traumatic brain injury, individuals often proceed through a series of intake methods and food consistencies to accomplish a transition from tube to oral feeding (Ylvisaker & Logemann, 1985). Camp and Kalscheur (1994) offered several examples of common foods and preparation tips for increasing textures within oral-motor intervention. Intervention involves a gradual but steady progression along the texture continuum as the child displays oral-motor skills (e.g., sucking, vertical chewing, lateral chewing, and eventually rotary movements). Liquid intake may be easier with heavy substances (e.g., milkshakes) than with thin, clear substances (e.g., broth) (Camp & Kalscheur, 1994). In any case, the progression recommended is from easiest to most difficult levels as oral-motor skills improve.

Positioning Techniques A third technique entails positioning the child to increase the likelihood that the larynx will close sufficiently to protect the airway during and after swallowing. An upright sitting position usually is the most efficient because it takes advantage of gravity forces to assist peristalsis and muscle function of the esophagus. Flexing the head forward to tuck the chin or, in cases of unilateral paralysis, tilting the head sideways are potentially useful methods of reducing aspiration. An angled-neck bottle or adapted cup or straw can assist with maintaining neck flexion during drinking (Wolf & Glass, 1992; Ylvisaker & Logemann, 1985).

Behavior Management Techniques Behavior management, the fourth approach listed, has been implemented primarily for functional swallowing disorders. Behavioral interventions typically include shaping intake of progressively larger bites and/or more textured foods as well as positive reinforcement of food acceptances and swallowing (e.g., Johnson & Babbitt, 1993; Luiselli & Gleason, 1987). In addition, antecedent stimuli or negative reinforcement procedures have been investigated, as exemplified by the following studies.

Lamm and Greer (1988) demonstrated the effectiveness of shaping and reinforcement procedures in combination with a continuum of antecedent prompts for interventions for three infants with swallowing problems. The authors' clinical descriptions suggested that, at the time of intervention, the problems presented as conditioned refusal to swallow rather than as physiological impairment. All three children had severe developmental disabilities that had precluded swallowing prior to corrective surgery, none had a history of swallowing after surgery, and their young ages (10–13 months at the outset of intervention) limited the range of techniques available for use. The prompts, which were implemented as needed from least to most intrusive forms, ranged from verbal cues to partial physical assistance to a physical stimulus (touching the right posterior portion of the tongue) that elicited swallowing.

In another case study of functional swallowing problems, a sibling was enlisted to model eating and receiving of reinforcement for an 18-month-old child with swallowing refusal (Greer, Dorow, Williams, McCorkle, & Asnes, 1991). This child had a history of gastroesophageal reflux, which had been treated by surgical implantation of a gastrostomy tube. After swallowing impediments were corrected, however, the child refused to accept food orally. In preparation for intervention, the target child's 5-year-old sister initially practiced eating in a slow, deliberate manner, for which she received praise and token reinforcement after each bite. During intervention meals, the sibling modeled eating a bite and receiving reinforcement, alternating with food offers and contingent reinforcement directed to the target child. The intervention package was implemented at home by the child's mother and resulted in independent oral intake in approximately 1 week, which compares favorably with the lengthy intervention regimens (several weeks or months) often needed to establish oral feeding after extended tube use.

Negative reinforcement and escape extinction procedures also have been included within behavior management programs to facilitate swallowing. (These procedures are explained in more detail in Chapter 4). In a negative reinforcement paradigm, the swallowing response is strengthened by removing an aversive stimulus, which had been presented following food refusal or expulsion, contingent on swallowing. In swallowing interventions, the aversive stimulus usually consists of physical guidance (also called jaw prompting or forced feeding) to induce swallowing (Ahearn et al., 1996; Riordan et al., 1984). An alternative procedure entails re-presenting ejected food or holding food to the child's mouth until it is accepted (Ahearn et al., 1996; Hoch, Babbitt, Coe, Krell, & Hackbert, 1994). This technique in effect precludes the child's avoidance of the food, thereby giving rise to the term escape extinction. As described in Chapters 4 and 6, structured behavioral interventions that include negative reinforcement or escape extinction techniques in combination with positive reinforcement have been found effective in enhancing oral intake in children with functional swallowing disorders. Because of the intrusive aspects of negative reinforcement and escape extinction procedures, however, professional consultation is essential to ensure that the child is capable of swallowing and that the techniques are used correctly.

In discussing intervention considerations for swallowing disorders, the issue of involving caregivers in the intervention (listed in Table 8.1 as Point 2 of "General aspects") again bears special mention. There are many advantages to creating a therapeutic alliance with parents. As Ylvisaker and Weinstein (1989) noted in discussing pediatric rehabilitation following brain injury, parents can provide valuable insights into a child's personal likes and abilities, which can be used in tailoring intervention. The feeding period also is a good opportunity to familiarize parents with new communication modes for a child with a brain injury. A more instrumental level of parent involvement occurs when parents serve as primary intervention agents (e.g., Greer et al., 1991; Lamm & Greer, 1988). Involving parents in swallowing intervention, however, has potential difficulties, as parents are likely to experience distress and may use recommended procedures inconsistently when faced with their child's swallowing resistance (Blackman & Nelson, 1987; Linscheid, Oliver, Blyler, & Palmer, 1978). Thus, as discussed in Chapter 4, the manner and extent to which parents are included in intervention must be considered thoughtfully—particularly when a child presents with frustrating and potentially life-threatening feeding delays. In some cases, it may be helpful to consider a less intensive role for parents that still involves them actively as part of the intervention team. As an alternative, parent training may occur after the child begins to respond to therapeutic strategies (Ahearn et al., 1996).

Oral-Sensory Disorders

Another problem area often reported in children with oral-motor impairments concerns sensory reactions to oral stimulation. Morris and Klein (1987) described four types of sensory problems: hyperreaction, hyporeaction, sensory defensiveness, and sensory overload. Hyperreaction involves a stronger-than-typical response to a specific sensation, which is suggested by a tonic bite reflex when something touches the child's teeth or by an easily elicited gag reflex. Hyporeaction refers to a weaker-than-typical response to stimuli, such as failure to show anticipation at the sight or smell of food or failure to initiate oral movement when food is placed in the mouth. Sensory defensiveness, a particular type of hyperreactive response, involves a guarded and emotionally charged quality of responding to sensory stimulation, such as pulling back forcefully and crying when food touches the mouth, which suggests that sensory input is perceived as unpleasant or dangerous. Sensory overload refers to distractible and/or hyperreactive responses to stimuli, such as looking in the direction of irrelevant noises, which suggest confusion in response to sensory input.

Atypical sensory reactions are assumed to relate to sensory processing problems, which, in turn, presumably are caused by deviations in neurological functioning (Walter, 1994). One of the difficulties for clinicians, however, is interpreting the actual sensations experienced by the child based on the observed reactions. In addition to central nervous system dysfunction, some sensory difficulties may be a function of medications, emotional arousal, motor fatigue, previous oral-tactile experiences, or other factors (Wolf & Glass, 1992). From a behavioral perspective, the responses involved in "sensory defensiveness" suggest a learning history in which eating has been associated with negative experiences. "Hyporeaction," likewise, may indicate the presence of weak motivational variables associated with absence of learning experiences or perhaps positive avoidance of food-related stimuli. A behavioral conceptualization may suggest interventions that differ from those that follow from a sensory integration perspective, as discussed in more detail in the following section. Given the uncertainty in judging sensations and neurological or other causes for sensory problems, intervention often involves a trial-and-error process of discovering what works for an individual child.

Interventions to reduce overreaction to oral-sensory input, which have been labeled variously as "neurophysiological facilitation," "oral-motor stimulation therapy," or "sensory integration," usually entail some common features (Morris & Klein, 1987; Sobsey & Orelove, 1984; Wolf & Glass, 1992). Intervention techniques include the following: 1) reducing unpleasant oral-tactile experiences (e.g., routine procedures involved in placing or changing feeding apparatus) as much as possible; 2) applying gentle pressure or massage to the child's gums and teeth during oral stimulation exercises, providing only as much oral contact as the child accepts; 3) providing slow vestibular stimulation during or before mealtimes using activities such as rocking, swinging, and rolling; 4) presenting food and drink opportunities in a rhythmic pattern to coincide with child's pace of intake or using anticipatory cues (e.g., touching the mouth, verbal prompts) with food offers; 5) using music or other calming stimuli to make mealtimes more pleasant and relaxing; and 6) using guided imagery (e.g., focusing on positive visual images or sensations), relaxation, or meditation activities to enhance concentration and to reduce distraction during meals. For children with underreactivity to oral stimulation, recommendations center around observing the levels and types of stimulation the child currently discriminates. Using present response patterns as a starting point, food presentation can be tailored to build on the child's skills.

Whereas all of the aforementioned strategies fit within Point 4 of "Neurodevelopmental aspects" of intervention options listed in

Table 8.1, it is worth noting that several of these neurophysiological or sensory integration interventions are similar to those that might be derived from a behavioral perspective. For example, oral desensitization is akin to the behavioral technique of systematic desensitization (as described in Chapter 4), and guided imagery frequently is an element of relaxation training provided in behavior therapy interventions for a wide variety of psychophysiological disorders (Dolgin & Jay, 1989).

Although oral-motor stimulation is widely used by occupational, physical, and speech-language therapists for children with oral-sensory problems, little research has been conducted with this approach. Sobsey and Orelove (1984) provided one of the few research demonstrations in which they implemented a neurophysiological facilitation package with four children (ages 3–12 years) with severe to profound mental retardation and other developmental disabilities. Intervention was conducted by teachers as part of daily classroom activities, and data from lunch observations showed systematic improvements in most oral skills (e.g., increased lip closure and rotary chewing, reduced spilling) following training.

Aspects of oral stimulation therapy also have been integrated into behavioral intervention for children with oral sensitivity and food selectivity problems. For example, Luiselli and Gleason (1987) developed a program for improving oral consumption in children with multiple disabilities involving the following components: 1) feeding demands (e.g., forced feeding) were eliminated from meals so as not to provoke resistance or agitation; 2) pleasurable stimulation (e.g., rocking) was made available on a noncontingent basis for a pretraining period and then on a contingent basis for cooperation during meals; and 3) requirements for oral consumption were introduced gradually using shaping procedures. The elimination of feeding demands in this behavior program corresponds to the reduction of unpleasant oral-tactile experiences, which is a common feature of sensory integration programs, and rocking exemplifies the provision of slow vestibular stimulation, which is another common feature of sensory integration programs. Using a single-subject design, Luiselli and Gleason (1987) demonstrated the effectiveness of the intervention package with one child, and Luiselli (1993) replicated this finding with two other children; however, the independent role of oral-sensitivity or sensory integration aspects of the program was not examined.

Oral-sensitivity problems are recognized as one of the biggest challenges for feeding therapists (Wolf & Glass, 1992), and further research in this area is definitely needed. In particular, many techniques have been described within this intervention approach, yet the relative effectiveness of different components is not known.

The preceding discussion provides a review of oral-motor feeding problems and of environmental intervention strategies. The case illustration that follows describes the coordination of behavioral intervention with concurrent therapies for a child with a well-defined oral-motor disability. Chapter 7 provides further discussion of the impact of medical aspects of treatment (i.e., gastronomy tube, surgery) on feeding issues.

■ ■ ■

CASE 8.1. A CHILD WITH PIERRE ROBIN SEQUENCE
NAME: Krista
AGE AT INTERVENTION: 5 years, 5 months

BACKGROUND

Krista is a child with Pierre Robin sequence, a congenital condition characterized by an abnormally small jaw. Krista had her nutritional needs met largely by a gastronomy tube that was placed when she was 4 months of age; a tracheostomy was performed at about the same time. Krista had undergone mandibular reconstruction at 4 years, 6 months. Her jaw had been wired closed for 2 months following surgery, and she had been referred for oral-motor intervention for reduced jaw movement. Although oral-motor intervention had improved jaw mobility and her ability to chew, lateralize, and otherwise process solid foods, her intake of both solids and liquids remained poor.

Observations of eating showed a child who dawdled and who used many social diversionary tactics during mealtimes. She verbally rejected food, played with food, offered food to others, and frowned during consumption of food. She required frequent prompting to swallow the food in her mouth, and there was a question of whether this pattern represented oral hyposensitivity or a stalling tactic. A modified barium swallow showed her swallow to be within normal limits. She has age-appropriate self-feeding skills, but her parents often resorted to feeding her to speed up the meal, which typically lasted for more than an hour. Parent interaction during the meal was characterized by coaxing, noncontingent talk, and modeling of food intake. Her parents acknowledged that heated disputes about meal management were common at home.

A nutritional assessment indicated that about 75% of Krista's caloric needs were met by gastronomy tube feeds and that oral intake was highly variable, ranging between 200 and 400 kilocalories per day. Her weight for age was at the 50th percentile, and her height was at the 75th percentile. There was a question of lactose intolerance, which narrowed her nutritional therapy options. Krista ate mainly sweet, soft-textured foods. Rice was a major component of the family diet, but the texture of this food was especially challenging. Krista was the oldest of three children of professionally successful parents, both immigrants from Taiwan. Her mother had recently become unemployed and was—with visiting nurses—the primary feeder during the day. Feeding and limit setting were roles that appeared to be difficult for the mother.

FORMULATION

Multiple factors appeared to influence Krista's feeding difficulties: limited experience with eating for the first 5 years of life, residual oral-motor difficulties, possible alterations in the experience of food intake resulting from tracheostomy, continued reliance on alternative sources of nutrition with resulting dissociation of appetite reduction and eating, constraint on dietary therapy due to possible lactose intolerance, cultural dietary factors, and maladaptive feeding practices.

INTERVENTION

The following mealtime guidelines were developed in a series of biweekly family sessions with a behavioral psychologist and a nutritionist. Sessions initially included both parents and were subsequently attended by the mother and by a visiting nurse. The major components of the plan were as follows: 1) systemic exposure to novel foods, 2) a consistent meal schedule, including time-limited meals, 3) differential consequences for eating, and 4) gradual reduction of gastronomy feeds. The plan that follows included general mealtime guidelines and also incorporates specific changes that were introduced during the course of intervention. Krista continued to attend oral-motor therapy sessions during this time, and there was frequent communication between the speech-language pathologist and the behavioral psychologist throughout the case.

1. Meal pattern
   - Provide three meals and one or two snacks each day.
   - Schedule meals and snacks at a regular time.
   - Allow 35 minutes for lunch and dinner, 30 minutes for breakfast, and 15 minutes for snacks.
2. Types of food
   - Provide a regular diet, with an emphasis on soft-textured, high-calorie foods.

- Continue exposure to a broad range of textures.
- Offer prune juice (previously provided by gastronomy) to be taken orally, as needed.
- Reduce amount of rice in her current diet (because rice is especially difficult for Krista to process orally), or mash rice with a fork before offering it to her.
- Offer one can of Pediasure after dinner.
- For gastronomy feeds, offer one feed of 240 milliliters of Pediasure at midnight.

3. Meal setting
   - Eat meals as a family.
   - Make one parent (or nurse) responsible for feeding during each meal. Other adults at the table should ignore her attempts to interact with them when this interferes with a steady rate of intake.

4. Utensils
   - Use regular utensils.
   - Provide liquids in a regular cup, with or without a straw.

5. Mealtime behavior
   a. Always praise *acceptance* of food.
   b. Have Krista fill in her food chart after she has finished a designated portion of food. Use the food chart symbols as tokens, which can be exchanged for activity rewards (e.g., watching a favorite videotape, taking a bike ride, gaining extra storytelling time, taking a trip to a favorite place), or use quarters as rewards for successful meals.
      - Let Krista choose the reward she may earn before the beginning of the meal from a "menu" of rewards.
      - It is very important that rewards not be available, except when Krista earns them.
   c. If Krista does not have a successful meal, do not permit her to immediately become involved in an activity that is interesting or amusing to her. Try having her sit in an "uninteresting" part of the house (e.g., no toys, no one to talk with) for 30 minutes.
   d. Define a successful meal as follows:
      - Breakfast: 40 pieces of rice cereal in 30 minutes.
      - Lunch and dinner: 2 ounces of each soft food (e.g., Spaghettios, apple sauce) within 35 minutes. Meal durations will be decreased gradually, and the amount of intake required for reward will be increased.
   e. When appropriate, allow Krista to select the menu *before* the meal, but do not permit her to change the menu *after* the meal

has started. Do not leave the table to prepare other foods for her after the meal has started.

   f. If Krista throws food or utensils, then ignore her.
   g. If Krista plays with food, then ignore this unless it occurs for longer than 15–30 seconds; then direct her attention back to taking food into her mouth.

6. Other

   • Feeds will be decreased gradually, beginning with discontinuation of one of the night feeds. After all gastronomy feeds have been discontinued, the program will reduce reliance on high-calorie liquids during the day.
   • Weight and intake will be monitored to ensure that Krista is substituting oral intake for the discontinued gastronomy feeds.

OUTCOME

Over a period of 6 months, Krista was weaned from dependence on tube feeds, and her weight remained stable. She also increased the variety of foods that she accepted and was expressing more spontaneous interest in eating. These outcomes were not achieved easily, as the family had difficulty implementing mealtime guidelines consistently, even though they understood them well. Biweekly sessions were often devoted to reviewing the rationale for each component of the intervention program, providing reassurance that Krista could indeed sustain herself on oral feeding although she had residual oral-motor problems, and trouble-shooting issues common to behavioral interventions (e.g., reinforcer satiety).

■ ■ ■

SELF-FEEDING IMPAIRMENTS

Self-feeding refers to a child's voluntary actions to independently transport food or liquid to the mouth using a feeding utensil (e.g., spoon, fork, cup) or fingers (Luiselli, 1989). The following section describes problems that can arise in acquisition or maintenance of independent feeding skills and introduces interventions to enhance self-feeding skills.

Problems and Etiologies

Self-feeding entails a sequence of motor skills, as exemplified in spoon-feeding—grasping the spoon, scooping up food, directing the spoon to the mouth, inserting it in the mouth, then removing it, and returning it to the bowl. A typically developing child acquires basic skills for "messy" self-feeding by 12–15 months of age and masters more refined eating skills by 24 months of age (Christophersen & Hall, 1978). Advanced feeding skills sometimes are included in the definition of self-feeding as well. For example, keeping one's mouth closed when chewing, using a napkin, and cutting food with a knife have been targeted in some self-feeding programs (Sisson & Dixon, 1986a, 1986b).

Self-feeding skills often are delayed in children with neuromuscular conditions (e.g., cerebral palsy, spina bifida, traumatic brain injury), global developmental disorders (e.g., mental retardation, autism), and/or sensory impairments (e.g., visual, auditory). As with oral-motor skills, self-feeding may be affected by impairments in neuromotor functions and integration, muscular weakness, or difficulties with imitative and receptive language abilities involved in learning motor skills (Stevenson, 1995). Children with multiple sensory impairments are likely to have particular difficulties with acquiring independent skills because they have restricted sensory modalities (Sisson, Van Hasselt, & Hersen, 1987).

Children who do not feed themselves must be fed by others, which places heavy demands on caregivers (Luiselli, 1989). Johnson and Deitz (1985) found that parents of children who have physical developmental disabilities spend an average of 3.5 hours per day in feeding activities, compared with less than 1 hour (0.8) per day for children without disabilities. Because of the extensive caregiver time involved, children who lack self-feeding skills may be restricted to intervention programs equipped to provide one-to-one supervision. In addition, children without self-feeding skills often miss out on opportunities for motor and socialization activities involved in mealtimes. Given these factors, self-feeding can be viewed as an important "entry skill" for many other learning activities.

Self-feeding delays may be accompanied by social and behavioral difficulties, such as disruptive eating habits, atypical eating rates, or stereotypic movements during mealtimes. As a result, intervention frequently focuses on reducing inappropriate mealtime behaviors and improving mealtime "etiquette" along with establishing self-feeding (e.g., Leibowitz & Holcer, 1974; Luiselli, 1988a, 1988b; Stimbert, Minor, & McCoy, 1977). Programs directed mainly at these qualitative aspects of feeding are discussed later in the section on social and behavior delays.

INTERVENTIONS FOR INCREASING SELF-FEEDING SKILLS

Self-feeding interventions embody several features introduced earlier in this chapter, which correspond to the basic neurodevelopmental, behavioral, and general characteristics of interventions for building oral-motor skills (see Table 8.1).

Neurodevelopmental Aspects

Self-feeding requires coordination of musculature in the head, upper torso, arms, and hands in order to bring food to the mouth without excessive spilling. Thus, it is important to establish a stable, well-supported seating position that leaves the hands free to manipulate food utensils. Specialized seating systems or feeding positions (e.g., a standing table, extra cushions, a wheelchair tray to provide elbow support) may be useful for children with inadequate sitting balance or uncontrolled motor movements (Morris & Klein, 1987).

The central objective of a self-feeding program is to develop sufficient fine motor control and coordination to transport food to the mouth independently. Techniques for accomplishing this objective include altering the properties of food or method by which food is presented. With regard to the form of presentation, food can be puréed, thickened, or cut in appropriately sized pieces to make it easier for the child to handle. With regard to the method of presentation, adaptive feeding utensils can simplify grasping utensils and balancing food in transit. For example, spoons are available that have deeper bowls, utensils are made with wider or longer handles, and plates are constructed with an extended outer ridge to accommodate self-feeding (Kosowski & Sopczyk, 1985; Morris & Klein, 1987).

Behavioral Aspects

Behavior management techniques are a mainstay of self-feeding programs, and numerous studies document the effectiveness of behavioral approaches (see reviews by Luiselli, 1989; Sisson & Van Hasselt, 1989). Most programs entail a combination of verbal instructions, modeling, shaping, fading, physical guidance, and/or positive reinforcement procedures (as described in more detail in Chapter 4). One study comparing modeling and physical guidance procedures for training children with severe mental retardation to use feeding utensils confirmed the superiority of physical guidance (Nelson, Cone, & Hanson, 1975). Physical prompts and reinforcement are virtually always included in behavioral self-feeding programs. Physical guidance is needed to establish the chain of motor responses (e.g., grasping food, bringing it to mouth) involved in the self-feeding sequence, and reinforcement (in the form of social praise, preferred food, tokens, or sensory stimulation) is used to strengthen self-feeding steps as they are acquired.

Several variations on physical prompting procedures have been used in self-feeding programs, including backward chaining

(Berkowitz, Sherry, & Davis, 1971; MacArthur, Ballard, & Artinian, 1986) and graduated guidance (e.g., Stimbert et al., 1977). In backward chaining, independent responding is established first for the final step of the feeding sequence (e.g., placing the fork back on the plate after the child takes a bite). The child initially is guided through the entire feeding sequence; as independent skill is acquired for the last step, physical guidance is faded for this step, and training then begins for the next-to-last step in the sequence, and so forth, in reverse order. Graduated guidance involves progressively decreasing the extent of manual support (e.g., full to partial guidance to touch only) and the distance from the child's hand (e.g., directly touching the child's hand, then the wrist, forearm, elbow, upper arm, and shoulder) until the child is performing the self-feeding sequence independently (Sisson & Van Hasselt, 1989). Although little research has examined the relative effectiveness of different physical prompting procedures, each employs a systematic, step-wise approach to skill development based on the child's performance.

Luiselli's (1993) single-subject analysis of teaching a child basic self-feeding skills illustrated several relevant aspects of a behavioral approach. (A second case in the same report, which dealt with refinement of existing feeding skills, is discussed in the section entitled "Interventions for Social and Behavioral Delays.") A 7-year-old girl, who had severe mental retardation and was legally deaf and blind was trained in self-feeding by her classroom teacher. Because of her motor limitations, the girl ate a puréed diet and used an adapted plate with an extended outer ridge throughout the study. Previous activities in the classroom showed that the girl enjoyed receiving sensory stimulation in the form of 3–5 seconds of illumination from a flashlight directed at her face, so brief activation of the flashlight was used as a reinforcing stimulus in this study.

Baseline observations of the girl determined that she was capable of completing the final two steps of the self-feeding sequence (removing the spoon from her mouth and returning it to the plate) independently, which suggested the appropriateness of a backward chaining procedure. Training consisted of physical prompting, prompt fading, and contingent reinforcement within a backward chaining format. Training focused first on inserting the spoon into her mouth, the step prior to the two that she could complete independently. After 12 training sessions, she performed this step consistently and also showed generalized acquisition of the prior step in the feeding sequence (transporting the spoon from the plate to her mouth). The next stage of training was directed at scooping food from the plate, which resulted in independent performance of this step as well as generalized acquisition of the initial step in the chain: grasping the spoon. Follow-up probes at 1, 6, and 8 months of age indicated maintenance of self-feeding in the girl's school dining room.

Luiselli's (1993) study is notable for several positive features: the clear yet simple system of documenting self-feeding steps, demonstration of successful training effects and generalization in a controlled experimental design, documentation of maintenance in the typical dining room setting, application to a child with severe and multiple developmental disabilities, and use of a regular caregiver as teacher. Her parents reported that, on acquiring the skill at school, the girl readily began eating independently at home as well. In contrast to lengthy and complicated training protocols sometimes used in experimental programs, the current program involved only 2 hours of teacher training. Together with the positive results of other studies (e.g., Luiselli, 1989; Sisson & Van Hasselt, 1989), Luiselli's (1993) study suggested that behavior management is a viable method for teaching basic self-feeding skills to people with severe developmental disabilities.

General Aspects

Regardless of the intervention approach, self-feeding programs should include some basic characteristics to increase the likelihood of success.

Preliminary Behavioral Assessment As noted in Point 1 of Table 8.1's "General aspects" of feeding intervention programs, teaching self-feeding involves starting intervention at the child's current functioning level. Given the complexity of cognitive and motor problems in children with developmental disabilities who do not feed themselves, it often is difficult to tell whether a child has the prerequisite skills to proceed with self-feeding (Linscheid, 1988). Morris and Klein (1987) suggested the following indications that a child may be ready to take more responsibility in feeding: 1) shows anticipation of the next bite; 2) shows an eagerness to participate in the mealtime process; 3) displays food preferences; 4) enjoys playing with food; and 5) reaches toward food, spoon, or cup and attempts to bring it to the mouth. These are indications, however, of motivation to eat rather than evidence that the child actually has the prerequisite skills. Thus, behavioral assessment is a necessary part of intervention planning for self-feeding. Assessment should focus on the child's self-feeding repertoire and preliminary skills (e.g., ability to grasp a spoon, pick up food with fingers, and show minimal control of motor movements involved in hand–mouth transport) (Luiselli, 1989), and it may include systematic evaluation of responding to different foods and textures (Munk & Repp, 1994; Reilly, Skuse, Mathisen, & Wolke, 1995). Issues and strategies for behavioral assessment are discussed further in Chapter 3.

Communication and Monitoring MacArthur et al. (1986) reported on a self-feeding case that illustrates the relevance of the other two general features of self-feeding interventions listed in Table 8.1: 1) communicating procedures with home caregivers and 2) monitoring the child's nutritional and health status. The child in MacArthur et al.'s study was a $3^{1}/_{2}$-year-old boy with autistic behaviors and severe developmental delays who showed a lack of expressive language, intermittent responsivity to simple verbal requests, and limited engagement with the physical and social environment. The boy reportedly had some skills required for self-feeding but displayed them inconsistently. In fact, prior to the study, a 5-month pattern of feeding resistance at home and at school had resulted in medical concerns regarding the boy's dehydration and weight loss. Intervention was initiated first at school, with his teacher serving as feeding therapist. The behavior management program consisted of backward chaining with prompts, gradual fading of prompts, verbal praise for appropriate eating, brief time-out for screaming and other disruptive behaviors, and gentle massage of the boy's elbow when he resisted prompts by stiffening his arm. Intervention resulted in increased independent eating and decreased disruptive behavior at school, although some inconsistency was seen, especially after interruptions because of illness or vacations. No improvements, however, occurred in the boy's eating patterns at home, despite the fact that his mother had observed intervention at school and that the intervention program had been discussed with her. The boy's mother eventually requested training in behavior management procedures, and she began implementing them at home, which resulted in improved eating at home.

MacArthur and colleagues' (1986) study underscored the need for systematic parent training in some cases, as opposed to reliance on informal observation and discussion of treatment, in order to produce generalized change in a child's feeding patterns. It also illustrates the need for medical monitoring during feeding treatment. Illness and concomitant deteriorations in feeding behavior recurred as problems for brief periods throughout the study, but they reportedly were less serious than prior to behavioral intervention. Despite the difficulties encountered, this research also demonstrated the effectiveness of behavior management procedures for accomplishing self-feeding in a child with severe developmental disabilities.

The case illustration that follows offers another example of systematic parent training directed at strengthening self-feeding skills in a child with developmental delays. This case concerns a child who could feed himself but who had been discouraged by his parents from doing so because of his highly selective eating habits. The period after intervention focused on broadening the child's diet and parent training shifted to increasing the child's independent feeding skills. This case also provides an example of an empirical evaluation of feeding intervention, involving repeated home-based observations of mealtimes.

■   ■   ■

CASE 8.2. SELF-FEEDING IMPAIRMENTS AND TEXTURE SELECTIVITY
NAME: Frank
AGE AT INTERVENTION: 4 years

BACKGROUND

Frank is one of three children who participated, with their mothers, in an applied research evaluation of a home-based model of feeding intervention (Werle, Murphy, & Budd, 1993). Frank was referred to the program by an outpatient psychology clinic because of ongoing problems with texture selectivity and delayed feeding skills. Prior to Frank's referral for the study, the referring psychologist had begun a parent training program directed at addressing general behavior management problems, but the training had stalled when the parents reported continuing difficulties implementing suggested procedures (particularly time-out) at home. Because feeding problems presented as a significant concern, Frank and his parents were referred to the home-based intervention program.

Frank's birth had entailed a premature forceps delivery after 36 hours of labor. He was jaundiced at birth and remained in intensive care for 5 days. Frank's mother remembered him as being a "difficult baby." He developed formula intolerance during infancy and did not show progression in eating beyond foods of puréed texture. Medical explanations for Frank's feeding problems had been ruled out. Psychological testing indicated overall developmental delays in all areas. Frank was ambulatory, showed expressive and receptive language skills at approximately the 2-year age level, could follow simple directions, and was capable of independent self-feeding (using fingers, spoon, and cup).

Prior to intervention, Frank's mother described him as very active, fussy, and noncompliant. She reported that, when presented with foods that were not mixed in a blender or were not strained, Frank would often refuse, cry, and attempt to leave his seat or run from the table. Frank vomited or gagged on occasion during meals; however, interdisciplinary assessment revealed no oral-motor impairments that might account for the pattern. Because of Frank's feeding difficulties, his mother fed him separately from the parents and Frank's 2-year-old sister. Although Frank was capable of feeding himself, his mother spoon-fed him most items and entertained Frank with books or toys during meals. She reported having given up offering him solid foods and instead fed Frank smooth textures (e.g., pudding) or those with only small lumps (e.g., mashed bananas). Preschool teachers reported that, because of Frank's food refusal at school, they had discontinued serving him lunch. Instead, Frank's mother fed him a snack immediately after school. Frank's diet contained several high-calorie items, such as milkshakes, and his growth and nutrition were considered adequate.

FORMULATION

Frank's feeding problems were assumed to have originated from multiple factors. His birth difficulties and stressful neonatal period suggested the possibility of neurological damage, which—together with overall developmental impairments—complicated the acquisition of typical feeding skills. Parental reactions to these difficulties appear to have inadvertently maintained maladaptive feeding patterns. Although Frank ate a sufficient amount of food and showed relatively little resistance, the specialized circumstances of Frank's eating were developmentally inappropriate, and his selective habits had eliminated him from school meals and family meals. Behavioral intervention was designed to help Frank accomplish two changes: 1) increase the proportion of coarse textures in Frank's diet, and 2) increase the extent to which Frank used independent feeding skills.

INTERVENTION

Systematic parent training was provided to Frank's mother to teach her behavior management skills for use during mealtimes. The initial nine sessions focused on texture training; the following six sessions focused on self-feeding skills. Training took place in Frank's home, and videotapes of home mealtimes were used to monitor progress. Parent training methods included instruction, discussion, handouts, role plays, behavior rehearsal during mealtimes, verbal feedback after meals, and periodic videotape review. The key ingredients of training were as follows:

Texture Training

1. Provide educational information on child nutrition (e.g., expected types and amounts of different food groups).
2. Provide suggestions on how to introduce more textured foods in small quantities (e.g., placing small bits of fruit or vegetable in junior foods to produce "chunky" items, offering cubed soft fruits or cheeses that were "chewy" items).
3. Provide clear, specific prompts (e.g., "Take a bite") when offering a bite of more coarsely textured food.
4. Use verbal and physical praise and other rewards (e.g., preferred foods, interactive games) for cooperation with eating.
5. Ignore disruptive behaviors such as crying or refusing and then re-offering food.
6. Follow food expulsions or attempts to leave the table with a mild corrective procedure (e.g., saying "no" in a firm voice and physically blocking the child's attempts to leave the meal area).
7. Use brief time-out (in which the mother left the table or rotated the child's chair away from the table for 30–60 seconds) as a means of interrupting continued disruptive behavior.

Self-Eating Training

1. Suggest how to arrange the environment for self-eating opportunities (e.g., giving Frank a plate or a bowl containing food that he could feed himself, placing a fork and/or a spoon at the table for Frank's use).
2. Provide clear, specific prompts for self-eating (e.g., "Try a bite of peaches") before offering physical assistance.
3. Use verbal and physical praise and other rewards for self-initiated feeding (e.g., "You did that all by yourself—great!").
4. Continue the feeding procedures used in texture training.

Outcome

Parent training was successful in accomplishing feeding objectives for Frank and in improving his mother's behavior management skills. Frank's progress in food intake in videotaped mealtime observations is shown in Figure 8.1. Three phases of the study are denoted: Baseline (BL); Texture Training (TR1); and Self-Eating Training (TR2). The top graph displays Frank's intake of textures that he generally accepted before intervention, namely "smooth" (e.g., pudding, puréed

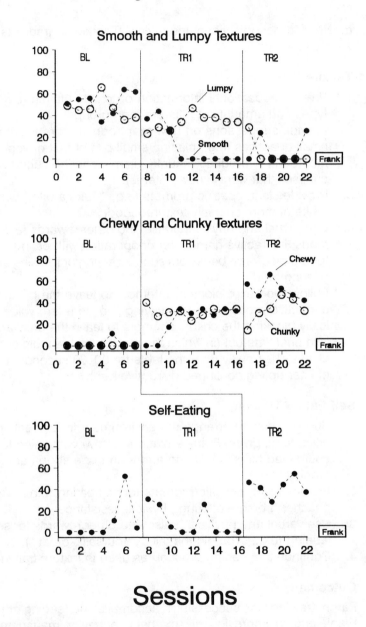

Figure 8.1. Percentage of Frank's intake of four texture categories (smooth, lumpy, chewy, chunky) and self-eating of total bites accepted across sessions. The top graph displays the proportion of smooth and lumpy textures, the middle graph displays the proportion of chewy and chunky textures, and the bottom graph shows the percentage of self-eating of total bites eaten. (BL = Baseline, TR1 = Training on food variety or texture, TR2 = Training on self-eating.) (From Werle, M.A., Murphy, T.B., & Budd, K.S. [1993]. Treating chronic food refusal in young children: Home-based parent training. *Journal of Applied Behavior Analysis, 26,* 430; reprinted by permission.)

foods) or "lumpy" (e.g., cottage cheese, mashed fruits). The middle graph displays Frank's intake of coarser textures ("chunky" and "chewy"), which increased when training was provided during TR1 and continued to increase further during TR2. The bottom graph shows Frank's self-eating, which occurred infrequently in BL and TR1 and then increased systematically when intervention was initiated for self-eating skills in TR2.

Although intervention accomplished some important changes, the process was interrupted when Frank's mother was hospitalized for an extended period for surgery. Had intervention continued, training would have been directed toward further strengthening Frank's independent feeding, fading special toys and activities out of mealtimes, and integrating Frank into family and school meals.

■ ■ ■

SOCIAL AND BEHAVIORAL DELAYS

A host of feeding patterns commonly seen in people with developmental disabilities are identified as problematic primarily because they violate social norms of mealtime etiquette (Ginsberg, 1988; Luiselli, 1989). The next section describes social and behavioral delays in feeding, reasons for these problems, and common intervention techniques.

Problems and Etiologies

Social and behavioral delays that have an impact on feeding include disruptive behaviors, stereotypic response patterns, and inappropriate eating rates. Examples are excessive sloppiness in handling food; eating with one's fingers without regard to food type; putting one's mouth directly on the plate or eating spilled food; stealing food from others' plates; having overly active or distractible eating patterns; crying or talking excessively during mealtimes; rocking, hand-flapping, or eye poking in a repetitive manner; and eating at an overly fast or slow pace.

Some of the etiquette-violating behaviors directly involve properties of food, which may set the occasion for the problems, whereas others (e.g., crying, self-stimulatory behaviors) may be as likely to occur during other child activities; thus, the latter group are less appropriately referred to as feeding problems per se, although they may require intervention during meals. In addition to the above examples of problematic behaviors, pica, rumination, and extreme selectivity of food types and textures also may be attributed to delays in social and behavioral feeding skills. Because pica, rumination, and extreme selectivity of food are covered in other chapters (5 and 9), only food selectivity is touched on briefly in this section to illustrate its overlap with disruptive feeding behaviors.

Qualitative aspects of feeding included within the rubric of mealtime etiquette usually relate to the social acceptability of mealtimes rather than to their nutritional adequacy. When displayed by individuals older than toddler age, aberrant social and behavior habits are considered inappropriate because they are unpleasant for other meal participants and because they may be dangerous to the child. Considering that mealtimes are a key social activity in most cultures, children who lack basic social skills related to feeding are likely to be excluded from family and group mealtimes, thus further limiting their opportunities for socialization and learning.

There are several possible reasons for delayed social and behavior skills around feeding. Significant cognitive, emotional, and sensory impairments associated with many developmental disabilities reduce children's capacity to learn developmentally appropriate social skills. Some disabilities (e.g., autism, fragile X syndrome) are associated with particular impairments in social and behavior patterns, and other disabilities are associated with impulsive or aggressive tendencies (Gourash, 1986). Sensory impairments such as blindness or deafness limit learning opportunities in the affected modalities (Sisson et al., 1987). In typically developing children, vicarious learning (i.e., learning via informal observation of others' behavior and its antecedents and consequences) is a major mechanism for transmission of social norms. Children with developmental disabilities, however, often fail to benefit from observational experiences, particularly without direct training and practice (Bandura, 1969).

Another factor contributing to social and behavioral delays is the learning impact of experience during mealtimes (Iwata, Riordan, Wohl, & Finney, 1982; Linscheid, 1992). Feeders may provide attention for a child's inappropriate behavior (e.g., exclaiming, "Don't you throw that!" when the child threatens to toss his plate on the floor), or they may lower their expectations for appropriate behavior (e.g., allowing a child with poor motor coordination to eat with her hands), thereby inadvertently strengthening socially inappropriate behavior patterns. Behavior mismanagement often has been implicated as a factor in the delays observed in children's social and behavioral feeding skills (see Chapter 4). Misplaced social contingencies are presumed to operate in combination with other etiological factors such as developmental impairments, biological conditions, or aversive conditioning (as described in Chapter 1 and exemplified in the Case 8.3).

In addition to developmental and learning explanations for social and behavioral delays in feeding, biological effects of medication, brain injury, or other organic conditions may alter a child's responsiveness to basic regulatory functions such as appetite. In these cases, a child's disruptive behaviors may be motivated by the desire to avoid or, conversely, to obtain food. Also, although motor impairments play a more obvious role in oral-motor and self-feeding delays than in social and behavioral delays, decreased muscle control contributes to some inappropriate feeding behaviors. For example, motor coordination problems increase the likelihood of food spillage (Cipani, 1981) and complicate the use of feeding utensils, so it is logical that children would opt to eat with their hands.

The likelihood that children with developmental disabilities will display general social and behavior problems is considerably higher than for typically developing children. For example, Schroeder, Mulick, and Schroeder's (1979) review of epidemiological studies found prevalence rates for behavior disturbances (e.g., physical aggression, temper tantrums, self-injury, stereotypic responses, noncompliance) of 20%–40% for people with mental retardation compared with around 5% for the general population. These behaviors are understandably distressing to caregivers, and they exact a heavy toll on family functioning (Budd, 1988). Given that mealtimes account for a sizable portion of daily activity, it is important to foster social and behavior skills related to feeding.

INTERVENTIONS FOR SOCIAL AND BEHAVIORAL DELAYS

Ginsberg (1988) pointed out that, although many feeding-related problems in people with developmental disabilities are attributable to nonpsychosocial factors, a majority of interventions entail application of behavior management procedures. This is especially true with respect to interventions addressing social and behavioral feeding delays in children. The features of a neurodevelopmental approach cited previously in Table 8.1 have limited relevance to intervention for social and behavior problems except to establish that the prerequisite skills exist for target responses. Instead, a central objective of intervention for social and behavioral feeding problems is to increase socially acceptable behaviors and to decrease deviant behavior patterns. Behavioral intervention features and general characteristics of feeding intervention outlined in Table 8.1 remain relevant to intervention for social and behavioral delays.

The following pages summarize common interventions for three types of social and behavioral delays related to mealtimes: disruptive behaviors, stereotypic response patterns, and inappropriate eating rate. Prior to the review of interventions, a case example of behavioral intervention for a child with social and behavioral impairments secondary to acquired brain injury (ABI) is described.

■ ■ ■

CASE 8.3. ACQUIRED BRAIN INJURY/
SOCIAL AND BEHAVIORAL IMPAIRMENTS
NAME: Jacob
AGE AT INTERVENTION: 7 years

BACKGROUND

Jacob was seen for feeding problems in a pediatric rehabilitation hospital subsequent to sustaining ABI in a motor vehicle–pedestrian accident. Prior to the accident, he was living at home with his mother, who was separated from Jacob's father. At the time, Jacob was attending a special education program in public school because of learning problems that, as reported by his mother, appeared to be consistent with ADHD. Otherwise, Jacob was a healthy child and had no history of significant feeding difficulty.

Immediately following his accident, Jacob was minimally responsive. He would open his eyes to a voice but was unable to follow simple commands. An initial electronic brain scan was negative but after an episode of apnea, a second brain scan showed diffuse cerebral edema, which was treated aggressively. Subsequent neurological tests showed an increased signal in the globus pallidus and inferior gyrus, which was consistent with small hemorrhages.

On admission to the pediatric rehabilitation facility, Jacob was not speaking, was intolerant of touch, made no eye contact, and refused to eat. Within a few days of admission, he began to use single words, which had no apparent connection to his situation. His speech, as it returned, was often explosive, and he frequently made negative comments about family members. He attended to objects but not to people, was echolalic (used repetitive vocalizations) and perseverative, and had frequent and extended periods of agitation. Episodes of agitation, as well as an absence of safety awareness, resulted in the frequent application of physical and mechanical restraints.

Jacob refused to eat and was sustained with nasogastric feeds. During an interdisciplinary feeding evaluation, he was noted to be orally hypersensitive and to avoid touch to any part of the body. A feeding program, based on frequent (4–5 times per day), structured exposure to a variety of foods and liquids, as well as modeling of eating and drinking, was instituted, as was oral-motor therapy to treat oral defensiveness. Tube feeds also were reduced by 25% during this phase of treatment. This combination of interventions and treatments was not immediately successful, and tube feeds were reinstated at full strength. Although feeding sessions were frequently cancelled or terminated because of episodes of extreme agitation, Jacob's aversion to eating was gradually reduced.

Within a week, he began—in response to a model—to blow bubbles in apple juice with a straw and then to take sips of juice with a straw. He also took an interest in finger-feeding, at first graham crackers and then dry cereal. During the first 2 weeks of the treatment and intervention program, he would usually expel any food or drinks that he sampled. Over the following weeks, however, he began to retain and swallow sampled foods and then began to sample a wider variety of finger foods, including french fries and pieces of hamburger. Tube feeding was again decreased in 25% increments and seemed to promote appetite. His mother was included in feeding sessions at this point. Jacob was soon taking all of his nutrition by mouth.

Two months following his injury, however, Jacob's feeding patterns showed an opposite problem: His oral consumption had increased sufficiently for him to be described as hyperphagic. If left unattended with food, he would stuff his mouth with food, swallow without chewing, eat with his hands, perseveratively request high-fat foods that were not in his diet, leave the table with food in his hands, and throw food that did not interest him. Throughout this phase of his recovery from ABI, Jacob's meals were frequently interrupted by food throwing, spitting, and aggressive behavior (hitting or kicking the feeder).

FORMULATION

Jacob's behavioral repertoire, including behavior related to feeding, was assumed to be strongly determined by organic factors related to his ABI, which, on the basis of electronic imaging studies, was thought to be diffuse. During recovery from ABI, Jacob's relationship to food changed from extreme aversion to hyperphagia, whereas his social behavior was consistently disinhibited, impulsive, and aggressive. Jacob's problems with mealtime conduct were consistent with his behavior problems in other social contexts. Behavioral intervention was designed to help Jacob to regulate appetite in the presence of food and to relearn social rules related to food consumption.

INTERVENTION

The following plan was designed to 1) promote appropriate eating rate; 2) decrease inappropriate behavior (e.g., spitting, throwing food) during mealtimes; and 3) maintain intake of a balanced, low-fat diet required to manage Jacob's weight.

Eating Rate

1. Jacob should be seated at a table for meals. He may need to be restrained in his chair.
2. Jacob will be offered the meal that is on his daily menu, which calls for a low-fat diet.
3. The meal should be in Jacob's view, but it should not be placed directly in front of him. At this point, the feeder must control the rate at which food is presented.
4. Jacob should be allowed to choose among the foods in front of him. Do not respond to requests for foods that are not available during the scheduled meal.
5. Jacob should be offered single bites (e.g., one spoonful) of each food. Hand him the spoon with the food, wait for him to completely swallow each bite, take the spoon from him, then offer him another bite. The same procedure should be used for finger foods. For example, break off a small piece of banana, hand it to him, and wait until his mouth is clear before offering him the next piece.

Throwing and Spitting Food

1. Remove food for 30 seconds for the first instance of throwing and spitting behaviors. Then present Jacob with the opportunity to eat again. If food throwing or spitting recurs, then remove food for 1 minute, then 2 minutes.
2. When he has refused, thrown, or spit a food three times, discontinue presentation of that food or drink. When he has eaten or eliminated all foods and drinks, discontinue meal.

OUTCOME

Because, during this phase in his recovery, food had become powerfully reinforcing to Jacob, the frequency of spitting and throwing food decreased rapidly, and these episodes were rare after 1 week of intervention. For the same reason, eating rate was more difficult to modify, and Jacob continued to require paced feeding throughout the meal for 2–3 weeks. After this time, mealtime restraint was discontinued, prompts became less necessary, and the plate was placed in front of Jacob after he had taken a few bites of the meal. The proximity of adult supervision was gradually faded, and Jacob was introduced to structured mealtimes with other children. At discharge from the hospital, approximately 6 months following his accident and 3 months after the intervention, Jacob was able to sit at meals with other children and required only periodic intervention from an adult to remind him to moderate his eating rate.

■ ■ ■

Disruptive Behaviors

Numerous behaviors have been categorized as inappropriate during mealtimes, such as screaming, spitting, throwing food, getting out of the chair, playing with food, licking the table or the floor, or letting food fall out of the mouth (Stimbert et al., 1977). Children with mild to moderate developmental impairments often display disruptive behaviors such as crying, throwing food, or excessive talking (Palmer et al., 1975; Thompson & Palmer, 1974). Positive counterparts to disruptive behaviors, which typically occur infrequently prior to intervention, include correct utensil use, food acceptance, and oral consumption. Disruptive behaviors precipitated by feeding cues (e.g., crying or turning away from the spoon) often are defined as food refusal (e.g., Duker, 1981; Hoch et al., 1994; Riordan et al., 1984). There is considerable overlap in the intervention literature dealing with extreme food selectivity and with social and behavioral delays, so sections of Chapter 5 are relevant to the review of inappropriate mealtime behaviors.

Most programs targeting disruptive mealtime behaviors also include procedures for strengthening alternative response patterns. Behavior management techniques to increase desired skills consist of instructions, modeling, fading, shaping, prompting, prompt fading, and reinforcement, which are the methods described previously in this chapter under the review of self-feeding interventions (see also reviews by Luiselli, 1989; Sisson & Van Hasselt, 1989). Usually, positive techniques alone are found to be insufficient to reduce disruptive behaviors (Hoch et al., 1994), so intervention typically includes some disciplinary procedures as well.

Behavior programs for reducing inappropriate feeding behaviors often rely on variations of time-out in conjunction with various positive techniques. Several studies (e.g., Barton, Guess, Garcia, & Baer, 1970; Sisson & Dixon, 1986a) found that interventions that included brief time-out effectively reduced inappropriate feeding behaviors in children with severe disabilities. Duker (1981), however, demonstrated that a package including overcorrection was substantially more effective than a package using time-out for treating disruptive and food refusal behaviors in a 10-year-old boy in an institution.

Still, other programs combine both time-out and overcorrection techniques in feeding intervention. For example, in treating six children who were in institutions and who had severe to profound mental retardation, Stimbert and colleagues (1977) employed manual guidance and social praise to teach appropriate self-feeding, along with a time-out procedure, in which a food tray was removed from a child's reach for 30 seconds contingent on inappropriate behavior. They also employed restitutional overcorrection when needed as a back-up procedure for inappropriate behavior. Overcorrection consisted of a loud reprimand (e.g., "No throwing"), guidance to correct the consequences of inappropriate behavior (e.g., having the child clean up the thrown food), and practice of the appropriate alternative behavior (e.g., correctly scooping and transporting food to the mouth three times) before a child was allowed to return to eating. The package resulted in substantial reductions in inappropriate behavior for all children, although the lengthy training period (mean of 173 sessions per child) raises questions about treatment efficacy.

Stereotypic Response Patterns

Children with sensory impairments, autism, or severe to profound mental retardation often engage in repetitive movements that appear to be sustained by organismic variables. Rocking, hand-flapping, and echolalia exemplify self-stimulatory patterns, whereas head banging and hand biting exemplify self-injurious patterns. Although these behaviors are not feeding problems per se, they can impede functional eating responses, disrupt the mealtime situation, and, in some cases, cause physical damage.

A variety of behavioral approaches have been employed successfully to decrease stereotypic response patterns (LaGrow & Repp, 1984). Intervention for stereotypic responses during mealtimes usually consists of a combination of positive reinforcement for desired responses together with extinction, time-out, or physical prompting techniques contingent on stereotypic behaviors. Leibowitz and Holcer (1974) reported on the successful use of praise and food reinforcement, plus mild negative contingencies (e.g., withdrawal of attention and food, time-out in the form of an unspecified period of lights-out) to increase self-feeding and decrease stereotypic behaviors in a 4-year-old child in a hospital.

Luiselli (1988a, 1993) demonstrated the effectiveness of intervention that includes an interruption procedure to decrease stereotypic behaviors (e.g., shaking utensils, tapping the table) and to increase independent self-feeding in two boys who were deaf and blind and had mental retardation. The interruption procedure consisted of gently stopping self-stimulatory responses and guiding the boys' hands into an appropriate position at the table or in their lap. In one case (Luiselli, 1988a), the boy received prompts consisting of a light tap on the elbow if he did not initiate self-feeding within 10 seconds of the last swallow, and he also earned preferred edibles for independent feeding responses. In the other case (Luiselli, 1993), social praise was provided contingent on correct feeding. Both interventions resulted in substantial increases in independent feeding.

Facial screening is a related procedure that has been used to modify self-stimulatory and self-injurious behaviors in children with developmental disabilities. Horton (1987) demonstrated successful application of facial screening to decrease repetitive spoon banging during classroom mealtimes in an 8-year-old girl with severe mental retardation. The procedure consisted of placing a terry cloth bib over the girl's face for 5 seconds contingent on the target behavior, along with stating "No bang" when initiating the procedure. This technique is far milder than alternative, more aversive techniques (e.g., electric shock, lemon juice) that have been used for more serious maladaptive behaviors than spoon banging, and thus it would seem to merit empirical evaluation as an approach with severe behavior problems that interfere with feeding. Stereotypic behavior, however, presents primarily in people with autism or severe mental retardation, and it rarely is confined to mealtimes. Thus, intervention procedures for this problem have limited application to feeding problems in general.

Inappropriate Eating Rate

The third general category of social and behavioral delays involves eating at an improper pace. Of the scant research on this topic, most has focused on excessively rapid eating, although one case (Luiselli, 1988b) concerns a child with overly slow eating. Favell, McGimsey, and Jones (1980) reported that fast eaters are common in residential facilities for individuals with severe or profound mental retardation. They identified 17 of 60 (28%) individuals (adults and children) in one facility who ate their entire meal in 1–3 minutes, sometimes consuming more than 20 bites per minute. Overly rapid eating poses acute health risks from vomiting or aspiration; by contrast, overly slow eating poses ongoing health risks of FTT and malnutrition.

Intervention approaches for improper eating rate include paced prompts (i.e., physical guidance to initiate or inhibit eating responses within predefined time intervals) and progressive fading of

prompts, sometimes combined with reinforcement. Favell and colleagues (1980) investigated an intervention package composed of
reinforcing short pauses (i.e., 1–2 seconds) with praise and preferred
food, shaping progressively longer pauses, providing manual
prompts to the hand to inhibit eating when the individual waited
less than the minimum pause interval, and gradual fading of
prompts. This package successfully reduced eating rates in four individuals at the residence from 20–24 bites to 6–8 bites per minute.

In another residential intervention program, Luiselli (1988b)
also used paced prompts and prompt fading to decrease eating rate
in an 8-year-old girl with multiple developmental disabilities. The
prompting procedure differed from Favell et al. (1980) in that after
each bite the girl's hand was guided back to the table and held there
for 5 seconds. After the effects of intervention were demonstrated,
physical guidance was used only when the girl attempted another
bite within the 5-second period. Intervention resulted in a reduction
of eating from approximately six bites to two bites per minute.

Another example of paced prompts and prompt fading limited
the amount of food available on a 10-year-old boy's plate to reduce
eating rate. Knapczyk (1983) initially gave the child single bites of
food and instructed him to eat them and then set down his spoon.
After substantially reducing eating rate with this procedure, the
amount of food offered at once was gradually increased to the size
of an entire meal, which effectively faded the paced prompts. The
intervention was successful in decreasing eating rate, and it also
eliminated the boy's habit of bringing the spoon to his mouth without food on it. Knapczyk proposed that the child's eating prior to intervention could be characterized as stereotypic responding because
he engaged in nearly continuous cycles of scooping and bringing
food to his mouth, but often he did not put food on the spoon.

Luiselli (1988b) extended the use of paced prompts to the problem of overly slow eating rate with a 13-year-old female who had
multiple developmental disabilities and who took longer than 1 hour
to eat meals. Intervention consisted of providing physical guidance
whenever 40 seconds elapsed without the initiation of a feeding response. Guidance involved prompting the girl to pick up food or a
utensil and bring it to her mouth and then allowing the girl to place
the food in her mouth. Intervention resulted in a modest but consistent increase in eating rate, from a mean of one bite per minute in
baseline to one and a half bites per minute during intervention.

It is interesting to note that few studies regarding social and
behavioral feeding delays have involved regular caregivers—particularly parents—in intervention. Many of the investigations were con-

ducted in residential settings during the 1970s and early 1980s and usually focused on individuals with severe disabilities. This research, however, is valuable in demonstrating the functional effects of behavior management techniques on feeding problems, and thus it laid the groundwork for subsequent research in outpatient settings. It is notable, however, that the studies rarely took an interdisciplinary or multidisciplinary approach to feeding problems, and little information was provided on medical or nutritional variables related to treatment. In clinical practice and applied research, interventions more often incorporate these characteristics and include home caregivers in the treatment and intervention programs (Luiselli, 1989).

SUMMARY

This chapter has surveyed the research and clinical literature on interventions for children with significant delays in feeding skills. Feeding delays frequently occur concomitant with a host of developmental disabilities or ongoing health conditions, including congenital anomalies, neuromotor dysfunction, global developmental disorders, and/or sensory impairments. Three major areas of feeding delays are oral-motor, self-feeding, and social and behavior skills. Neurodevelopmental intervention techniques emphasize working from a whole-body perspective, normalizing muscle tone and movement patterns, using adaptive equipment, and incorporating sensory experiences to enhance feeding. Behavioral intervention focuses on arranging antecedent stimuli, providing consistent positive and negative consequences contingent on feeding responses, altering intervention using shaping and fading procedures, and using systematic desensitization to pair eating with neutral or positive events. General features of feeding intervention—irrespective of conceptual approach—include beginning at the child's current skill level and advancing intervention based on child performance, communicating about intervention with regular caregivers, and monitoring the child's health status throughout the process.

REFERENCES

Accardo, P.J., & Whitman, B.Y. (1996). *Dictionary of developmental disabilities terminology.* Baltimore: Paul H. Brookes Publishing Co.

Ahearn, W.H., Kerwin, M.E., Eicher, P.S., Shantz, J., & Swearingin, W. (1996). An alternating treatments comparison of two intensive interventions for food refusal. *Journal of Applied Behavior Analysis, 29,* 321–332.

Babbitt, R.L., Hoch, T.A., & Coe, D.A. (1994). Behavioral feeding disorders. In D.N. Tuchman & R.S. Walter (Eds.), *Disorders of feeding and swal-*

lowing in infants and children: Pathophysiology, diagnosis, and treatment (pp. 77–95). San Diego: Singular.

Bandura, A. (1969). Modeling and vicarious processes. In *Principles of behavior modification* (pp. 118–216). New York: Holt, Rinehart & Winston.

Barton, E.S., Guess, D., Garcia, E., & Baer, D.M. (1970). Improvement of retardates' mealtime behaviors by timeout procedures using multiple baseline techniques. *Journal of Applied Behavior Analysis, 3,* 77–84.

Berkowitz, S., Sherry, P.J., & Davis, B.A. (1971). Teaching self-feeding skills to profound retardates using reinforcement and fading procedures. *Behavior Therapy, 2,* 62–67.

Blackman, J.A., & Nelson, C.L.A. (1987). Rapid introduction of oral feedings to tube-fed patients. *Journal of Developmental and Behavioral Pediatrics, 8,* 63–67.

Brown, J.E., Davis, E., & Flemming, P.L. (1979). Nutritional assessment of children with handicapping conditions. *Mental Retardation, 17,* 129–132.

Budd, K.S. (1988). Behavioral parent training for families of developmentally disabled children: A behavioral medicine perspective. In D.C. Russo & J.H. Kedesdy (Eds.), *Behavioral medicine with the developmentally disabled* (pp. 229–238). New York: Plenum.

Butterfield, W.H., & Parson, R. (1973). Modeling and shaping by parents to develop chewing behavior in their retarded child. *Journal of Behavior Therapy and Experimental Psychiatry, 4,* 285–287.

Camp, K.M., & Kalscheur, M.C. (1994). Nutritional approach to diagnosis and management of pediatric feeding and swallowing disorders. In D.N. Tuchman & R.S. Walter (Eds.), *Disorders of feeding and swallowing in infants and children: Pathophysiology, diagnosis, and treatment* (pp. 153–185). San Diego: Singular.

Christophersen, E., & Hall, C.L. (1978). Eating patterns and associated problems encountered in normal children. *Issues in Comprehensive Pediatric Nursing, 3,* 1–16.

Cipani, E. (1981). Modifying food spillage behavior in an institutionalized retarded client. *Journal of Behavior Therapy and Experimental Psychiatry, 12,* 261–265.

DiScipio, W.J., & Kaslon, K. (1982). Conditioned dysphagia in cleft palate children after pharyngeal flap surgery. *Psychosomatic Medicine, 44,* 247–257.

Dolgin, M.J., & Jay, S.M. (1989). Pain management in children. In E.J. Mash & R.A. Barkley (Eds.), *Treatment of childhood disorders* (pp. 383–404). New York: Guilford Press.

Duker, P.C. (1981). Treatment of food refusal by the overcorrective functional movement training method. *Journal of Behavior Therapy and Experimental Psychiatry, 12,* 337–340.

Eicher, P.M. (1997). Feeding. In M.L. Batshaw (Ed.), *Children with disabilities* (4th ed., pp. 621–641). Baltimore: Paul H. Brookes Publishing Co.

Favell, J.E., McGimsey, J.F., & Jones, M.L. (1980). Rapid eating in the retarded: Reduction by nonaversive procedures. *Behavior Modification, 4,* 481–492.

Ginsberg, A.J. (1988). Feeding disorders in the developmentally disabled population. In D.C. Russo & J.H. Kedesdy (Eds.), *Behavioral medicine with the developmentally disabled* (pp. 21–41). New York: Plenum.

Gisel, E.G. (1994). Oral-motor skills following sensorimotor intervention in the moderately eating-impaired child with cerebral palsy. *Dysphagia, 9,* 180–192.

Gisel, E.G. (1996). Effect of oral sensorimotor treatment on measures of growth and efficiency of eating in the moderately eating-impaired child with cerebral palsy. *Dysphagia, 11,* 48–58.

Gisel, E.G., Appelgate-Ferrante, T., Benson, J., & Bosma, J.F. (1996). Oral-motor skills following sensorimotor therapy in two groups of moderately dysphagic children with cerebral palsy: Aspiration vs nonaspiration. *Dysphagia, 11,* 59–71.

Gisel, E.G., Lange, L.J., & Niman, C.W. (1984). Tongue movements in 4- and 5-year-old Down's syndrome children during eating: A comparison with normal children. *The American Journal of Occupational Therapy, 38,* 660–665.

Gisel, E.G., & Patrick, J. (1988, February 6). Identification of children with cerebral palsy unable to maintain a normal nutritional state. *Lancet,* 283–286.

Gourash, L.F. (1986). Assessing and managing medical factors. In R.P. Barrett (Ed.), *Severe behavior disorders in the mentally retarded: Nondrug approaches to treatment* (pp. 157–205). New York: Plenum.

Greer, R.D., Dorow, L., Williams, G., McCorkle, N., & Asnes, R. (1991). Peer-mediated procedures to induce swallowing and food acceptance in young children. *Journal of Applied Behavior Analysis, 24,* 783–790.

Hoch, T.A., Babbitt, R.L., Coe, D.A., Krell, D.M., & Hackbert, L. (1994). Contingency contacting: Combining positive reinforcement and escape extinction procedures to treat persistent food refusal. *Behavior Modification, 18,* 106–128.

Horton, S.V. (1987). Reduction of disruptive mealtime behavior by facial screening: A case study of a mentally retarded girl with long-term follow-up. *Behavior Modification, 11,* 53–64.

Iwata, B.A., Riordan, M.M., Wohl, M.K., & Finney, J.W. (1982). Pediatric feeding disorders: Behavioral analysis and treatment. In P.J. Accardo (Ed.), *Failure to thrive in infancy and early childhood: A multidisciplinary approach* (pp. 297–329). Baltimore: University Park Press.

Johnson, C.B., & Deitz, J.C. (1985). Time use of mothers with preschool children: A pilot study. *The American Journal of Occupational Therapy, 39,* 578–583.

Johnson, C.R., & Babbitt, R.L. (1993). Antecedent manipulation in the treatment of primary solid food refusal. *Behavior Modification, 17,* 510–521.

Kerwin, M.E., Osborne, M., & Eicher, P.S. (1994). Effect of position and support on oral-motor skills of a child with bronchopulmonary dysplasia. *Clinical Pediatrics, 33,* 8–13.

Knapczyk, D.R. (1983). Use of teacher-paced instruction in developing and maintaining independent self-feeding. *Journal of The Association for the Severely Handicapped, 8,* 10–16.

Kosowski, M.M., & Sopczyk, D.L. (1985). Feeding hospitalized children with developmental disabilities. *American Journal of Maternal and Child Nursing, 10,* 190–194.

LaGrow, S.J., & Repp, A.C. (1984). Stereotypic responding: A review of intervention research. *American Journal of Mental Deficiency, 88,* 595–609.

Lamm, N., & Greer, R.D. (1988). Induction and maintenance of swallowing responses in infants with dysphagia. *Journal of Applied Behavior Analysis, 21,* 143–156.

Leibowitz, J.M., & Holcer, P. (1974). Increasing food variety and texture: Building and maintaining self-feeding skills in a retarded child. *The American Journal of Occupational Therapy, 28,* 545–548.

Lewis, J.A. (1982). Oral motor assessment and treatment of feeding difficulties. In P.J. Accardo (Ed.), *Failure to thrive in infancy and early childhood: A multidisciplinary approach* (pp. 265–295). Baltimore: University Park Press.

Linscheid, T.R. (1988). The role of development and learning in feeding disorders. In D.E. Russo & J.H. Kedesdy (Eds.), *Behavioral medicine with the developmentally disabled* (pp. 43–48). New York: Plenum.

Linscheid, T.R. (1992). Eating problems in children. In C.E. Walker & M.C. Roberts (Eds.), *Handbook of clinical child psychology* (2nd ed., pp. 451–473). New York: John Wiley & Sons.

Linscheid, T.R., Oliver, J., Blyler, E., & Palmer, S. (1978). Brief hospitalization for the behavioral treatment of feeding problems in the developmentally disabled. *Journal of Pediatric Psychology, 3,* 72–76.

Logemann, J.A. (1986). Treatment for aspiration related to dysphagia: An overview. *Dysphagia, 1,* 34–38.

Luiselli, J.K. (1988a). Behavioral feeding intervention with deaf-blind, multihandicapped children. *Child and Family Behavior Therapy, 10,* 49–62.

Luiselli, J.K. (1988b). Improvement in feeding skills in multihandicapped students through paced-prompting interventions. *Journal of the Multihandicapped Person, 1,* 17–30.

Luiselli, J.K. (1989). Behavioral assessment and treatment of pediatric feeding disorders in developmental disabilities. In M. Hersen, R.K. Eisler, & P.M. Miller (Eds.), *Progress in behavior modification* (Vol. 24, pp. 91–131). Beverly Hills: Sage Publications.

Luiselli, J.K. (1993). Training self-feeding skills in children who are deaf and blind. *Behavior Modification, 17,* 457–473.

Luiselli, J.K., & Gleason, D.J. (1987). Combining sensory reinforcement and texture fading procedures to overcome chronic food refusal. *Journal of Behavior Therapy and Experimental Psychology, 18,* 149–155.

MacArthur, J., Ballard, K.D., & Artinian, M. (1986). Teaching independent eating to a developmentally handicapped child showing chronic food refusal and disruption at mealtimes. *Australia and New Zealand Journal of Developmental Disabilities, 12,* 203–210.

Morris, S.E., & Klein, M.D. (1987). *Pre-feeding skills: A comprehensive resource for feeding development.* Tucson, AZ: Therapy Skill Builders.

Munk, D.D., & Repp, A.C. (1994). Behavioral assessment of feeding problems of individuals with severe disabilities. *Journal of Applied Behavior Analysis, 27,* 241–250.

Nelson, G.L., Cone, J.D., & Hanson, C.R. (1975). Training correct utensil use in retarded children: Modeling vs. physical guidance. *American Journal of Mental Deficiency, 80,* 114–122.

Palmer, S. (1978). Nutrition and developmental disorders: An overview. In S. Palmer & S. Ekvall (Eds.), *Pediatric nutrition in developmental disorders* (pp. 21–24). Springfield, IL: Charles C Thomas.

Palmer, S., & Horn, S. (1978). Feeding problems in children. In S. Palmer & S. Ekvall (Eds.), *Pediatric nutrition in developmental disorders* (pp. 107–129). Springfield, IL: Charles C Thomas.

Palmer, S., Thompson, R.J., & Linscheid, T.R. (1975). Applied behavior analysis in the treatment of childhood feeding problems. *Developmental Medicine and Child Neurology, 17,* 333–339.

Perske, R., Clifton, A., McLean, B.M., & Stein, J.E. (Eds.). (1977). *Mealtimes for severely and profoundly handicapped persons: New concepts and attitudes.* Baltimore: University Park Press.

Pipes, P.L., & Glass, R.P. (1993). Developmental disabilities and other special health care needs. In P.L. Pipes & C.M. Trahms (Eds.), *Nutrition in infancy and childhood* (5th ed., pp. 344–373). St. Louis: Times Mirror/Mosby College Publishing.

Reilly, S., & Skuse, D. (1992). Characteristics and management of feeding problems in young children with cerebral palsy. *Developmental Medicine and Child Neurology, 34,* 379–388.

Reilly, S., Skuse, D., Mathisen, B., & Wolke, D. (1995). The objective rating of oral-motor functions during feeding. *Dysphagia, 10,* 177–191.

Riordan, M.M., Iwata, B.A., Finney, J.W., Wohl, M.K., & Stanley, A.E. (1984). Behavioral assessment and treatment of chronic food refusal in handicapped children. *Journal of Applied Behavior Analysis, 17,* 327–341.

Schroeder, S.R., Mulick, J.A., & Schroeder, C.S. (1979). Management of severe behavior problems of the retarded. In N.R. Ellis (Ed.), *Handbook of mental deficiency, psychological theory, and research* (Rev. ed., pp. 341–366). Hillsdale, NJ: Lawrence Erlbaum Associates.

Schuberth, L.M. (1994). The role of occupational therapy in diagnosis and management. In D.N. Tuchman & R.S. Walter (Eds.), *Disorders of feeding and swallowing in infants and children: Pathophysiology, diagnosis, and treatment* (pp. 115–129). San Diego: Singular.

Shprintzen, R.J. (1992). The implications of the diagnosis of Robin sequence. *Cleft Palate Craniofacial Journal, 29,* 205–209.

Sisson, L.A., & Dixon, M.J. (1986a). A behavioral approach to the training and assessment of feeding skills in multihandicapped children. *Applied Research in Mental Retardation, 7,* 149–163.

Sisson, L.A., & Dixon, M.J. (1986b). Improving mealtime behaviors through token reinforcement: A study with mentally retarded, behaviorally disordered children. *Behavior Modification, 10,* 333–354.

Sisson, L.A., & Van Hasselt, V.B. (1989). Feeding disorders. In J.K. Luiselli (Ed.), *Behavioral medicine and developmental disabilities* (pp. 45–73). New York: Springer-Verlag.

Sisson, L.A., Van Hasselt, V.B., & Hersen, M. (1987). Psychological approaches with deaf-blind persons: Strategies and issues in research and treatment. *Clinical Psychology Review, 7,* 303–328.

Sobsey, R., & Orelove, F.P. (1984). Neurophysiological facilitation of eating skills in children with severe handicaps. *Journal of The Association for Persons with Severe Handicaps, 9,* 98–110.

Stevenson, R.D. (1995). Feeding and nutrition in children with developmental disabilities. *Pediatric Annals, 24,* 255–260.

Stimbert, V.E., Minor, J.W., & McCoy, J.F. (1977). Intensive feeding training with retarded children. *Behavior Modification, 1,* 517–530.

Thompson, G.A., Jr., Iwata, B.A., & Poynter, H. (1979). Operant control of pathological tongue thrust in spastic cerebral palsy. *Journal of Applied Behavior Analysis, 12,* 325–333.

Thompson, R.J., & Palmer, S. (1974). Treatment of feeding problems: A behavioral approach. *Journal of Nutrition Education, 6,* 63–66.

Tuchman, D.N., & Walter, R.S. (1994). Disorders of deglutition. In D.N. Tuchman & R.S. Walter (Eds.), *Disorders of feeding and swallowing in infants and children: Pathophysiology, diagnosis, and treatment* (pp. 53–75). San Diego: Singular.

Walter, R.S. (1994). Issues surrounding the development of feeding and swallowing. In D.N. Tuchman & R.S. Walter (Eds.), *Disorders of feeding and swallowing in infants and children: Pathophysiology, diagnosis, and treatment* (pp. 27–35). San Diego: Singular.

Werle, M.A., Murphy, T.B., & Budd, K.S. (1993). Treating chronic food refusal in young children: Home-based parent training. *Journal of Applied Behavior Analysis, 26,* 421–433.

Wolf, L.S., & Glass, R.P. (1992). *Feeding and swallowing disorders in infancy: Assessment and management.* Tucson, AZ: Therapy Skill Builders.

Ylvisaker M., & Logemann, J. (1985). Therapy for feeding and swallowing disorders following head injury. In M. Ylvisaker (Ed.), *Head injury rehabilitation: Children and adolescents* (pp. 195–209). Boston: College-Hill.

Ylvisaker, M., & Weinstein, M. (1989). Recovery of oral feeding after pediatric head injury. *The Journal of Head Trauma Rehabilitation, 4,* 51–63.

Zausmer, E., & Pueschel, S.M. (1978). Feeding the young child with Down syndrome. In S.M. Pueschel (Ed.), *Down syndrome: Growing and learning* (pp. 114–120). Kansas City, KS: Andrews and McMeel.

9 | Children Who Eat the Wrong Things

Pica and Rumination

This chapter considers two early childhood feeding disorders—pica and rumination—in which the chief concern is the ingestion of *inappropriate substances* or "eating the wrong things." The problem of extreme selectivity, in which children eat an inappropriately *narrow range* of foods, is covered in Chapter 5.

Whether a substance is considered to be appropriate for ingestion is not entirely determined by its nutritive content. The distinction between "food" and "nonfood" and between edible and nonedible substances is, to a great extent, socially determined and culturally transmitted. Some nutritive substances (e.g., beef, pork, insects) are considered to be edible in some cultures but not in others, and the ingestion of some entirely nonnutritive substances (e.g., dirt) is sanctioned in some cultures (Parry-Jones & Parry-Jones, 1992). This chapter focuses primarily on disorders of inappropriate intake that have negative health consequences, regardless of whether the ingested substances are "edible."

PICA

The discussion of pica often is complicated by the fact that the eating disorder has been studied in three distinct populations: typically developing infants and toddlers, children and adults with severe or profound disabilities, and specific adult populations such as rural women in the southern United States for whom some forms of pica (e.g., eating laundry starch during pregnancy) are a traditional and culturally sanctioned practice (Lacey, 1990). The following discussion focuses on pica in children.

Definition

The *Diagnostic and Statistical Manual of Mental Disorders, Fourth Edition* (DSM-IV) (American Psychiatric Association, 1994) defines *pica* as a childhood eating disorder characterized by the developmentally inappropriate and persistent eating of nonnutritive substances for a period of at least 1 month. The DSM-IV diagnostic criteria for pica explicitly exclude culturally sanctioned eating practices.

The term *pica* historically has been used more broadly to include the consumption of socially marginal foods (e.g., raw potatoes, tomato seeds, ice) and also to refer to a compulsive craving for specific foods that are both culturally appropriate and nutritive (e.g., peanuts, pickled olives) (Lacey, 1990; Parry-Jones & Parry-Jones, 1992). Thus, the term *pica* is sometimes used to reference a dimension of eating behavior (i.e., craving or compulsion) without regard to the characteristics of the ingested substance. An elaborate nomenclature has evolved to classify cravings for specific substances. For example, "geophagia" refers to a craving for dirt, "pagophagia" to a craving for ice, "amylophagia" to a craving for starch, and "gooberphagia" to a craving for peanuts. These cravings could be considered forms of differentiated *hyperphagia,* which is discussed in Chapter 10. Childhood pica is usually undifferentiated and does not typically have the characteristics of a specific craving (Robischon, 1971), but there are exceptions to this general rule (Korman, 1990). Barltrop (1966), in a study of pica prevalence in children between the ages of 1 and 6 years, found that pica is more likely to be selective in older children.

Consequences and Associated Conditions

Pica is a disorder with significant, potentially life-threatening, health consequences. Children have been known to ingest paper in various forms (e.g., newspaper, wallpaper, cardboard), clothing (e.g., hats, gloves), dirt (including pebbles and glass fragments), toiletries (e.g., soap, toothbrushes, sponges), wall plaster, tobacco products, and writing products (e.g., crayons, pencils, erasers) (Barltrop, 1966). Pica can cause intestinal obstruction, parasitic infection, and poisoning. Children with pica who live in homes with high concentrations of lead are at risk for lead poisoning. High blood levels of lead can cause intellectual impairments and, in sufficient concentrations, severe encephalopathy and death. Eating lead paint chips is the primary source of lead intoxication in children (Pueschel, 1988). Other pica-related sources of lead poisoning include mouthing newspapers, chewing on toothpaste tubes with high lead content, eating dirt with high lead content, and chewing on imported toys with leaded paint (Pueschel, Cullen, Howard, & Cullinane, 1977).

Prevalence

The prevalence of pica in children has been documented in numerous studies. Robischon (1971) reviewed a number of studies, one of which reported a pica prevalence of between 32% and 50% of children 1–2 years of age and another of which reported a pica prevalence of 21% in a population of children 30–31 months of age. Robischon's (1971) own study found a prevalence of 37% in a population of low-income, urban, African American children.

The prevalence of pica is age dependent. Barltrop (1966) found a steady decline, from 35% to 6%, in the prevalence of pica in children between the ages of 1 and 4 years. Although pica does not persist in most children, it is interesting to note that Marchi and Cohen (1990) found that pica at an early age is a predictor for later bulimia nervosa. Marchi and Cohen (1990) speculated that pica may be indicative of a general tendency toward indiscriminant or uncontrolled eating behavior. A study of pica in a rural obstetric population found that 33% of adult patients with pica had a history of childhood pica (Smulian, Motiwala, & Sigman, 1995).

Etiology

There are multiple, competing hypotheses regarding the etiology of pica. The absence of a consensus is not entirely surprising given the heterogeneity of the populations in which pica has been studied. One would not necessarily assume, for example, that the consumption of laundry starch during pregnancy would be under the control of the same variables as the ingestion of paint chips in toddlers. Pica in children has been attributed to several broad classes of causal variables: diet (e.g., nutritional deficiencies), child constitution (e.g., developmental lags, sensory reinforcement), caregiver competence (e.g., maternal deprivation), and systemic factors (e.g., impoverished home environments).

Some children who engage in pica have been found to be deficient in certain nutrients, especially iron and zinc (Lacey, 1990). One potential explanation for this finding is that nutritional deficiencies cause pica by inducing a craving for specific substances. An alternative explanation for a correlation between mineral deficiency and pica is that the consumed substances could interfere with the absorption of trace mineral. Some support for the nutritional deficiency hypothesis is provided by case studies that have reported reductions in pica when children are treated with iron supplements, but other studies have failed to obtain this effect (Danford, 1982; Lacey, 1990). Furthermore, childhood pica is seldom selective, and the nonnutritive substances that children consume are not usually rich in iron, zinc, or any other specific nutrient.

A variety of psychological and environmental hypotheses have been advanced as explanations for pica. It has been argued that pica is an oral fixation that serves as relief of anxiety for children with absent or inadequate mothers (Millican, Layman, Lourie, & Takahashi, 1968). A related hypothesis suggests that some cases of pica may represent a form of obsessive-compulsive disorder (Zeitlin & Polivy, 1995). Support for the psychogenic etiology of pica is limited to clinical case studies.

Pica, and behaviors closely related to pica (e.g., mouthing), have been shown to be inversely correlated with environmental quality measured on a number of different dimensions. For example, Pueschel et al. (1977) found that several social and environmental conditions—including absence of a father in the home, an unstable home situation, and a house in poor repair—were significantly more likely in a group of children with increased lead burden secondary to pica as compared with a matched control group. Madden, Russo, and Cataldo (1980) found that mouthing—a behavior often correlated with pica—occurred more frequently in impoverished environments, relative to environments in which either group play or enriched individual play was available.

Pica that occurs during the course of mouthing objects is generally considered to be normative in infants up to the ages of 18–24 months. When pica persists beyond this stage, it is sometimes interpreted as a sign of developmental delay (Nelson, 1995). Pica in adults with mental retardation is sometimes conceptualized as a developmental lag—that is, as the persistence of hand-to-mouth behaviors that are part of the normal sequence of development (Robischon, 1971). It also has been argued that pica may be maintained by its sensory consequences (Favell, McGimsey, & Schell, 1982); for example, a child who eats paint chips may do so because the associated oral sensations (e.g., "crunchiness") are enjoyable. Some studies have reported commonalities in texture, taste, and other properties of the substances consumed by children with pica (Danford, 1982), but the sensory attributes of pica substances have not been studied extensively.

Intervention

There are relatively few empirical studies of interventions to reduce pica in otherwise healthy, young children. Because pica in infants and toddlers can be anticipated during the course of normal child development and because the probability of pica diminishes with increasing age, there is always a question of whether pica behavior justifies parent or professional concern and whether it requires "treatment." When concerns are raised during health supervision visits, testing the child for lead levels, counseling increased parental supervision, and emphasizing home "childproofing" are often recommended (Nelson, 1995). Robischon (1971), writing from a nursing perspective, argued for the following: 1) developing interview techniques to better identify children with pica, 2) educating professionals to observe child behavior for pica-related behavior, and 3) monitoring children with gross motor delays—a possible risk factor associated with persistent pica—more closely. Madden et al. (1980) suggested, on the basis of their study of environmental influences on child mouthing behavior, that environmental enrichment—in the form of group activities, toys, and social contact—may be helpful in preventing pica. Enrolling children in child care, training mothers in infant stimulation, and using toy-lending libraries are recommended as ways to implement environmental enrichment. Most of these recommendations are directed at preventing or reducing the health and developmental risks associated with pica, not at eliminating the behavior itself.

As discussed in the section on Etiology, there are several studies supporting the use of iron supplements in children with pica, in particular those children who are also iron deficient, but empirical support for the efficacy of nutritional therapies for pica is generally weak (Danford, 1982). Children with pica should always be tested for lead levels and be treated appropriately.

Behavior Modification Interventions The majority of intervention studies for persistent pica use behavior modification procedures that manipulate the antecedents and consequences of pica or a related behavior (e.g., mouthing). A comprehensive review of published behavioral interventions for pica (Bell & Stein, 1992) found that self-protective devices (e.g., arm restraints, helmets), physical restraints, overcorrection (teaching correct behavior through exaggerated practice), contingent aversive stimulation (e.g., water mist, ammonia, lemon juice), and differential reinforcement procedures all have been used, with varying degrees of success, to reduce pica. The majority of the interventions reviewed by Bell and Stein (1992) were employed in studies with adults with moderate to profound mental retardation. The following discussion focuses on representative intervention studies with children.

Finney, Russo, and Cataldo (1982) described an intervention program for four young children, ages 2–5 years, who had been hospitalized for lead poisoning and who showed high baseline rates of pica. The basic intervention, conducted while the children were inpatients, consisted of discrimination training and of differential reinforcement of other behavior (DRO). An additional procedure, overcorrection, was used with two of the four children. The interventions were conducted in a small observation room in which nonedible substances, including simulated paint chips made of flour and water, were distributed. During the discrimination training phases, children were reinforced for correct verbal identification of five edible substances (e.g., cookies) and for five nonedible substances (e.g., paint chips). The substances were presented in random order, and each child was asked, "What is this?" and, "Should you put this in your mouth?" If discrimination training failed to eliminate pica behavior, the DRO intervention was initiated. During this intervention, the children were reinforced when they did not place nonedible substances in their mouths during a specified and gradually increasing interval. If the discrimination training and DRO procedures did not succeed in eliminating pica, then an overcorrection procedure was implemented after parental permission had been obtained. This consisted of brushing the child's teeth for 1 minute, using a toothbrush dipped in an astringent mouthwash, whenever pica behavior occurred.

Discrimination training, by itself, resulted in slight decreases in pica behavior in two of the four children but was ineffective in the remaining two children. When DRO was added to the intervention, pica behavior was eliminated in two children, and the addition of overcorrection resulted in elimination of pica in the remaining children. Parents were then trained in the use of the behavioral procedures and were asked to implement them at home. Blood lead levels remained low in all children in the year following discharge.

Another use of discrimination training to treat pica was reported by Fisher et al. (1994). This inpatient treatment study used empirically derived consequences to reward children for eating food only in the presence of a discriminative stimulus (a plate on a placemat) and to punish pica behaviors. Three children with pica, from 3 to 5 years of age, were assessed to determine reinforcer preferences and the potency of punishers for each child. Suppression (but not complete elimination) of pica was achieved rapidly in a baited analogue situation, similar to that used in the Finney et al. (1982) study, and then generalized to a living unit in the hospital, and finally to the child's home. Low rates of pica were sustained for 9 months following discharge from the hospital. Fisher et al. (1994) speculated that the behavioral assessment of the potency of reinforcers and punishers may enhance the effectiveness of pica interventions.

Physical restraint contingent on pica-related behavior also has been described in some individual case studies, often as one element in a multicomponent intervention package (Paniagua, Braverman, & Capriotti, 1986). Physical restraint typically involves holding the child's arms to his or her side when pica or pica-related behavior occurs. The duration of holding is usually brief (10–30 seconds). This procedure has the advantage of simplicity but may result in physical resistance by the child. Whether physical restraint, by itself, can function as an effective intervention for pica is unknown.

Empirically validated behavioral interventions for pica have been utilized, for the most part, in hospital or residential environments that employ staff trained in implementing behavior modification procedures. The efficacy of these procedures in outpatient, parent-mediated interventions is not as well established.

Clinical guidelines for the evaluation of and methods for intervention for pica are summarized in Table 9.1. The following case study illustrates the use of suppressive techniques, discrimination training, and reinforcement of alternative behavior in a parent-mediated outpatient intervention package.

■ ■ ■

CASE 9.1. A CHILD WITH PICA
NAME: Sally
AGE AT INTERVENTION: 4 years

BACKGROUND

Sally, a 4-year-old girl with Down syndrome and moderate mental retardation, was referred by her pediatrician for the assessment and treatment of excessive mouthing and pica. She was the only child of middle-class parents, both of whom came to the initial evaluation and agreed to participate in a parent-mediated intervention. Sally's parents reported a 3-year history of mouthing, chewing, and ingesting inedible objects. Sally was especially likely to chew plastic objects, tap her teeth with spoons, eat sand at the beach, and consume crayons whenever they were available. Mouthing and pica appeared to be stimulus bound, tending to occur whenever favored inedible objects were present. Sally had previously received treatment for pica from an occupational therapist who conceptualized the problem as one of oral hyposensitivity. Oral stimulation therapy, including the use of a plastic gum massager, was provided during individual therapy sessions conducted at Sally's preschool program.

Table 9.1.   Clinical guidelines for evaluation and intervention for pica

EVALUATION
- Is pica developmentally expected? Is it persistent?
- What are the immediate health risks?
- Has the child been evaluated for lead poisoning?
- Is there evidence of nutritional deficiency?
- Can access to ingested substances be controlled by the child's caregiver?
- Does the child select specific nonnutritive substances, or is pica indiscriminate?
- If pica is specific, do the preferred substances have common sensory properties?
- What (if any) conditions appear to precipitate pica?
- What is the quality of the home environment and other resources for developmental stimulation?

INTERVENTION
- If pica is developmentally expected, lead levels are normal, and other health risks are negligible, counsel the following:
  - Increased parental supervision
  - Removal of environmental hazards
  - Environmental enrichment
- If there is evidence of nutritional deficiency, provide appropriate nutrition therapy.
- If pica is not developmentally expected, or persists for more than one month, add explicit discrimination training (i.e., reinforce child for correct identification of edible and nonedible substances) to the preceding interventions.
- If discrimination training is not completely effective, develop a contingency management program with the following elements:
  - If child is unable to discriminate accurately between foods and nonfoods, reinforce for ingestion under tight stimulus control (e.g., only eating food on plates).
  - Reinforce the child for behavior inconsistent with pica.
  - Encourage alternative, appropriate forms of oral stimulation.
  - Consider using a negative consequence (e.g., overcorrection, brief physical restraint) for each instance of pica.

FORMULATION

Sally's mouthing, chewing, and pica were assumed to be self-stimulatory. She appeared to derive intense oral satisfaction from these behaviors. Pica was partially selective, as some substances (crayons, plastic, and sand) were preferred over others. Complex texture rather than taste appeared to be a common sensory attribute of some preferred substances. An intervention strategy was devised as follows: 1) Provide negative social consequences for pica and mouthing, 2) include explicit discrimination training, and 3) encourage alternative forms of oral stimulation.

INTERVENTION

The following behavioral guidelines were negotiated with Sally's parents and were shared with her preschool teacher:

1. Whenever Sally is observed to bring objects to her mouth (either her lips or teeth), use a loud, authoritative (but not angry) "no mouthing" command. If mouthing does not cease within 2–3 seconds of the command, then repeat the command and hold Sally's hands to her side for 5–10 seconds. Use the same intervention if Sally places her fingers into her mouth for more than 1–2 seconds.
2. If Sally is found with an object *entirely in* her mouth, then remove the object; show her the object, saying "no eating" in an authoritative voice; and take her to time-out for 5 minutes.
3. These interventions should be used across all settings by everyone who interacts with Sally.
4. In addition, Sally's mother will conduct special discrimination sessions with Sally, which will focus on teaching appropriate crayon use. During these 5- to 10-minute sessions, scheduled several times per week, Sally's mother will do the following: 1) model appropriate crayon use, 2) prompt crayon use (both physically and verbally), 3) praise appropriate crayon use, and 4) use a loud "no mouthing" command if crayons are brought to the mouth, as in intervention number 1.
5. To provide additional opportunities for appropriate oral stimulation, chewy and crunchy-textured snacks (e.g., apples, granola bars, popcorn, raw vegetables) should be provided between meals.
6. The effects of these interventions will be reviewed every 2 weeks.

OUTCOME

Sally's parents reported a sharp decrease in pica and mouthing across all settings within 2 weeks. Because pica could occur when Sally was alone, her parents were asked to arrange several unobtrusive observations each week. During these semistructured observations, the opportunity to engage in pica was arranged, and Sally did not know she was being observed. Pica was suppressed relative to baseline during these observations as well. Sally's taste for crayons was more difficult to discourage and was suppressed only in the presence of an adult, so Sally's access to crayons continued to be controlled. Sally's mother also noted that Sally seemed to be unable to use crayons appropriately, and this was believed to be related to her stage of cognitive development. Her parents believed that providing crunchy snacks was an especially important part of the program and believed that Sally would often seek crunchy snacks as substitutes for mouthing materials.

■ ■ ■

RUMINATION

Rumination, the ingestion of previously consumed foods, is a disorder of inappropriate intake that, as with pica, is associated with significant negative health consequences. Like pica, rumination occurs in several disparate clinical populations: infants, children and adults with mental retardation, and normally functioning adults. The following sections focus on rumination in infants and children.

Definition

Rumination refers to the persistent regurgitation and reconsumption of previously eaten food. The DSM-IV defines *rumination* as a disorder of infancy or childhood, characterized by the repeated regurgitation and rechewing of food for a period of at least 1 month following a period of normal functioning (American Psychiatric Association, 1994). Furthermore, the ruminative behavior must not be due to an associated gastrointestinal (GI) or other general medical condition. Because rumination in children is sometimes difficult to differentiate clinically from vomiting and related GI disorders, the next section provides discussion of some issues related to the differential diagnosis of rumination.

Differential Diagnosis

Although rumination and vomiting may be found concurrently in the same child, the two phenomena are different in a number of important ways. *Vomiting,* the forceful expulsion of stomach contents through the mouth, is a common symptom with many causes (Hanson & McCallum, 1985). Vomiting often is associated with acute, time-limited illness but also may occur secondary to congenital anatomical defects, various GI diseases (e.g., Crohn's disease, gastroenteritis), inborn errors of metabolism, central nervous system dysfunction, and oral-motor dysfunction. The physiology of vomiting includes sudden contraction of abdominal muscles, descent of the diaphragm, and relaxation of the lower esophageal sphincter in a reflexive sequence mediated by a vomiting center in the medulla (Whitehead & Schuster, 1985). Although vomiting is reflexive, some of the muscle groups involved in vomiting are under voluntary control, providing the basis for "learned vomiting" (Whitehead & Schuster, 1985).

Rumination, on the contrary, is always voluntary and usually not directly associated with acute illness or disease. It is not accompanied by nausea and, in fact, commonly appears to be pleasurable to the ruminator. The manifest pleasure associated with rumination is what distinguishes it from other forms of learned vomiting. Rumination may be obviously self-induced using the fingers or other objects placed in the mouth, but it also may be self-elicited in less visible ways, including tongue movements and voluntary contraction of the stomach muscles.

Rumination also should be clearly distinguished from *gastroesophageal reflux* (GER), an involuntary, spontaneous return of stomach contents into the esophagus (see Chapters 2 and 7). In addition to being involuntary, GER does not necessarily result in regurgitation, a critical feature of both rumination and vomiting. Nevertheless, an association between GER and rumination is sometimes reported (Shepard, Wren, Evans, Lander, & Ong, 1987), and it is sometimes suggested (Woolston, 1991) that GER may be the physiological substrate on which learning and psychosocial factors act to produce ruminative behavior.

Finally, rumination can be distinguished from *childhood psychogenic vomiting,* an apparently rare disorder that is thought to occur during periods of frustration or anxiety and may be reinforced by affording escape from anxiety-inducing situations (Kanner, 1972). Childhood psychogenic vomiting also may have a cyclical pattern, occurring several days in succession and then subsiding for months at a time (Reinhart, Evans, & McFadden, 1977). Psychogenic vomiting is more prevalent in young and middle-age adults than in children and is five times more prevalent in females than in males (Morgan, 1985). By contrast, the onset of rumination usually occurs in infancy, and the prevalence of rumination is apparently higher in males than in females (Mayes, Humphrey, Handford, & Mitchell, 1988). The diagnosis of childhood psychogenic vomiting is often complicated because both psychological and physiological factors (e.g., GI hypomotility) frequently contribute to vomiting in the same child (Gonzalez-Heydrich, Kerner, & Steiner, 1991).

Table 9.2 summarizes some features that differentiate rumination, vomiting, psychogenic vomiting, and GER. These differences constitute part of the basis of a "bedside" differential diagnosis. Workup of possible organic factors for vomiting should always be pursued (see Chapter 2).

Table 9.2. Some distinctions among rumination, vomiting, psychogenic vomiting, and GER

Symptom or population	Rumination	Vomiting	Psychogenic vomiting	GER
Nausea	No	Yes	No	Seldom
Subjective distress	No	Yes	No	Often
Voluntary	Yes	No	Yes	No
Gastric contents expelled	No	Yes	Yes	Seldom
Volume expelled (per bout)	Small	Large	Usually small	Varies
Postprandial	Usually	Sometimes	Sometimes; may also interrupt meals	Often
Weight loss	Sometimes	Acute	Seldom	Sometimes
Ages and developmental conditions	Infants; children and adults with severe/ profound mental retardation	All	Typically young adults; typically female; rare in middle childhood	All; common and usually benign in infancy

Consequences Children who ruminate are at risk for dehydration, electrolyte imbalance, weight loss, malnutrition, dental problems, esophageal inflammation, aspiration, increased transmission of disease (e.g., viral hepatitis), social ostracism, developmental regression, and interference with educational programming. In some cases, rumination can be life threatening (Kanner, 1972; Sajwaj, Libet, & Agras, 1974).

Prevalence There have been no systematic studies of the prevalence of infantile rumination. Kanner (1972) reported that .07% of infants admitted to an acute-care pediatric hospital displayed rumination. Prevalence estimates in institutions for people who have mental retardation have been considerably higher, with a prevalence of 6% reported by Singh (1981) and a prevalence of 9.6% reported by Ball, Hendricksen, and Clayton (1974). In a literature review of 66 published cases, Mayes et al. (1988) found that the incidence of rumination was more than five times higher in males than in females. This differential incidence held both for rumination in infants, for whom developmental delay was rarely specified, and for individuals of various ages who have mental retardation.

Etiology

The etiology of ruminative behavior is largely a matter of speculation. Although it is occasionally suggested (Herbst, Friedland, & Zboralske, 1971) that rumination is caused solely by organic factors (e.g., hiatal hernia), it is more often assumed that psychosocial factors such as caregiver competence (e.g., dysfunctional maternal–child relationship), interaction (e.g., misplaced social contingencies), or some interaction of these variables with illness (e.g., GER) are responsible for the emergence of this feeding disorder.

Disturbed Mother–Infant Relationship For many years, maternal deprivation or a dysfunctional parent–child relationship was the most widely suspected cause of rumination in infants and children with no obvious organic problems. The high prevalence of rumination in infants in institutions (by implication, an environment characterized by total maternal deprivation) and the clinical observation that some mothers of infant ruminators presented as anxious, depressed, immature, or mechanical in their interactions were used to support the view that a disordered maternal–child relationship was responsible for rumination (Richmond, Eddy, & Green, 1958; Sauvage, Leddet, Hameury, & Barthelemy, 1985). The parents of many infant ruminators, however, present as capable, warm, and nurturant (Lavigne, Burns, & Cotter, 1981). Furthermore, as is noted in previous chapters, causation cannot safely be inferred from a correlation between parent characteristics and childhood eating disorders. For example, Sauvage et al. (1985) observed many mothers of infant ruminators to be over-anxious and depressed, but whether these maternal emotional characteristics are the cause or the result of infant rumination is not clear.

Social and Sensory Reinforcement It also has been argued that ruminative behavior is learned and maintained by differential reinforcement (Lavigne et al., 1981). Rumination may be strengthened (positively reinforced) if it effectively recruits social attention or if it serves to avoid or terminate some negative event (e.g., the departure of a caregiver). Ruminative behavior also may be strengthened if it produces pleasurable sensory consequences (e.g., the oropharyngeal stimulation of reconsuming a meal), a process sometimes called self-reinforcement or sensory reinforcement. The view that rumination is self-reinforcing is consistent with the observation that the occurrence of the behavior does not seem to depend on the presence of a caregiver and that the child appears to derive intense pleasure from the act of ruminating.

These etiological hypotheses are not mutually exclusive. For example, both an organic predisposition and caregiver factors might provide the context in which ruminative behavior becomes reinforcing to the child. A child with GER may regurgitate more frequently and, therefore, have more opportunities to "discover" that rumination can provide social or sensory reinforcement. The same child is more likely to find rumination pleasurable if other sources of stimulation and reinforcement (e.g., parental nurturance) are less available. Anxious parental interactions during feeding can influence GI functioning (e.g., by decreasing GI motility) and, thereby, increase the likelihood of regurgitation (Fleisher, 1994). It also has been suggested that specific biological mechanisms, such as the release of endogenous opiates (endorphins), may underlie both maternal–infant attachment and the seemingly addictive pleasures of rumination (Blinder, Goodman, & Goldstein, 1988; Chatoor, Dickson, & Einhorn, 1984). According to this hypothesis, infants are physiologically dependent on their mothers for endorphin stimulation and a disruption of infant–mother attachment leads to endorphin withdrawal. Infants with a propensity for or a history of reflux and vomiting discover that rumination also releases endogenous opiates. For these infants, rumination becomes the biological equivalent of maternal attachment.

Intervention

A broad range of intervention modalities have been used for rumination in infants and young children. Therapeutic nurturing, contingency management (using either positive or negative consequences), modified feeding techniques, and satiation all have received some empirical support and are discussed in this section.

Therapeutic Nurturing The most frequently reported intervention for infantile rumination is the planned therapeutic provision of some type of "intense nurturing" to correct a perceived deficiency in the parent–child relationship. Therapeutic nurturing is undertaken during hospitalization and usually includes the following elements: 1) provision of a mother "surrogate," most often a nurse; 2) intensive, noncontingent social attention directed to the child for most of the day; 3) individual parent and family psychotherapy; and 4) modeling of infant nurturing techniques (Blinder et al., 1988; Franco, Campbell, Tamburrino, & Evans, 1993). Although therapeutic nurturing is frequently reported to be effective, it is an often lengthy, relatively expensive intervention. It is also a multi-element intervention, and the individual treatment elements are often poorly defined and their necessity and efficacy not empirically established.

One exception is a study by Whitehead, Drescher, Morrill-Corbin, and Cataldo (1985) that empirically demonstrated the effectiveness of a simple holding treatment for rumination in young children. This technique calls for holding the child for a designated period of time (e.g., 10 minutes) before, during, and after a meal. Substantial decreases in rumination were achieved within a few days using this intervention with three children. Time-out was required to suppress rumination in a fourth child. Whitehead et al. (1985) argued that holding is the effective component of many of the therapeutic nurturing studies using surrogate mothers. As they pointed out, scheduled holding is not a technique that easily lends itself to the treatment of rumination in older children or adults.

Contingency Management Both reinforcing consequences and punishing consequences have been used in interventions for rumination. Several critical reviews published in the 1980s provide a detailed consideration of the empirical studies, many of which were conducted with adults with mental retardation (Holvoet, 1982; Starin & Fuqua, 1987). The following discussion emphasizes some representative studies with children.

Reinforcement Procedures There are surprisingly few published studies that provide convincing demonstrations of the clinical efficacy of positive reinforcement procedures to reduce or eliminate rumination. Two types of interventions have been evaluated: DRO and differential reinforcement of incompatible behavior (DRI). DRO reinforcement schedules program reinforcement after some designated interval in which the undesirable behavior has *not* occurred. For example, a ruminating child might be reinforced with praise or with an edible reward after each 1-minute interval in which rumination has not occurred. In a DRI schedule, reinforcement is programmed to occur whenever behavior that is *incompatible* with rumination occurs. For example, a child who self-induces rumination by placing a finger in her mouth might be rewarded for stacking blocks or for some other form of play that requires use of both hands. Mulick, Schroeder, and Rojahn (1980) investigated the use of both DRO and DRI schedules of reinforcement in the intervention for a 15-year-old boy with Down syndrome. DRI was found to be superior to DRO in this study, but neither procedure resulted in the complete cessation of rumination. O'Neil, White, King, and Carek (1979) also obtained moderate decreases in ruminative behavior using a DRO schedule with a 2-year-old girl with mental retardation. Barmann (1980) achieved clinically meaningful reductions in ruminative vomiting in a 6-year-old boy with profound mental retardation by using a DRO schedule of vibratory stimulation, contingent on the absence of hand-mouthing.

There are no published studies supporting the use of positive reinforcement procedures alone as an intervention technique for infantile (children younger than 2 years old) rumination. There are several possible reasons for this. First, rumination in infants can be life threatening, and this special urgency may argue for the use of more intensive procedures, which might be expected to have rapid effects. Second, positive reinforcement procedures require that the child be observed continuously, even when the events of concern are not in evidence. This can be difficult to arrange. Third, the types of reinforcers that are commonly available for infants may not compete effectively with the self-reinforcing value of rumination.

Punishment Procedures   The majority of contingency management studies have used some type of punishment contingent on rumination. Electric shock, aversive taste, time-out, and verbal reprimands all have been used with varying degrees of success. Electric shock has been used with infants, children, and adults; all of the published studies using electric shock with infants (Cunningham & Linscheid, 1976; Lang & Melamed, 1969; Linscheid & Cunningham, 1977; Toister, Condron, Worley, & Arthur, 1975) report total or substantial decrease in rumination within a few days and a complete absence of rumination at follow-up. Use of electric shock appears to be a rapid and effective procedure for eliminating rumination in infants, and it could be considered in life-threatening cases in which other treatments have failed. Electric shock is not, however, well-accepted by parents or professional staff.

The use of aversive tastes (e.g., lemon juice, hot pepper sauce) contingent on rumination also has been frequently employed (Becker, Turner, & Sajwaj, 1978; Sajwaj et al., 1974). Although use of aversive tastes may appear to be more benign than electric shock, this intervention is generally reported to be less successful (Whitehead & Schuster, 1985).

Time-out from reinforcement is a relatively benign punishment procedure in which social attention is withdrawn contingent on inappropriate behavior (see Chapter 4). Madison and Adubato (1984) described an outpatient intervention used in the elimination of rumination in a 15-month-old boy with GER, using response contingent withdrawal of parental attention, signaled by a loud click and the word "no." Withdrawal of social attention also was used in an inpatient intervention with a 9-month-old girl, described by Wright, Brown, and Andrews (1978). Nursing staff in this study were instructed to leave the room immediately when rumination occurred and not to clean the child until 3 minutes had elapsed. Parents then were trained in the use of this procedure and were asked to use it after discharge.

Another minimally intrusive and easily implemented form of aversive stimulation is a loud "no." This was one component in the intervention used by Madison and Adubato (1984). Lavigne et al. (1981) also described a successful intervention that included a loud "no," as did Chatoor et al. (1984).

Modified Feeding Techniques   Variations in feeding techniques have been reported to decrease rumination in some studies conducted with individuals who have mental retardation. Ball et al. (1974) reported on an intervention that encouraged more "active" participation in feeding with two boys who had profound mental retardation. Specific techniques to increase active participation included playing "tug-of-war" with the nipple of the bottle, tapping the spoon on the teeth to stimulate biting, moving the lip of the cup around the lips, and encouraging active biting and chewing.

Alteration of feeding rate by spacing eating (dividing each of the regular three meals into five portions, separated by 15 minutes each) and by using prompts and differential reinforcement to encourage moderate bites of food and swallowing between bites have been shown to reduce vomiting in adults who have mental retardation (Azrin, Jamner, & Besalel, 1987). In Azrin et al.'s (1987) study, two of the three participants ruminated as well as vomited, but rumination was not directly measured in this study. Spaced eating may be effective because the gastric volume of each meal is reduced or because oral satisfaction is increased by the interventions directed at bite size and at moderated eating rate.

Satiation   Satiation refers to a decrease in the probability of a response resulting from free access to the reinforcer maintaining that response. Use of satiation to eliminate rumination involves providing the individual with unlimited amounts of food during or after a meal until eating is voluntarily discontinued. Successful use of this intervention with adults who have mental retardation was first reported by Jackson, Johnson, Ackron, and Crowley (1975), but the variables responsible for the effectiveness of satiation have not yet been fully explicated. Some dietary variables that appear to be important—but not sufficient—factors in satiation are meal size (Rast, Johnston, Drum, & Conrin, 1981), the caloric density of the meal (Rast, Johnston, Ellinger-Allen, & Drum, 1985), and increased food texture/consistency (Johnston, Greene, Vazin, Rawal, & Chung, 1990).

Satiation interventions have been accomplished by 1) simply providing unlimited portions of the regular meal, 2) providing double portions, 3) providing unlimited starches (e.g., mashed potatoes, bread) during and/or after meals, 4) providing foods with specific textures or consistencies (e.g., peanut butter) during and/or after meals, and/or 5) providing between-meal "snacks" (e.g., milkshakes).

Excessive weight gain is one obvious potential side effect of satiation. Because many chronic ruminators are underweight, this is an initially desirable outcome, but in the longer term, excessive weight gain is a potential drawback. Two approaches have been taken to deal with the problem of excessive weight gain: Lobato, Carlson, and Barrera (1986) used low-calorie foods (e.g., fresh fruits and vegetables, diet soda, diluted fruit juice) to limit weight gain; two other studies (Clauser & Scibak, 1990; Yang, 1988) successfully used fading (gradual reduction) of the amount of food offered during satiation.

As of this writing, there have been no reports describing the successful use of satiation for rumination with children who do not have mental retardation or with infant ruminators. It is unclear whether satiation simply has not been tried or, as Mayes et al. (1988) suggested, that distinct etiologies are responsible for rumination in these different populations, and one would therefore not expect satiation to be effective with "psychogenic rumination." Table 9.3 summarizes clinical guidelines for the evaluation of and intervention for rumination.

The following case illustrates the use of a satiation procedure in treating rumination in a child hospitalized for chronic rumination and vomiting.

■ ■ ■

CASE 9.2. INPATIENT TREATMENT OF A CHILD WITH RUMINATION
NAME: Billy
AGE AT INTERVENTION: 4 years, 11 months

BACKGROUND

At birth, Billy weighed 7 pounds, 10 ounces. Although he had an uneventful 38-week gestation, his neonatal course was complicated by hypotonia and repeated episodes of cyanosis during feeding, for which he was hospitalized. An extensive workup failed to define any specific cause for Billy's feeding difficulties, and he was discharged home. At age 5 months, he continued to be a "poor feeder" who had difficulty coordinating sucking with breathing but who managed to

Table 9.3. Clinical guidelines for evaluation of and intervention for rumination

EVALUATION
- Is the child ruminating? Have alternative diagnoses (e.g., vomiting, psychogenic vomiting, GER) been ruled out?
- Has there been an adequate medical workup and optimal management of any concurrent organic conditions?
- What are the associated health risks (e.g., dehydration, electrolyte imbalance), and are they appropriately managed?
- Do associated health risks call for hospitalization?
- If rumination is diagnosed, then which factors contribute to the behavior?
  - Quality of parent–child interaction?
  - Reinforced by caregiver attention?
  - Reinforced by avoidance or termination of negative event?
  - Reinforced by sensory factors (self-stimulatory)?
  - If self-stimulatory, which property of the behavior seems to be reinforcing?

INTERVENTION
- Scheduled holding or other appropriate therapeutic nurturing intervention should be considered as the intervention of first choice for infant rumination.
- Parent–child interaction therapies should be implemented, if needed.
- If therapeutic nurturing is ineffective, or if rumination is maintained by social contingencies, consider time-out and/or a loud verbal reprimand.
- If rumination appears to be maintained by sensory consequences and does not respond to scheduled holding, consider a satiation procedure or modified feeding techniques.
- If contributory factors are unclear, or if other interventions have been ineffective, and health or social risks are significant, consider use of other contingent negative consequences.

gain weight at a satisfactory rate. Billy was also described as an unusually sleepy baby who had poor eye contact and who "hated to be held." At age 7 months, his weight and length were at the 50th percentile; but his developmental age was estimated to be between 1 and 4 months. Brain imaging studies conducted at that time revealed diffuse abnormalities, more evident on the right side than on the left, and he was given a provisional diagnosis of cerebral atrophy of unknown etiology. Billy's subsequent developmental progress was very slow, but there was no evidence of regression. His cognitive skills at the time of the intervention for rumination were estimated to be in the 4- to 8-month range, and his communication skills were especially limited. He also presented with hyperactivity, multiple stereotypic behaviors (e.g., spinning, hand posturing), labile mood, and atypical social interaction. Billy's parents presented as loving and very concerned but periodically overwhelmed. There was no evidence of parent–child disturbance or significant family dysfunction. Billy had always lived at home and now received special education services in the public school system.

Billy's history of vomiting and rumination had originated with frequent spitting up during feeding in infancy; reconsumption of vomitus had become an established habit by the age of 7 months. Many interventions, including anti-reflux medications, frequent holding, and DRO, had been tried over the past 4 years; but none had been successful. Despite chronic rumination, Billy was usually able to gain weight at a satisfactory rate. He did have occasional periods of poor weight gain and had sustained a 15-pound weight loss prior to this intervention. He was able to eat any food with a ground texture and also small bites of soft table food that did not require chewing. He drank whole milk as well as a variety of juices, and his diet was occasionally supplemented with high-calorie formulas. There was no history of food intolerance or food sensitivity. Billy's self-feeding skills were delayed; for example, he could drink independently from a bottle but was unable to drink independently from a cup or to use a spoon to feed himself. Observation during hospitalization revealed rumination to be primarily a postprandial phenomenon, occurring more than 150 times, on the average, after each meal. Rumination frequency and duration were higher after meals with solid food than after liquid meals.

FORMULATION

Billy's rumination had no apparent social function and appeared to be self-stimulatory. Billy would mouth endlessly on objects and ingest nonnutritive substances indiscriminately and appeared to be powerfully reinforced by oropharyngeal stimulation of any kind. He always seemed ravenously hungry, did not appear to be readily sated by age-appropriate food portions, and appeared blissfully happy during meals and during bouts of rumination. The frequency and duration of rumination was unaffected by social context. It was hypothesized that postprandial rumination served to "prolong" the preceding meal, providing repeated oral stimulation as well as recurrent satiety sensations. It was possible that Billy's ruminative behavior had been strengthened, over the course of several years, by a "vicious cycle" in which rumination led to weight loss, weight loss led to increased hunger, and increased hunger resulted in the increased value of regurgitating and reconsuming meals. Satiation seemed a promising intervention because it promised to break the cycle by minimizing hunger and by maximizing oral stimulation.

INTERVENTION

There were several phases of treatment. The first, to decrease vomiting, was a dietary intervention that involved limiting Billy's diet to high-calorie formula (which seemed to result in less rumination) and adding cornstarch to the formula. The assumption was that thickened feeds would be more difficult to regurgitate and, if regurgitated, would be less likely to be accidentally expelled. The cornstarch was added to a carbohydrate-free formula to maintain nutritional balance in Billy's diet. This dietary intervention succeeded in dramatically reducing the amount of expelled vomitus but had little effect on rumination.

A brief satiation period, following unlimited feeding of mashed potatoes after each meal, was then tried but found to be ineffective. A subsequent behavioral analysis found that rumination would decrease when meal frequency was increased. Hourly meals of formula with cornstarch were then instituted until Billy's rumination was virtually eliminated. At this point, small portions of solid foods were gradually reintroduced into the diet. Solid foods were offered in small bites, with a 10- to 15-second interval between bites, a technique that served to prolong each meal and to maximize oral stimulation.

OUTCOME

Figure 9.1 shows the frequency of rumination as a function of meal frequency when Billy's meals consisted of formula plus cornstarch. Meals scheduled every hour (Q1 in Figure 9.1) resulted in less rumination than meals scheduled every 4 hours (Q4) or every 2 hours (Q2). Fig-

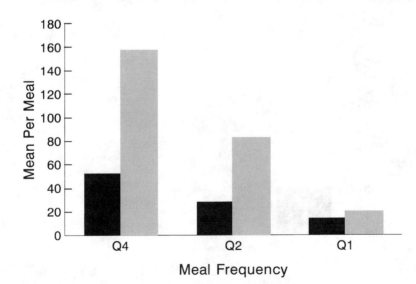

Figure 9.1. Frequency of postprandial rumination (formula and cornstarch) as a function of meal frequency. (Key: ■, duration; ▓, frequency.)

ure 9.2 shows the same meal frequency effect after solid meals were re-introduced. Billy continued on a schedule of hourly "meals" of formula with cornstarch and three meals daily of his usual diet, using the technique of paced feeding. Over the course of several weeks, Billy no longer finished all of the bottles of formula he was offered, and he would occasionally reject them altogether, indicating that he was indeed becoming sated. Billy regained the weight that he had lost prior to hospitalization and was discharged with the recommendation that he continue to be offered formula with cornstarch every hour, as well as for breakfast, lunch, and dinner, using the paced-feeding technique. This intervention was well accepted by Billy's family and continued to be effective in minimizing rumination and supporting appropriate weight gain after discharge from the hospital.

■ ■ ■

SUMMARY

Pica and rumination are feeding disorders of inappropriate intake with significant potential health consequences. Pica, the persistent ingestion of nonnutritive substances, is relatively common between the ages of 18 and 36 months but is increasingly rare thereafter. Ru-

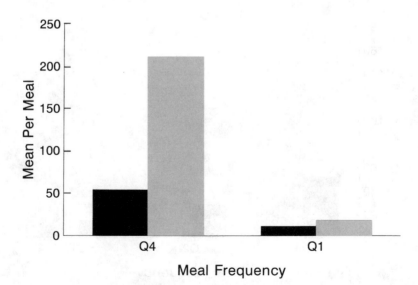

Figure 9.2.   Meal frequency effect of postprandial rumination (solid foods) after re-introduction of solid meals. (Key: ■, duration; ■, frequency.)

mination, the voluntary ingestion of previously consumed foods, is relatively rare at any age. As with early childhood disorders of insufficient, selective, or excessive intake, disorders of inappropriate intake benefit from a biobehavioral conceptualization and intervention. Behavioral interventions, including differential reinforcement, punishment, and stimulus-control procedures, have been applied to both pica and rumination with variable success. Nutritional supplements, environmental enrichment, and discrimination training are additional potentially useful interventions for pica. Rumination is reported to respond to therapeutic nurturing, contingency management, modified feeding techniques, and satiation.

REFERENCES

American Psychiatric Association. (1994). *Diagnostic and statistical manual of mental disorders* (4th ed.). Washington, DC: Author.

Azrin, N.H., Jamner, J.P., & Besalel, V.A. (1987). The rate and amount of food intake as determinants of vomiting. *Behavioral Residential Treatment, 2,* 211–221.

Ball, T.S., Hendricksen, H., & Clayton, J. (1974). A special feeding technique for chronic regurgitation. *American Journal of Mental Deficiency, 78,* 486–493.

Barltrop, D. (1966). The prevalence of pica. *American Journal of Diseases of Children, 112,* 116–123.

Barmann, B.C. (1980). Use of contingent vibration in the treatment of self-stimulatory hand-mouthing and rumination vomiting behavior. *Journal of Behavior Therapy and Experimental Psychiatry, 11,* 307–311.

Becker, J.V., Turner, S.M., & Sajwaj, T.E. (1978). Multiple behavioral effects of the use of lemon juice with a ruminating toddler-age child. *Behavior Modification, 2,* 267–268.

Bell, K.E., & Stein, D.M. (1992). Behavioral treatments for pica: A review of empirical studies. *International Journal of Eating Disorders, 11,* 377–389.

Blinder, B.J., Goodman, S.L., & Goldstein, R. (1988). Rumination: A critical review of diagnosis and treatment. In B.J. Blinder, B.F. Chaitlin, & R. Goldstein (Eds.), *The eating disorders: Medical and psychological bases of diagnosis and treatment* (pp. 315–329). New York: PMA Publishing.

Chatoor, I., Dickson, L., & Einhorn, A. (1984). Rumination: Etiology and treatment. *Pediatric Annals, 13,* 924–929.

Clauser, B., & Scibak, J.W. (1990). Direct and generalized effects of food satiation in reducing rumination. *Research in Developmental Disabilities, 11,* 23–36.

Cunningham, C.E., & Linscheid, T.R. (1976). Elimination of chronic infant ruminating by electric shock. *Behavior Therapy, 7,* 231–234.

Danford, D.A. (1982). Pica and nutrition. *Annual Review of Nutrition, 2,* 303–322.

Favell, J.E., McGimsey, J., & Schell, R. (1982). Treatment of self-injury by providing alternate sensory activities. *Analysis and Intervention in Developmental Disabilities, 2,* 83–104.

Finney, J.W., Russo, D.C., & Cataldo, M.F. (1982). Reduction of pica in young children with lead poisoning. *Journal of Pediatric Psychology, 7,* 197–207.

Fisher, W.C., Piazza, C.C., Bowman, L.G., Kurtz, P.F., Sherer, M.R., & Lachman, S.R. (1994). A preliminary evaluation of empirically derived consequences for the treatment of pica. *Journal of Applied Behavior Analysis, 27,* 447–457.

Fleisher, D.R. (1994). Functional vomiting disorders in infancy: Innocent vomiting, nervous vomiting, and infant rumination syndrome. *Journal of Pediatrics, 125,* S84–S94.

Franco, K., Campbell, N., Tamburrino, M., & Evans, C. (1993). Rumination: The eating disorder of infancy. *Childhood Psychiatry and Human Development, 24,* 91–97.

Gonzalez-Heydrich, J., Kerner, J.A., & Steiner, H. (1991). Testing the psychogenic vomiting diagnosis: Four pediatric patients. *American Journal of Diseases of Children, 145,* 913–916.

Hanson, J.S., & McCallum, R.W. (1985). The diagnosis and management of nausea and vomiting: A review. *The American Journal of Gastroenterology, 80,* 210–218.

Herbst, J., Friedland, G.W., & Zboralske, F.F. (1971). Hiatal hernia and rumination in infants and children. *Journal of Pediatrics, 78,* 261–265.

Holvoet, J.F. (1982). The etiology and management of rumination and psychogenic vomiting: A review. In J.H. Hollis & C.E. Meyers (Eds.), *Life threatening behavior: Analysis and intervention* (pp. 29–77). Washington, DC: American Association on Mental Deficiency.

Jackson, G.M., Johnson, C.R., Ackron, G.S., & Crowley, R. (1975). Food satiation as a procedure to decelerate vomiting. *American Journal of Mental Deficiency, 80,* 223–227.

Johnston, J.M., Greene, K., Vazin, T., Rawal, A., & Chung, S. (1990). Effects of food consistency on ruminating. *The Psychological Record, 40,* 609–618.

Kanner, L. (1972). *Child psychiatry* (4th ed.). Springfield, IL: Charles C Thomas.

Korman, S.H. (1990). Pica as a presenting symptom in childhood celiac disease. *American Journal of Clinical Nutrition, 51,* 139–141.

Lacey, E.P. (1990). Broadening the perspective of pica: Literature review. *Public Health Reports, 105,* 29–35.

Lang, P.J., & Melamed, B.G. (1969). Case report: Avoidance conditioning therapy of an infant with chronic ruminative vomiting. *Journal of Abnormal Psychology, 74,* 1–8.

Lavigne, J.V., Burns, W.J., & Cotter, P.D. (1981). Rumination in infancy: Recent behavioral approaches. *International Journal of Eating Disorders, 1,* 70–82.

Linscheid, T.R., & Cunningham, C.E. (1977). A controlled demonstration of the effectiveness of electric shock in the elimination of chronic infant rumination. *Journal of Applied Behavior Analysis, 10,* 500.

Lobato, D., Carlson, E.I., & Barrera, R.B. (1986). Modified satiation: Reducing ruminative vomiting without excessive weight gain. *Applied Research in Mental Retardation, 7,* 337–347.

Madden, N.A., Russo, D.C., & Cataldo, M.F. (1980). Environmental influences on mouthing in children with lead intoxication. *Journal of Pediatric Psychology, 5,* 207–216.

Madison, L.S., & Adubato, S.A. (1984). The elimination of ruminative vomiting in a 15-month-old child with gastroesophageal reflux. *Journal of Pediatric Psychology, 9,* 231–239.

Marchi, M., & Cohen, P. (1990). Early childhood eating behaviors and adolescent eating disorders. *Journal of the American Academy of Child and Adolescent Psychiatry, 29,* 112–117.

Mayes, S.D., Humphrey, F.J., Handford, H.A., & Mitchell, J.F. (1988). Rumination disorder: Differential diagnosis. *Journal of the American Academy of Child and Adolescent Psychiatry, 27,* 300–302.

Millican, F.K., Layman, E.M., Lourie, R.S., & Takahashi, L.Y. (1968). Study of an oral fixation. *Journal of the American Academy of Child Psychiatry, 7,* 79–107.

Morgan, H.G. (1985). Functional vomiting. *Journal of Psychosomatic Research, 29,* 341–352.

Mulick, J.A., Schroeder, S.R., & Rojahn, J. (1980). Chronic ruminative vomiting: A comparison of four treatment procedures. *Journal of Autism and Developmental Disorders, 10,* 203–213.

Nelson, K. (1995). Feeding problems. In S. Parker & B. Zuckerman (Eds.), *Behavioral and developmental pediatrics: A handbook of primary care* (pp. 143–148). Boston: Little, Brown.

O'Neil, P.M., White, J.L., King, C.R., & Carek, D.J. (1979). Controlling childhood rumination through differential reinforcement of other behavior. *Behavior Modification, 3,* 355–372.

Paniagua, F.A., Braverman, C., & Capriotti, R.M. (1986). Use of a treatment package in the management of a profoundly mentally retarded girl's pica and self-stimulation. *American Journal of Mental Deficiency, 90,* 550–557.

Parry-Jones, B., & Parry-Jones, W.L. (1992). Pica: Symptom or eating disorder? A historical assessment. *British Journal of Psychiatry, 160,* 341–354.

Pueschel, S.M. (1988). On effective prevention of mental retardation. In D.C. Russo & J.H. Kedesdy (Eds.), *Behavioral medicine with the developmentally disabled* (pp. 201–209). New York: Plenum.

Pueschel, S.M., Cullen, S.M., Howard, R.B., & Cullinane, M.M. (1977). Pathogenetic considerations of pica in lead poisoning. *International Journal of Psychiatry in Medicine, 8,* 13–24.

Rast, J., Johnston, J.M., Drum, C., & Conrin, J. (1981). The relation of food quantity to ruminative behavior. *Journal of Applied Behavior Analysis, 14,* 121–130.

Rast, J., Johnston, J.M., Ellinger-Allen, J., & Drum, C. (1985). Effects of nutritional and mechanical properties of food on ruminative behavior. *Journal of the Experimental Analysis of Behavior, 44,* 195–206.

Reinhart, J.B., Evans, S.L., & McFadden, D.L. (1977). Cyclic vomiting in children: Seen through the psychiatrist's eye. *Pediatrics, 59,* 371–377.

Richmond, J.B., Eddy, E., & Green, M. (1958). Rumination: A psychosomatic syndrome of infancy. *Pediatrics, 22,* 49–54.

Robischon, P. (1971). Pica practice and other hand–mouth behavior and children's developmental level. *Nursing Research, 20,* 4–16.

Sajwaj, T., Libet, J., & Agras, S. (1974). Lemon juice therapy: The control of life-threatening rumination in a six-month old infant. *Journal of Applied Behavior Analysis, 7,* 557–563.

Sauvage, D., Leddet, I., Hameury, L., & Barthelemy, C. (1985). Infantile rumination: Diagnosis and follow-up study of twenty cases. *Journal of the American Academy of Child Psychiatry, 24,* 197–203.

Shepard, R.W., Wren, J., Evans, S., Lander, M., & Ong, T.H. (1987). Gastroesophageal reflux in children. *Clinical Pediatrics, 26,* 55–60.

Singh, N.N. (1981). Rumination. In N.F. Ellis (Ed.), *International review of research in mental retardation* (Vol. 10, pp. 139–182). New York: Academic Press.

Smulian, J.C., Motiwala, S., & Sigman, R.K. (1995). Pica in a rural obstetric population. *Southwestern Medical Journal, 88,* 1236–1240.

Starin, S.P., & Fuqua, R.W. (1987). Rumination and vomiting in the developmentally disabled: A critical review of the behavioral, medical, and psychiatric treatment research. *Research in Developmental Disabilities, 8,* 575–605.

Toister, R.P., Condron, C.J., Worley, L., & Arthur, D. (1975). Faradic therapy of chronic vomiting in infancy: A case study. *Journal of Behavior Therapy and Experimental Psychiatry, 6,* 55–59.

Whitehead, W.E., Drescher, V.M., Morrill-Corbin, E., & Cataldo, M.F. (1985). Rumination syndrome in children treated by increased holding. *Journal of Pediatric Gastroenterology and Nutrition, 4,* 550–556.

Whitehead, W.E., & Schuster, M.M. (1985). *Gastrointestinal disorders: Behavioral and physiological basis for treatment.* New York: Academic Press.

Woolston, J.L. (1991). *Eating and growth disorders in infants and young children.* Beverly Hills: Sage Publications.

Wright, D.F., Brown, R.A., & Andrews, M.E. (1978). Remission of chronic ruminative vomiting through the reversal of social contingencies. *Behaviour Research and Therapy, 16,* 134–136.

Yang, L. (1988). Elimination of habitual rumination through strategies of food satiation and fading: A case study. *Behavioral Residential Treatment, 3,* 223–234.

Zeitlin, S.B., & Polivy, J. (1995). Coprophagia as a manifestation of obsessive-compulsive disorder: A case report. *Journal of Behavior Therapy and Experimental Psychiatry, 26,* 57–63.

Children Who Eat Too Much

Obesity and Hyperphagia

10

Children who "eat too much" usually come to the attention of health care professionals because questions are raised about the possible negative health consequences of overeating (chiefly obesity) or, less frequently, because there is concern that conspicuous overeating may be symptomatic of pathology (e.g., as in Prader-Willi syndrome [PWS]). Both of these clinical issues are addressed in this chapter, but obesity—because of its higher prevalence and its recognized association with negative medical sequelae—receives more detailed coverage. It should be noted at the outset that the question of whether obese children do, in fact, "eat too much" is a matter of ongoing debate.

PEDIATRIC OBESITY

The imperative to intervene with children who eat selectively, who are underweight, or who eat the wrong things usually exceeds the clinical urgency associated with childhood obesity. Indeed, there is controversy over whether overweight children should be treated at all (see Mallick, 1983; Wooley & Garner, 1994). There are several reasons for the relative hesitancy to treat childhood obesity. First, the consequences of both overeating and obesity are delayed. A relatively small imbalance of daily energy intake can result in obesity. For example, a 3-year-old boy with a weight-for-age at the 50th percentile can attain a weight-for-age above the 95th percentile within a year by consuming as few as 80 excess kilocalories per day—the energy in an single apple. "Excesses" of this magnitude easily go unnoticed until they have had time to accumulate. The negative health consequences of obesity in childhood are also largely delayed, compared with the more immediate health risks of obesity in adults. Second, there is evidence that obesity, at least in infancy and

343

in early childhood, has a high rate of spontaneous remission (Dietz, 1984). This supports the often-heard advice that children who are obese will "grow out of it." Third, because there is considerable evidence that genetic factors significantly predispose an individual to obesity, as well as discouraging independent evidence about the long-term efficacy of weight management programs for adults, the utility of intervening with children can be and has been questioned. Fourth, there is growing concern about the potential psychological risks of child weight management. Body image dissatisfaction and preoccupation with body weight are pervasive in Western cultures, and children—especially adolescent females—are at increasing risk for developing eating disorders, which are engendered by fears of becoming fat and the pursuit of unattainable ideal body types (Brownell & Wadden, 1991).

Whether overeating or obesity in children should be considered a pediatric feeding or eating disorder also is controversial. Woolston (1991) has commented on the absence of a code for obesity in the revised third edition of the *Diagnostic and Statistical Manual of Mental Disorders* (DSM-III-R) (American Psychiatric Association, 1987), and this has not changed in the fourth edition, DSM-IV (American Psychiatric Association, 1994). DSM-IV, however, does list research criteria for a Binge-Eating Disorder (see the section entitled Etiology: Emotional Factors in this chapter).

Despite the lack of consensus, a strong case can be made for intervening to reduce the social and health risks associated with pediatric obesity. Epstein (1990) has advanced several reasons why interventions for children who are obese should be considered: 1) Many children who are overweight are at risk for becoming obese adults, and treatment at an early age may help prevent adult obesity; 2) because children have a shorter history of maladaptive eating patterns than adults, their behavior may be easier to change; 3) it is easier to mobilize social support for intervention in childhood, because parents can be involved in treatment; and 4) whereas adults can become less obese only by losing weight, children also can achieve the same result by maintaining weight and by growing taller.

Perhaps most important, behavioral intervention for childhood obesity appears to be relatively effective. For at least some children (about 30%), weight loss can be maintained for periods of at least 10 years (Epstein, Valoski, Wing, & McCurley, 1994). The relative success of the child weight management interventions summarized by Epstein et al. (1994) stands in contrast to the discouraging results of similar interventions with adults (Brownell & Wadden, 1992) and suggests that there may be a narrow window of opportunity to intervene successfully with obesity. The components of successful pediatric weight management are reviewed after a discussion of the definition, prevalence, persistence, and etiology of childhood obesity.

Definition

Obesity, in both children and adults, is generally defined as an excess of body fat. Body fat, or adiposity, in children must be measured indirectly, and some measurement error is introduced with all widely used estimates of obesity. Many measures of adiposity, including radiography, determination of total body potassium, total body water, or body density determined by hydrostatic weighing, are too expensive and/or invasive for clinical practice (Kraemer, Berkowitz, & Hammer, 1990). The most widely used clinical measure of adiposity is relative body weight (RW). An RW that is 20% greater than the ideal body weight (IBW)—the median weight for height, age, and gender—is often the recommended criterion for obesity (Israel, 1990). One shortcoming of RW as a measure of obesity is that it is tied to a reference population, and the characteristics of the reference population may not be stable or completely representative. For example, the National Health and Nutrition Examination Survey, which forms the basis for the most widely used children's growth curves, has been criticized for oversampling from lower socioeconomic groups. An especially important consideration in evaluating pediatric obesity is that the reference population is thought to be growing rapidly more adipose (see the section entitled Prevalence).

Body mass index (BMI), which is also based on measures of weight and height, is another frequently used estimate of excess adiposity. BMI is defined as weight (in kilograms) divided by height (in meters) squared (W/H^2). For example, a child with a weight of 36.6 kilograms and a height of 1.2 meters would have a BMI of 25.4 ($36.6/[1.2]^2$). This measure normalizes weight-for-height, is independent of standard tables, and correlates reasonably well with other measures of adiposity (Foreyt & Goodrick, 1988). It is important to note that the relationship between BMI and age is not linear in childhood (Hammer, Kraemer, Wilson, Ritter, & Dornbusch, 1991). For example, a BMI of 18 for boys falls at about the 95th percentile for a 4-year-old and at about the 5th percentile for an 18-year-old. A BMI equal to or greater than the 85th percentile often is used to define obesity.

Measuring obesity by means of body weight and height is both convenient and practical. Body weight is a function of both lean muscle and fat, however, and it is possible to be overweight without being obese and to be obese without being overweight. Other measures are therefore sometimes required. Because most fat is distributed beneath the skin, measurement of skinfold, especially triceps skinfold, is another useful clinical measure of obesity. Norms for triceps and subscapular skinfold are available, and a triceps skinfold in excess of the 85th percentile is the generally accepted diagnostic criterion for obesity (Garn & Clark, 1976). In cases in which weight-for-height is marginal, skinfold measures should be considered to confirm the diagnosis. Skinfold measures are not, however, without their problems: It is difficult to obtain reliable skinfold measures, especially in children; and population norms are not ethnically representative (Foreyt & Cousins, 1989).

Obesity clearly varies in severity, and a classification of obesity on the basis of severity has been proposed by several investigators (Brownell & Wadden, 1991; Stunkard, 1992). For example, mild, moderate, and severe obesity are defined by percentages overweight of 20%–40%, 41%–100%, and more than 100%, respectively. These percentages correspond approximately to adult BMI scores of 27–30, 30.1–35, and greater than 35, respectively.

Prevalence

The prevalence of obesity in adults and in children has increased significantly in the United States. From 1976 to 1980, more than 25% of the U.S. adult population was overweight (BMI greater than the 85th percentile) (Kuczmarski, 1992). A comparable study of the U.S. population from 1988 to 1991 estimated that 35% of adults were overweight (Kuczmarski, Flegal, Campbell, & Johnson, 1994). The prevalence of obesity in children in the United States also is increasing. Gortmaker, Dietz, Sobol, and Wehler (1987) analyzed triceps skinfold data in surveys of children from 1963 to 1980. Obesity was defined as triceps skinfolds equal to or greater than the 85th percentile, and superobesity was defined as skinfolds equal to or greater than the 95th percentile. Gortmaker et al. (1987) found a 54% increase in obesity among children 6–11 years old and a 98% increase in superobesity in the same age group. Likewise, they found a 39% increase in the prevalence of obesity among children 12–17 years old and a 64% increase in the prevalence of superobesity. Prevalence depends on age and gender, with a higher prevalence (and prevalence increase) in boys than in girls during preadolescence and a higher prevalence (and prevalence increase) in females than in males after age 12 (Gortmaker et al., 1987). Troiano, Flegal, Kuczmarski, Campbell, and Johnson (1995) found that the number of children and adolescents who are overweight continues to increase steadily and that 22% of children and adolescents between the ages of 6 and 17 are obese (BMI above the 85th percentile). Some studies have found a higher prevalence of obesity in minority and low socioeconomic status populations (Kumanyika, 1993; Sobal & Stunkard, 1989).

Persistence

Persistence, the issue of whether a child who is obese will remain obese and whether children who are obese become obese adults has important implications for treatment. In general, the older the child, the greater the likelihood that obesity will persist. The rate of spontaneous remission is very high in infancy; the majority of infants who are found to be obese in the first year are no longer obese at age 4 years (Dietz, 1984). But childhood obesity increasingly predicts adult obesity as the individual grows older. The percentage of obese children who become obese adults increases from 41% at age 7 to about 70% at ages 10–13 years (Epstein, Wing, & Valoski, 1985). Persistence also depends on the severity of obesity; the greater the severity, the lower the probability of spontaneous remission. There is little chance of remission of obesity in children with an RW greater than 130% (Dietz, 1987).

Consequences

The health risks of obesity in adults have been well documented. Excess body weight and mortality (particularly from cardiovascular disease) are directly related, as are obesity and morbidity in the form of hypertension, elevated serum cholesterol, diabetes mellitus, gallbladder disease, osteoarthritis, gout, abnormalities of pulmonary functioning, and cancer (Manson et al., 1995; Pi-Sunyer, 1991). The direct medical costs of obesity in the United States are estimated to be about $50 billion per year (Wolf & Colditz, 1996). The health risks of obesity during childhood are not as clearly established. Significant health problems are less frequent in childhood and occur primarily in children with severe obesity. The medical complications of obesity in childhood and adolescence include orthopedic problems (e.g., slipped capital femoral epiphysis), respiratory problems (e.g., Pickwickian syndrome), diabetes mellitus, and hypertension (Dietz, 1987). Whether obesity in childhood predicts adult morbidity is also debated. A study of overweight children in Sweden found that body weight at puberty predicted mortality and cardiovascular disease 40 years later but that being overweight prior to puberty was not associated with adult morbidity or mortality (DiPietro, Mossberg, & Stunkard, 1994).

Social stigma secondary to negative stereotyping is perhaps the most reliable and immediate risk of being overweight in childhood. Children who are obese are often less popular with peers, are often discriminated against by adults, and often have poorer self-concepts than normal-weight peers (Foreyt & Goodrick, 1988). For example, Strauss, Smith, Frame, and Forehand (1985) found that teachers and peers perceived children who are obese to have more behavior problems and to be less liked than children who are not obese. Children who are obese sometimes are perceived negatively by members of their own families (Kinston, Loader, & Miller, 1988). Being overweight during adolescence is associated with reduced socioeconomic status, including fewer years in school, lower income, and decreased likelihood of marriage (Gortmaker, Must, Perrin, Sobol, & Dietz, 1993).

Etiology

Although the causes of obesity are not completely understood, it is generally accepted that obesity results from a positive energy balance, in which more calories are consumed than expended and that multiple biological and environmental factors significantly affect energy balance and weight regulation.

Biological Factors Biological accounts of obesity tend to implicate either genetic or homeostatic mechanisms. In addition, there are a number of biologically based syndromes associated with obesity.

Heritability The evidence for a strong genetic contribution to obesity comes from several sources. First, studies comparing adopted children with their biological and adoptive families have shown that children more closely resemble their biological parents in adiposity (Stunkard et al., 1986). Second, studies of identical twins raised apart have shown that heritability accounts for about 70% of the variance in BMI (Stunkard, Harris, Pedersen, & McClearn, 1990). How genes control excess adiposity, however, is not well understood. At the behavioral level, genetic influence could be expressed as inherited differences in appetite, sensory predisposition to specific food preferences, physical activity levels, or some interaction of these variables with congenital metabolic differences (Bouchard & Perusse, 1993).

Homeostasis Set point and fat cell theory describe two biological mechanisms that have been proposed to account for constraints on variation in body weight as caloric intake varies. Set point theory proposes that changes in basic metabolic processes operate to produce relatively constant body weight (Keesey, 1986). Each individual has a predetermined basal metabolic rate, the rate at which the body burns fuel. As caloric intake decreases, however, basal metabolism decreases (less fuel is burned), and body weight consequently tends to remain constant. The opposite occurs when caloric intake increases because thermic metabolism (the metabolic activity associated with digesting food) increases.

Fat cell theory derives from the finding that both the number and the size of fat cells can vary widely in individuals. Individuals who are mildly obese have the same number of fat cells as individuals who are not obese; it is an increase in the size of the fat cells that accounts for excess adiposity in the mildly obese. Both the size and the number of fat cells are greater in individuals with severe obesity. In severely obese individuals, the number of adipose cells may increase by a factor of 2 or 3. Caloric restriction can reduce the size of fat cells but not their number, thus placing constraints on the amount of weight reduction possible in people who are severely obese. The increase in the number of fat cells tends to occur in childhood, though it also may occur later in life (Sjostrom, 1980).

Specific Syndromes Associated with Obesity Heritability and homeostasis are biological mechanisms that influence weight regulation in all members of a species. In addition, there are a number of relatively rare conditions or syndromes that are associated with obesity. These include Alstrom syndrome, Cohen syndrome, Cushing syndrome, Frolich syndrome (hypothalamic tumors), Laurence-Moon-Bardet-Biedl syndrome, PWS (see the section entitled Hyperphagia for more details on PWS), and Stein-Leventhal syndrome (polycystic ovaries). These syndromes are shown in Table 10.1. Some endocrine disorders (e.g., growth hormone deficiency, hypothyroidism) are associated with short stature and mild to moderate obesity. Other disorders (e.g., myelodysplasia) that limit energy expenditure also may lead to obesity. According to Dietz (1987), the syndromes discussed in this paragraph account for less than 1% of all cases of childhood obesity.

Environmental Factors Multiple environmental factors influence the acquisition and maintenance of obesity. Some of these factors (e.g., changes in the national diet) potentially affect all children; other factors (e.g., social learning, eating style) may vary across individuals and families.

Cultural Dietary Practices The increasing prevalence of both child and adult obesity in the United States appears to argue strongly for the influence of environmental factors on the expression of obesity. There have been significant changes in the American diet during the 20th century—notably an increase in the avail-

Table 10.1. Syndromes associated with obesity

Syndrome	Common symptoms
Alstrom syndrome	Nerve deafness, hypogonadism, early blindness, adult-resolution obesity
Cohen syndrome	Truncal obesity, short stature, delayed puberty, hypotonia, mental retardation
Cushing syndrome	Short stature, truncal obesity, buffalo hump, hypertension, violaceous striae
Frohlich syndrome (hypothalamic tumor)	Headaches of increasing frequency or duration, ocular or neurological abnormalities, nausea and vomiting
Laurence-Moon-Bardet-Biedl syndrome	Hypogonadism, mental retardation, polydactyly (extra digits), late blindness
Prader-Willi syndrome	Short stature, truncal obesity, hyperphagia, hypotonia, mental retardation, hypogonadism, short hands and feet
Stein-Leventhal syndrome (polycystic ovaries)	Possible hirsutism, possible irregular menses, later amenorrhea

ability of foods rich in sugar and fat and a corresponding decrease in the consumption of complex carbohydrates—that have resulted in a net increase in the caloric density of the average meal (Brownell & Wadden, 1992). The percentage of calories consumed from fat is especially important because dietary fat is converted to body fat more efficiently than are carbohydrates. The ubiquity of fast-food restaurants that specialize in low-cost, high-fat meals and the relentless television marketing of foods high in sugar and fat to children contribute to what has been described as a "toxic food environment" (Brownell, 1994). Whether these very salient changes in national diet can completely account for the increasing prevalence in pediatric obesity is not clear. Nationally representative surveys indicate that the reported caloric intake of children 1–15 years of age has been static or declining since the early 1970s (Kennedy & Goldberg, 1995). Significant questions have been raised, however, about the accuracy of these and other surveys that use self-report to estimate dietary intake (Klesges, Eck, & Ray, 1995).

Inactivity   There has been a significant reduction in the amount of physical work required of the average individual since the 1800s, and it has been suggested that the increasingly inactive lifestyles of Americans may play a role in the growing prevalence of obesity in the United States (Brownell & Wadden, 1992). Data on the relationship between inactivity and childhood obesity are equivocal. Several studies have found that children and adolescents who are obese are less active than peers who are not obese, although others studies have failed to demonstrate this correlation (Foreyt & Cousins, 1989). Differences in the methods used to measure physical activity (e.g., self-report, observation, electronic monitoring), as well as other methodological differences, may account for differential outcome in these studies. Berkowitz, Agras, Korner, Kraemer, and Zeanah (1985) assessed physical activity in a group of 4- to 8-year-old children over a 24-hour period, using an ambulatory electronic activity monitor—a relatively reliable and objective measure. They found that childhood adiposity increased as amount of time engaged in high activity levels decreased, although the differences were small. Using a relatively sophisticated assessment of physical activity—the technique of doubly labeled water—Davies, Gregory, and White (1995) found a significant correlation between physical activity and body fat in a sample of preschool children.

Television   Children ages 6–11 years watch more than 23 hours of television per week (Nielsen Media Research, 1990), which is approximately the same amount of time they spend in school per week each year. Because television viewing represents a relatively recent change in the American lifestyle, it is natural to ask whether this factor contributes to the increasing prevalence of childhood obesity. Dietz and Gortmaker (1985) found that each hourly increment of television viewing by adolescents was associated with a 2% increase in the prevalence of obesity. Television viewing could foster obesity by affecting intake (either by influencing food choices or by encouraging excess intake during viewing) or by reducing the time available for activities that burn calories at a higher rate than television viewing. Klesges, Shelton, and Klesges (1993) provided evidence for yet another mechanism to account for the possible relationship between television viewing and obesity. Klesges et al. (1993) showed that both children who are obese and children who are not had lower resting metabolic rates while watching television than while at rest. Although these studies are suggestive, not all studies show that amount of television viewing is related to obesity (Robinson et al., 1993). Increased television viewing also could be the result of social rejection and diminished recreational opportunities secondary to obesity.

Television viewing also has been found to be a strong predictor of pediatric hypercholesterolemia (Wong et al., 1992). Children watching 2–4 hours of television per day were approximately twice as likely to have cholesterol levels of 200 milligrams per deciliter or greater as those children watching less than 2 hours per day; this risk was doubled when children watched in excess of 4 hours per day. Excess television viewing, in Wong's study, was a better predictor of hypercholesterolemia than was a positive family history of high cholesterol.

Eating Style   Several (but not all) studies support the contention that eating style differentiates children who are obese from children who are not obese. Agras and his colleagues (Agras, Kraemer, Berkowitz, Korner, & Hammer, 1987) found that a vigorous feeding style was associated with adiposity in a group of healthy infants observed from birth to 2 years of age. Vigorous infant feeding consisted of sucking more rapidly, at higher pressure, with a longer suck and burst duration, and at a shorter interval between bursts of sucking. High-pressure sucking at 2 and 4 weeks of age continued to predict adiposity at 3 years of age but not at 6 years of age (Agras, Kraemer, Berkowitz, & Hammer, 1990).

Eating style also has been found to differentiate older children who are obese from those who are not. Waxman and Stunkard (1980) studied eating behaviors at home and at school for brothers between the ages of 4.5 and 13 years. The brothers who were obese had shorter meals, had faster eating rates, and tended to eat everything on their plates, relative to their brothers who were not obese. Drabman, Hammer, and Jarvie (1977) found that children who were obese between first through sixth grades took more bites and chewed less than normal-weight controls.

Modeling/Social Effects   Simply eating in the presence of others may increase the amount of food consumed. Several studies with adult males and females have shown that more food is consumed when individuals eat in groups than when they eat alone (Logue, 1991). Children are more likely to consume food offered by adults when adults also are eating (Harper & Sanders, 1975). In a laboratory study that assessed the relationship between the eating behavior of parents and their 18-month-old children, Agras, Berkowitz, Hammer, and Kraemer (1988) found that a pattern of rapid eating in mothers and a pattern of prolonged eating in fathers were associated with a higher caloric intake in their children.

Parents can affect the likelihood of eating quite directly. For example, the probability that a child will consume food has been shown to be directly related to frequency of parent prompting (Klesges et al., 1983), with relative child weight positively correlated with prompt frequency. A less direct but potentially significant parental influence on child obesity was examined in a study by Johnson and Birch (1994) that investigated the relationship among children's ability to self-regulate appetite, adiposity, and parent feeding practices. Johnson and Birch found that 1) children with greater body fat were less able to accurately self-regulate appetite, and 2) children with less ability to self-regulate energy intake had mothers who were more controlling of child food intake (e.g., by encouraging children to eat only at mealtimes rather than when hungry).

Emotional Factors   Eating also may be influenced by emotional factors. Emotionally induced eating, also known as stress-induced eating, is thought to reduce negative emotions such as anxiety, depression, loneliness, or boredom. Empirical support for this hypothesis comes largely from uncontrolled clinical studies with adults who are obese—who often report emotionally induced eating—and from laboratory studies—primarily with college students, in whom emotional states are artificially induced (Ganley, 1989). A comprehensive review of the stress-induction hypothesis (Greeno & Wing, 1994) found only weak empirical support for the general effects of stress on eating and found stronger support that stress increases eating in restrained eaters (i.e., those actively attempting to manage weight). Whether pre-adolescent children who are obese are similarly affected by emotional factors and whether this has implications for the etiology of obesity in children who are not originally obese has yet to be established.

Although obesity itself is not classified as a mental disorder in the DSM-IV, increased appetite, weight gain, and dysregulated eating are among the DSM-IV criteria for other mental disorders, including depression and dysthymia. Also included in the DSM-IV are research criteria for Binge-Eating Disorder (American Psychiatric Association, 1994). This disorder is defined by recurrent episodes of binge eating characterized by the following: 1) eating more than normal amounts of food and 2) a sense of lack of control over eating during the episode. These episodes are associated with three or more of the following: 1) eating rapidly; 2) eating until uncomfortably full; 3) eating large amounts of food when not physically hungry; 4) eating alone due to embarrassment; and 5) having feelings of disgust, depression, or guilt after overeating. The onset of binge eating typically occurs in late adolescence or early adulthood (American Psychiatric Association, 1994). The prevalence of binge eating in preadolescent children is unknown but is probably extremely rare. Binge eating may be associated with dieting in adulthood (Wilson, 1993), but little is known about the relationship between caloric restriction and binge eating in childhood. (Excessive, binge-like eating also is discussed in the section entitled Hyperphagia.)

In conclusion, both biological and environmental factors strongly influence the expression of obesity, and it is often difficult to separate the effects of these variables. For example, eating rate and style, discussed here as environmental variables, can be transmitted from parent to child, but eating rate may itself be genetically influenced.

INTERVENTION

Weight reduction requires that individuals consume fewer calories than they expend. The modification of both energy intake and energy expenditure is the essence of obesity intervention for children as well as for adults. Dietary counseling, moderate caloric restriction, and prescribed increases in physical activity—supported by specific behavioral techniques—are regarded as the most conservative interventions. Very low calorie diets (VLCD), pharmacotherapy, and surgery are reserved for the most severe cases of obesity. Classification of the severity of obesity often is used to select an intervention. For example, Stunkard (1992) recommended that mild obesity (20%–40% overweight) be treated with conservative therapy, moderate obesity (41%–100% overweight) with VLCD plus behavior therapy, and severe obesity (greater than 100% overweight) with surgery. The selection of an intervention also may be guided by the presence of specific health risks such as high blood pressure or elevated cholesterol levels, morbid complications of obesity such as non–insulin-dependent diabetes, the presence of a family history of overweight, and child or family concerns about obesity (Dietz & Robinson, 1993).

Energy Intake

Dietary counseling for parents and children and prescribed caloric restriction are the principle strategies used to decrease child energy intake.

Dietary Counseling Nutrition counseling is often the first intervention triggered by the assessment of child obesity. Dietary counseling usually is based on a classification of foods into groups (e.g., dairy, meats, vegetables, fruits, breads, fats) as well as guidelines, which are expressed in portions or servings of how much of each food group should be consumed each day to achieve recommended dietary allowances of basic nutrients. Often this information is accompanied by exchange lists, which describe portions of different foods matched in calories and nutrients (carbohydrates, protein, fat) (Crocker, 1993). For example, 1 ounce of chicken is equivalent to $^1/_4$ cup of canned tuna; one small apple is equivalent to four halves of dried apricot.

The Traffic Light diet, developed by Epstein and his colleagues (Epstein, Wing, & Valoski, 1985), is an example of a food classification system that has been used in dietary counseling of children. This diet divides foods into 11 categories with each category assigned to one of three color groups: red, yellow, or green. These colors are derived from the traffic light and indicate the following: GO (green), eat as much as you want; CAUTION (yellow), eat in moderation; and STOP (red), do not eat. "Green" foods contain fewer than 20 calories per average serving and include foods such as asparagus and herbs and spices. "Yellow" foods are approximately 20 calories per serving (e.g., corn, apples, skim milk). "Red" foods exceed the caloric value of "yellow" foods and include scalloped potatoes, fruits in heavy syrup, donuts, and candy.

Prescribed Caloric Restriction   A wide range of structured diets have been prescribed to reduce weight in adults, ranging from conventional reducing diets of 1,000–1,200 kilocalories per day, designed to result in body weight loss of about 1% per week, to VLCDs, often in the range of 400–800 kilocalories per day (Wadden & Bartlett, 1992). Many popular diets may be inadequate or unsafe for adults and children. In the interests of preserving linear growth, prescribed diets for young children tend to be conservative. Any prescribed diet for children must provide sufficient calories and must preserve other nutrients required for growth.

Dietz (1987) recommended a diet balanced in nutrients that reduces energy intake by approximately 30% for most overweight children. More restrictive diets are recommended only for individuals who are severely overweight, defined as those exceeding 160% of IBW. For infants and young children, weight maintenance, or decelerated weight gain, rather than weight loss is often the goal of treatment (Dietz, 1984).

In a series of controlled behavioral weight management studies, Epstein, Wing, and Valoski (1985) incorporated structured diets for children in age groups of 1–5 years, 5–8 years, and 8 years and older. Children in these groups were placed on diets ranging from 900 to 1,300 kilocalories per day. Calorie limits for children in the 1–5 years age group were obtained by subtracting 200 calories from their typical intake. There was no evidence of linear growth deceleration in a 5-year follow-up of children treated with this diet (Epstein, McCurley, Valoski, & Wing, 1990).

The degree of prescribed caloric restriction depends, in part, on the age of the child. More aggressive diets have been used with older children and adolescents. Figueroa-Colon, vonAlmen, Franklin, Schuftan, and Suskind (1993) reported use of a protein-sparing modified fast (PSMF) diet, which was provided in a comprehensive weight management program for children ranging in age from 9 to

15 years that included behavior modification, aerobic conditioning, vitamin and mineral supplementation, nutrition education, and parent participation. This study compared the PSMF diet with a more conservative balanced hypocaloric diet of about 1,000 kilocalories per day. Half of the children were on the PSMF diet for 10 weeks before being placed on the balanced diet, whereas the other half were started and continued on the balanced diet. The PSMF diet group showed greater weight loss after 10 weeks than children on the more conservative diet, but there was no difference between groups after 14.5 months. Both groups experienced a transitory slowing of growth velocity at 6 months but recovered at 14.5 months—the point at which they also had recovered their baseline weight. The authors of the study advised that PSMF diets should not be used without medical supervision.

Energy Expenditure

Most weight management programs, for both children and adults, incorporate exercise programs to increase and maintain physical activity. Exercise has several potential benefits: It burns the calories consumed in food, it may help maintain lean body mass (which can be lost during diet alone), it may help maintain resting metabolic rate (which is reduced when caloric intake is decreased), and it appears to support the maintenance of weight loss (Saris, 1993). Types of exercise programs vary widely, ranging from relatively structured aerobic conditioning programs to lifestyle changes (e.g., taking the stairs rather than the elevator) that result in modest but sustained increases in energy expenditure.

Exercise plus diet and behavioral intervention has been found to produce superior weight loss maintenance in children when compared with the same intervention without exercise (Epstein, Wing, Woodall, et al., 1985). Lifestyle exercise and structured aerobic exercise appear to produce similar benefits during intervention, but lifestyle exercise produces greater weight loss maintenance over time (Epstein, Wing, Koeske, Ossip, & Beck, 1982; Epstein, Wing, Koeske, & Valoski, 1985). The advantage of lifestyle exercise presumably lies in increased adherence.

Behavioral Techniques

Behavior modification and cognitive-behavioral therapy techniques have become a staple of both adult and child weight management programs. A meta-analysis of 41 controlled treatment-outcome studies (Haddock, Shadish, Klesges, & Stein, 1994) concluded that child and adolescent weight management programs that include behavior modification techniques produce better treatment effects than weight loss programs not using these techniques. The most common components of behavioral interventions are stimulus control, self-monitoring, contingency management, cognitive restructuring, and relapse prevention. Strategies for including parents and other family members are also significant features of child weight management programs.

Tables 10.2 and 10.3 summarize some of the behavioral principles and guidelines commonly found in behavioral weight management manuals. The guidelines in Table 10.2 pertain to the parents of children with weight management problems, whereas the recommendations in Table 10.3 apply to children themselves. The application of some of these principles is illustrated in Case 10.1.

Stimulus Control   In the context of weight management, *stimulus control* refers to the tendency for specific settings to control or evoke eating or the impulse to eat because of a prior association with eating (Birch, McPhee, Sullivan, & Johnson, 1989). Sitting at the kitchen or dining room table, for example, properly evokes the impulse to eat. If eating occurs repeatedly in other contexts (e.g., in front of the television set), then those contexts also will evoke the desire to eat. Resisting the "urge to eat" becomes more difficult when multiple settings tend to elicit eating behavior. Parents are therefore counseled to provide meals at regular times and in a specific location (e.g., kitchen, dining room). Other recommendations that derive from the principle of stimulus control include storing high-calorie foods out of sight and not bringing serving dishes to the table.

Self-Monitoring   A common feature of many behavioral interventions is self-monitoring of critical information about the occurrence and context of symptoms and other health-related behaviors. In child weight management interventions, children are taught to record the type and the amount of food eaten; the time of day; where the food was eaten; and other facts relevant to eating, such as mood and the presence of other people during meals and snacks. Exercise is similarly self-monitored. Self-monitoring is usually begun early in the intervention process, with initial measurements providing baseline information, which can help shape intervention and against which the effects of intervention are measured. Monitoring for preschool children remains a parental responsibility, of course, but children 7 years of age and older can usually be taught to self-monitor. The reliability and validity of child self-monitoring has not yet been established (Foreyt & Goodrick, 1988); but self-monitoring is generally recognized to be an essential feature of obesity inter-

Table 10.2. Parents' behavioral weight management guidelines for children who are obese

STIMULUS CONTROL

Shopping
- Shop for food after eating.
- Shop from a list—avoid impulse buying.
- Avoid ready-to-eat foods.
- Buy more low-calorie foods.
- Do not carry more cash than needed for shopping list.
- Do not include child in food shopping trips.

Meal Management
- Store food out of sight.
- Offer/eat all food in the same place.
- Offer meals and snacks at scheduled times.
- Remove food from inappropriate storage areas in the house.
- Keep serving dishes off the table.
- Use smaller dishes and utensils (this will make food portions look larger).
- Do not have the television on during meals.
- Model moderate eating and choice of low-fat foods.

Holidays and parties
- Prepare child before parties (help him or her anticipate temptations).
- Offer your child a low-calorie snack before parties.
- Practice with your child polite ways that he or she can decline food.

REWARD
- Encourage child to ask for help from family and friends.
- Use praise and material rewards to reinforce sensible eating and increased physical ability.
- Use child's self-monitoring records as a basis for rewards.
- Do not use food as reward or punishment.

NUTRITION EDUCATION
- Learn nutritional value of foods.
- Help your child to make sensible food choices.

PHYSICAL ACTIVITY
- Encourage lifestyle changes that result in increased physical activity.
- Encourage and reward participation in an exercise program.
- Encourage participation in sports.
- Limit television viewing.

COGNITIVE RESTRUCTURING
- Avoid setting unreasonable goals for your child.
- Think about progress, not shortcomings.
- Avoid imperatives such as "always" and "never."
- Counter your child's negative thoughts with rational statements.
- Do not get discouraged by an occasional setback, and do not allow your child to become discouraged.

Adapted from Stunkard (1992) and Varni & Banis (1985).

Table 10.3. Behavioral weight management guidelines for children who are obese

STIMULUS CONTROL

Meal Management
- Eat all food in the same place.
- Eat meals and snacks at scheduled times.
- Do not buy snacks at school.
- Eat low-calorie snacks.
- Substitute exercise for snacking.

Holidays and parties
- Plan eating habits before parties.
- Eat a low-calorie snack before parties.
- Practice polite ways to decline food.

EATING BEHAVIOR
- Put utensil down between mouthfuls.
- Chew thoroughly before swallowing.
- Prepare foods one portion at a time.
- Leave some food on the plate.
- Do nothing else (e.g., read, watch television) while eating.

REWARD
- Negotiate with parents for praise and material rewards.
- Use self-monitoring records as a basis for rewards for specific behaviors.
- Solicit help from family and friends.

SELF-MONITORING

Keep a diary that includes the following:
- Time and place of eating
- Type and amount of food
- Who is present/How you feel
- Type and duration of exercise

COGNITIVE RESTRUCTURING
- Set reasonable weight goals/Avoid setting unreasonable goals.
- Think about progress, not shortcomings.
- Avoid imperatives such as "always" and "never."
- Counter negative thoughts with rational statements.
- Do not get discouraged by an occasional setback (e.g., during holidays).

Adapted from Stunkard (1992) and Varni & Banis (1985).

ventions, and adherence to recordkeeping has been found to be an important predictor of weight loss (Baker & Kirschenbaum, 1993).

Contingency Management The use of rewards and disincentives is a common ingredient of child weight management programs. For example, Aragona, Cassaday, and Drabman (1975) described a multicomponent parent-mediated treatment program using either response cost alone or response cost plus reinforcement. All parents were given response cost contracts, which allowed them to redeem money that they had deposited prior to treatment. Opportunity to redeem was dependent on attending sessions, bringing monitoring data to sessions, and having the child lose a predetermined amount of weight. The reinforcement plus response cost group also included parent training in reinforcement techniques and use of reinforcers for losing weight, reducing calorie intake, exercising, and following stimulus control techniques.

The use of immediate, concrete rewards may be especially important when working with younger children. Parent training in child behavior management was one component of a weight control intervention for children between the ages of 1 and 6 years (Epstein, Valoski, Koeske, & Wing, 1986). Parents were taught how to use modeling, praise, time-out, and extinction. "Star charts" were used to reinforce dietary compliance and exercise habits; for example, a star was earned for each meal at which "red" foods on the Traffic Light diet were avoided, with bonus stars available if no "red" foods were consumed all day. Stars also could be earned for walking a required distance.

Reinforcement procedures also have been used in teaching the educational components (e.g., nutrition education) of weight control programs (Epstein, Wing, & Valoski, 1985). Instructional material is divided into small, self-contained lessons; mastery of the material is assessed using quizzes; and the introduction of new lessons is contingent on the mastery of previous lessons.

Eating Rate Modification Weight management interventions for children frequently include recommendations to modify eating style. These recommendations are based on data indicating that many children who are obese have "high-density eating styles," including eating rapidly, taking large bites, and chewing each bite little or not at all (Drabman et al., 1977). Unless the size of food portions or meals is strictly limited, eating faster will result in ingestion of more food. If meal size is limited, the meal may be consumed before satiety ensues, leaving the child hungry at the end of the meal. This may result in additional, postmeal snacking. Children are usually counseled to reduce eating rate by chewing each bite thoroughly, deliberately pausing for 1–3 minutes at some point during the meal and putting utensils down between mouthfuls.

Cognitive Restructuring Children and adults who are obese often are given to dysfunctional beliefs that may maintain poor eating habits and interfere with weight management. Cognitive restructuring is a cognitive-behavioral technique directed at modifying dysfunctional thoughts and self-statements. People trying to manage weight often fall into a number of common cognitive "traps," including the following: 1) setting unrealistic weight loss goals, 2) dichotomous thinking ("I am either on my diet or off my diet"), or 3) "catastrophizing" ("Because I went off my diet today, I will never achieve my weight management goals"). Older children can be asked to monitor negative thoughts and can be taught to counter them with more rational, positive thoughts. For example, the previously mentioned thoughts could be countered with the following self-statements: "I ate a little more than I expected today, but that's because I was nervous about my exam. Next week, I can walk for 15 extra minutes on Tuesday and Thursday and that should help bring me closer to my goals."

Relapse Prevention Initial weight loss often occurs with deceptive ease in motivated individuals. Weight loss maintenance over a period of months and years, however, appears to be the exception rather than the rule. Specific maintenance strategies have been suggested to enhance the likelihood of long-term weight loss maintenance (Brownell & Wadden, 1992). These strategies include the following: 1) matching treatments and interventions to individuals, 2) extending the duration of intervention, 3) placing greater emphasis on exercise, 4) teaching specific coping skills, and 5) placing special emphasis on low-fat diets. Compassionate weight management intervention must be mindful of potential psychological risks (e.g., negative self-appraisal during relapse) and should include ongoing therapeutic support to children and their families to minimize those risks.

Parental Inclusion Parents play a major role in child energy intake by buying, preparing, and serving much of the food consumed by their children. Parents also influence child intake less directly by serving as models for consummatory and health-related behavior. It makes sense, therefore, to involve parents in child weight control interventions, and a number of studies have attempted to determine the best method for including parents. Whether parents attend child treatment sessions, are seen separately, or are not seen at all and whether the child alone or both the child and the parents are targets for weight control are among the factors that have been studied. A detailed comparison of individual studies of parental involvement leads to conflicting conclusions. Haddock et al. (1994) concluded, on the basis of a meta-analysis of 41 child weight management studies, that the level of parental participation does not significantly affect outcome. A 10-year treatment outcome study reported by Epstein and his colleagues (Epstein et al., 1994), however, found that targeting both the child and the parents for weight loss resulted in significantly greater weight loss than if the child alone were targeted and found that this superiority was maintained 10 years after treatment.

Developmental factors also may be important. It is difficult to imagine a credible treatment for younger children that does not include significant parental participation, whereas the treatment of adolescents who are obese may call for less direct parental roles (see Brownell, Kelman, & Stunkard, 1983). The inclusion of other family members (e.g., siblings, grandparents) may be useful in some cases, but the efficacy of incorporating extended family in child weight management programs has not yet been evaluated.

The following case illustrates the implementation of a weight management intervention with an 8-year-old girl.

■ ■ ■

CASE 10.1. A CHILD WITH OBESITY
NAME: Gloria
AGE AT INTERVENTION: 8 years

BACKGROUND

Gloria was the first of two children born to Hispanic parents who had recently immigrated to the United States from Central America. After a medical evaluation had ruled out organic causes of obesity, she was referred for nutrition counseling and behavioral weight management by her pediatrician. Her weight at the beginning of treatment was 36 kilograms, and her height was 122 centimeters. Her weight and weight-for-height exceeded the 95th percentile for girls her age, her weight was about 160% of IBW, and her BMI was 24.2. Both of Gloria's parents were overweight (her mother's weight was about 125% of IBW; the father's exact weight was unknown) and had apparently been so from early childhood. Gloria's younger brother also was overweight and was included in this intervention, but he is not discussed here. The parents had been separated for about a year, and Gloria, who expressed sadness about her parents' separation as well as worries about her future, had experienced weight gain acceleration correlated with this life stressor. Her weight had tracked at about the 75th percentile prior to her parents' separation.

Otherwise, Gloria was emotionally well-adjusted; her school work was above average, she had several close friends, and she was engaged to articulate interest in a variety of social activities. There was no evidence of depression or of body image disturbance. She denied binge eating; but she did snack frequently, especially after school. She did not articulate any negative feelings ameliorated by eating. A 3-day diet record suggested that she might be consuming 100–200 extra calories per day. High-fat snacks (e.g., potato chips) and school lunches with high fat content contributed to excessive caloric intake. Her life-style was judged to be relatively inactive, with normative amounts of time spent watching television.

The initial evaluation established that Gloria's mother would ben-efit from dietary counseling and that she was motivated to support her daughter's weight management efforts. Nutrition assessment also re-vealed that the family had some unusual dietary practices that were apparently common in their country of origin; for example, all mem-bers of the family were accustomed to adding copious amounts of sugar to their milk.

FORMULATION

Family stressors and cultural dietary factors contributed to the onset of Gloria's obesity; and because both parents had been overweight since early childhood, hereditary factors were suspected as well. A good deal of Gloria's excess weight had been acquired during the previous year and was apparently related to excess snacking, which may have been one of several coping strategies that evolved to deal with pa-rental separation. Gloria's mother also reported gaining weight during the prior year, and she may have inadvertently played a role (by mod-eling or by changes in the type, amount, or frequency of food offered) in her daughter's weight acceleration. Gloria's mother was appropri-ately concerned, but significant deficiencies in her understanding of basic nutrition left her poorly equipped to deal effectively with the chal-lenge of weight management.

INTERVENTION

Gloria and her mother were seen in biweekly sessions conducted col-laboratively by a registered dietitian and a pediatric psychologist. Indi-vidual psychotherapy sessions with Gloria were interspersed among sessions that included both professionals and family members. Inter-vention included the following:

1. *Goal setting* involved extensive discussion with both Gloria and her mother, as it soon became clear that Gloria had unrealistic expectations ("to be skinny") for weight management therapy. A goal of returning to Gloria's "premorbid" weight for age (75th per-centile) during the course of therapy was finally negotiated. Gloria and her mother were given the option of choosing weight mainte-nance as a goal, with the understanding that the negotiated goal could be reached in about 1.5–2 years with this strategy. This strategy was unacceptable to Gloria and her mother, and, in a

concession to keep the family in treatment, a weight-loss strategy calling for the loss of 1 pound per week was negotiated.

2. *Dietary counseling,* with an emphasis on basic principles of nutrition, was provided during each session. Counseling was mildly complicated by language issues. Many concepts required repetition and multiple exemplars. There was some culturally based resistance to recommendations for changing food preparation. Nutrition recommendations, therefore, were kept concrete and were provided in stages. Substituting fruits and vegetables for all snacks was the first recommendation. Reviewing the school lunch menu and substituting a turkey sandwich prepared at home for high-fat school lunches was the second major recommendation. Once these changes were firmly incorporated into Gloria's lifestyle, additional recommendations were made. Because Gloria was strongly motivated to lose weight, no additional rewards were negotiated for dietary compliance or for weight loss.

3. *Exercise counseling* was provided, and an exercise program was negotiated. Gloria and her mother agreed to walk for at least 30 minutes, 3 times per week. Television viewing was reduced by 50%. Meeting exercise goals and reducing television viewing was rewarded by offering Gloria her choice of videotapes to watch on weekends.

4. In *individual psychotherapy,* Gloria was encouraged to explore her feelings about her parents' separation. She was eventually able to articulate her fear of abandonment. With support she was able to openly discuss this fear with her mother and to receive appropriate reassurance.

OUTCOME

Gloria lost weight at the rate of about 1 pound per week for the first 2 months of treatment and lost about ½ pound per week for the remainder of the 6 months of intensive intervention. At a 9-month visit, she had lost a total of 8 kilograms and had achieved a BMI of 18.5, which is between the 75th and 90th percentile for girls her age. She agreed at this point to adjust her goal to weight maintenance. She was seen for brief follow-up visits at 12 months and at 15 months, continued to maintain her weight, and was subsequently discharged to her pediatrician for growth monitoring.

■ ■ ■

Medical Treatments

Several medications—chiefly centrally acting agents such as mazindol, dexfenfluramine, fenfluramine, phentermine, sertraline, and fluoxetine—suppress appetite and have been found to be superior to placebo controls in assisting with weight loss in adults (Goldstein & Potvin, 1994). The weight loss achieved with anorectic medication plateaus by 6 months, however, and all of the weight lost is regained when medication is discontinued (Guy-Grand, 1992). Thus, medication, if discontinued, confers no advantage over diet alone or over diet plus behavioral intervention in adults. It has been suggested that selected adults with obesity may benefit from lifelong treatment with medication, but pharmacotherapy for children with obesity is recommended only under strictly regulated experimental protocols (National Task Force on the Prevention and Treatment of Obesity, 1996).

The intervention of last resort is gastric bypass surgery (Kral, 1992). In this surgery, the lower part of the stomach is bypassed by disconnecting it from the upper part of the stomach and then attaching the intestine directly to the upper part. This results in a reduced gastric pouch, which induces early satiety. Surgical intervention with children usually is reserved for adolescents who weigh more than 200% of IBW or who are experiencing serious health complications resulting from obesity (Dietz, 1983).

Children with Developmental Disabilities

Obesity appears to be at least as prevalent in children with mental retardation as in children with normal intelligence, and the same etiological factors are thought to contribute to obesity in both populations (Burkhart, Fox, & Rotatori, 1988). Weight management programs for children with developmental disabilities are based on the modification of energy intake and energy expenditure and employ the same principles of caloric restriction, exercise promotion, and behavior modification discussed in previous sections of this chapter. Parent inclusion is especially important when working with children with developmental disabilities who are overweight, and the participation of teachers and other school staff can be very helpful as well.

Primary Prevention

Successful intervention with children who have become obese is an important element in a comprehensive strategy for the prevention of adult obesity. The primary prevention of child obesity—intervening *before* children become obese—has received little systematic study. In an early study, Pisacano, Lichter, Ritter, and Siegal (1978) described an intervention implemented with newborn infants in a private pediatric practice, which significantly reduced the prevalence of overweight by age 3 years. The intervention consisted primarily of counseling parents to reduce dietary fat by having the parents offer skim milk rather than whole milk after the age of 3 months. There have been no recent replications of this type of dietary intervention with infants. Dietary fat is essential for central nervous system maturation, and feeding skim milk before the age of 1 year and similar restrictions on dietary fat in infancy and early childhood are contraindicated as of this writing (Hardy & Kleinman, 1994). Considerable care must be taken in counseling parents regarding child intake of dietary fat, lest overzealous restrictions on dietary fat result in compromised growth (Lifshitz & Moses, 1989).

Discussions regarding the primary prevention of child obesity have focused on guidelines for counseling parents during pediatric office visits and on advocacy for relevant public health policy initiatives. Charney (1993) suggested that anticipatory guidance during health supervision visits focus on infants at high risk whose parents both are overweight. Common recommendations are breast-feeding, delaying the introduction of solid foods until 4–6 months of age, not using the bottle to pacify, offering reduced-fat milk after 12 months of age, limiting high-calorie snack foods, eating all meals at the table, not eating in front of the television, and establishing regular patterns of exercise for all members of the family. The efficacy of weight management recommendations made during pediatric office visits is unknown (Charney, 1993). Dietz (1986) advised a broad-based parent counseling strategy that includes attending to seemingly trivial sources of energy imbalance, reducing dietary fat, and discouraging television viewing. Public policies that encourage school programs to increase child physical activity, especially in winter, and legislation that bans food advertising directed at children are also recommended (Dietz, 1986). As mentioned previously, Brownell (1994) attributed the increasing prevalence of obesity to a "toxic food environment" and argued for significant public policy initiatives (e.g., placing taxes on high-fat foods, regulating food advertisements directed at children) to support the consumption of less-fattening foods. Clinical guidelines for the management of pediatric obesity are provided in Table 10.4.

HYPERPHAGIA

Although pediatric obesity is by far the most prevalent and significant eating problem involving the presumed overintake of food, other relatively rare and less adequately described disorders of excessive intake may come to the attention of the health care professional. This section reviews conspicuous excesses in eating that may or may not result in obesity.

Table 10.4. Pediatric obesity: Clinical guidelines

EVALUATION
- Is the child obese by objective standards?
  - Does percentage overweight equal or exceed 120%?
  - Is BMI greater than 85th percentile?
  - Are there other indications of excess adiposity?
  - How severe is the child's obesity?
- Has a thorough medical evaluation ruled out endocrinological abnormalities, syndromes associated with obesity, and other possible organic contributions to obesity?
- Have associated health risks (e.g., elevated blood cholesterol, hypertension, orthopedic problems) been adequately assessed?
- Are other family members obese?
- What is the course of the child's weight gain (e.g., gradual or sudden onset)?
- What is the likelihood of persistence (Generally a function of age and severity, with older, more severely obese children at greater risk)?
- What is the child's current dietary intake, as reflected in a 3-day food record? How is the child's diet affected by family nutrition beliefs and cultural factors?
- What is the activity level of the child and of other family members? What are their television viewing habits?
- What are the immediate psychosocial costs of obesity?
  - Is the child distressed (e.g., dysphoric mood, poor self-esteem, other emotional/behavioral problems)?
  - Is the child stigmatized by peers, family?
  - Are there academic problems?
  - Is there ongoing family stress/dysfunction?
- Is there evidence of body image distortion?
- How motivated are the child and family to pursue treatment?
- Has the child or family previously participated in weight management attempts? How will this affect motivation?
- Will at least one parent commit to active participation in treatment?

INTERVENTION
Medical management
- Treat associated health risks.
- Monitor linear growth and health of children on hypocaloric diets.
- Supervise treatment of adolescents on VLC diets.
Diet modification
- For infants and young children, weight maintenance, not weight loss, should be identified as the treatment goal.
- Emphasize reductions in dietary fats.
- Encourage simple, permanent changes in the child's and family's diet.
- For older children, prescribe balanced hypocaloric diet.
- For adolescents with severe obesity, consider VLC diet, under medical supervision.
Nutrition education
- Provide dietary education for parents and other relevant family members.
- Provide developmentally appropriate nutrition education for older children.

(continued)

Table 10.4. *(continued)*

Activity modification
- Design and prescribe exercise program, favoring lifestyle modification, adapted to family resources.
- Encourage participation in age-appropriate sports.
- Monitor and systematically decrease sedentary activities, such as television viewing.
- Encourage participation of both parents in all aspects of dietary and exercise programs.

Behavior modification/therapy
- Set realistic, compassionate treatment goals.
- Teach school-age children to self-monitor intake, exercise, and eating habits.
- Provide stimulus control recommendations (e.g., meals at regular times, regular locations).
- Provide eating rate recommendations.
- Reinforce behavior change (e.g., compliance with self-monitoring, activity modification) in children and parents.
- For school-age children, recommendations should take school meals into consideration (e.g., quality of typical school menu, time allowed for lunch).
- Provide cognitive restructuring for older children and parents.
- Monitor child and family psychosocial functioning: Provide reassurance, support, and other psychotherapeutic interventions, as needed.

Relapse prevention
- Provide extended treatment, for at least 1 year.
- Provide follow-up, for up to 5 years, with booster sessions, as indicated.

Organically Based Hyperphagia

PWS is a complex genetic disorder, first identified by Prader, Labhart, and Willi in 1956 (Cassidy, 1984). The chief characteristics of this disorder are listed in Table 10.5. Hyperphagia and obesity, the most salient and refractory symptoms of PWS, emerge in early childhood after a prior history of difficult feeding and failure to thrive, secondary to hypotonia. Obesity in individuals with PWS occurs as the result of both overeating (Holm & Pipes, 1976) and reduced energy expenditure (Davies & Joughin, 1993).

Children with PWS appear to have insatiable appetites and to eat indiscriminately. Given free access to food, energy intakes of more than 5,000 kilocalories per day have been reported in children with PWS (Holm & Pipes, 1976). Food stealing, hoarding, and consuming marginal foods (e.g., unthawed frozen food) are characteristic. Parental attempts to limit food intake often result in the acquisition of highly refined repertoires of covert and manipulative behaviors as well as overt expressions of resistance such as temper tantrums.

In a standardized presentation of an unlimited amount of food over a 1-hour time period, Zipf and Bernston (1987) compared the food intake patterns of children with PWS with intake patterns of a control group of children who were obese but who did not have

Table 10.5. Clinical features of Prader-Willi syndrome

Prenatal
   Decreased fetal movement
   Abnormal position at delivery
Infancy
   Hypotonia[a]
   Feeding problems[a]
   Failure to thrive
   Genital hypoplasia/cryptorchism
   Mild dysmorphism[a]
   Delayed motor development[a]
Childhood and adulthood
   Obesity/hyperphagia[a]
   Speech delay/poor articulation
   Intellectual impairment/school problems[a]
   Behavioral abnormalities
   Small hands and feet
   Strabismus/myopia
   Skin picking/decreased pain sensitivity
   Inability to vomit
   Scoliosis
   Mild short stature
   Abnormal pubertal development/hypogonadism[a]

Source: Cassidy (1984).
[a]Features considered essential for the diagnosis

PWS. Zipf and Bernston (1987) found no significant differences in rate of food consumed during the first 10 minutes, but children with PWS continued to eat for a much longer period of time than controls. Thus, when food is freely available, hyperphagia for children with PWS seems to be characterized by a delayed onset of satiety rather than by a conspicuously rapid eating rate.

Behavioral interventions to reduce obesity and to support normalized eating in children with PWS have met with limited success. Successful long-term maintenance appears to depend on placement in environments in which close supervision, controlled access to food, and a high degree of structure and support are available (Page, 1988). There is little evidence that individuals with PWS are able to self-manage weight or diet.

Hyperphagia also has been reported in children following surgery for craniopharyngioma. Skorzewska, Lal, Waserman, and Guyda (1989) described three cases of children between the ages of 5 and 12 years who developed abnormal food-seeking behavior postoperatively. Voracious appetite, food stealing, stealing money to buy food, obsessional thinking about food, having tantrums, and aggressive behavior in response to food removal were common in these individuals. Hyperphagia in these children was believed to result from postoperative hypothalamic damage and is reported to have responded poorly to either behavioral intervention or pharmacological treatment.

Psychogenic Hyperphagia

Demb (1991) described a subsample of 10 children with hyperphagia found in a population of 200 foster children. These children were reported by their foster mothers to have excessive appetite, a "driven quality" to consumption of food, an apparent lack of satiety, and frequent eating to the point of vomiting or gastric pain if limits were not placed on the availability of food. It is interesting to note that these children were not obese. The children ranged in age between 19 and 101 months at evaluation, had been in foster care for an average of 24 months, and all exhibited developmental delays and behavior problems in addition to hyperphagia. Mothers of the children had a high rate of drug and alcohol abuse, and Demb speculated that prenatal drug exposure may be implicated in producing hyperphagia.

Hyperphagia and bizarre eating behavior, including food stealing, hoarding, gorging, and eating marginal foods, also have been reported in children with psychosocial dwarfism (Woolston, 1991). These are children who show deceleration of linear growth in the absence of weight gain deceleration. Because children with psychosocial dwarfism often are discovered in disturbed psychosocial contexts and because dwarfism is often ameliorated when the children are removed from these situations, psychosocial dwarfism has been confused with nonorganic failure to thrive. It is important to emphasize, however, that these children are not malnourished, and excessive oral intake—rather than food refusal—is a cardinal behavioral feature of the disorder (see Chapter 6).

There have been no controlled studies of treatment for psychogenic hyperphagia in children. The following case describes a successful intervention with a child very similar to the foster children described by Demb (1991).

▪ ▪ ▪

CASE 10.2. A CHILD WITH HYPERPHAGIA
NAME: Jerome
AGE AT INTERVENTION: 1 year, 11 months

BACKGROUND

Jerome, a boy who was almost 2 years old and who lived in the custody of child protective services, was referred by his social worker for evaluation and treatment of hyperphagia. At the time of the evaluation, Jerome had lived in a foster home for 6 months subsequent to having been removed from the home of his biological parents. His biological father had been incarcerated for dealing in drugs, and his mother was reportedly a polysubstance abuser. Jerome had an older brother and a sister who had been physically and sexually abused. There was no evidence that Jerome himself had been abused nor was he obviously malnourished at the time he came to the attention of child protective services.

Jerome's history was provided by his social worker. Jerome reportedly ate and drank without satiety, had no strong taste preferences, would eat from the floor, and also would eat nonnutritive substances (e.g., lint, thread). During meals he would "wolf" food, and there was concern that eating was so impulsive that Jerome might choke on his food, although this had not yet occurred. Immediately after finishing his meal, he would begin to cry and attempt to take food from others at the table who had not yet finished their meals. He would cry when he observed food being offered to others and when food was taken from him, and he also would cry unpredictably. Jerome also cried continuously during supervised visitation with his biological mother, who would offer him food to console him. No sleep problems were reported. Jerome's weight and height were between the 10th and 25th percentiles for age. Dietary records were not available at the time of evaluation.

Jerome initially presented as subdued, shy, sad, and passive—a presentation consistent with elevated Social Withdrawal and Depression subscales on the Child Behavior Checklist (Achenbach, 1988) completed by his social worker. He did cry unpredictably during the interview, but he was able to console himself without special intervention. No indiscriminant mouthing was observed in a period of free play nor was there any evidence of pica. During a brief feeding observation, Jerome was offered a small cup of water and a piece of blueberry pie. He cried after finishing the cup of water, cried again when half of his portion of pie was removed, and cried again after finishing the pie. His actual ingestion of the pie was not unusually urgent.

FORMULATION

Jerome's diagnosis was complicated by some disparities between Jerome's observed behavior and the reports that accompanied him. He did not eat rapidly, take large bites, or engage in pica during the evaluation. His caloric intake, as inferred from his current weight, appeared to be within normal limits. Thus, he did not seem to be truly hyperphagic, but he gave the impression of hyperphagia because of his intense emotional and behavioral reactions to food. These reactions had presumably developed in a family context of food scarcity, emotional and physical neglect, competition for food, and the reinforcement of crying with food.

INTERVENTION

The following recommendations were provided for Jerome's foster mother:

1. Offer three meals and two well-defined snacks per day. Meals and snacks should be offered at approximately the same time each day.
2. For the time being, provide one-to-one supervision during meals a) to prompt less rapid eating, if necessary, and b) to provide assurance against the possibility of choking.
3. Try to pace family meals so that Jerome is the last to finish his meal. At the end of each meal, take Jerome from the dining area and engage him in play.
4. Jerome will benefit from being held and cuddled on a frequent and predictable basis. It may be especially useful to do this before meals.
5. Jerome may need help in differentiating between his emotional and physiological needs. Try to determine what his needs are when he cries or seems distressed without apparent reason (is he lonely, afraid, in pain?), and console him accordingly. Do *not* offer food or drink when Jerome cries unpredictably because it is not likely that he is crying because he is hungry or thirsty. It also will be necessary to set limits on his biological mother's reported tendency to console Jerome with food.

OUTCOME

Telephone follow-up with Jerome's foster mother indicated that she had followed the recommendations and that hyperphagia ceased to be a concern after 3–4 weeks. Jerome gradually became more cheerful, trusting, and socially engaging; but he required considerable individual attention, and he was becoming more overtly oppositional. Additional follow-up for child behavior management counseling was recommended and was provided through another agency.

■ ■ ■

SUMMARY

Children who eat too much, relative to energy expenditure, are at risk for becoming obese. Obesity has become an increasing public health concern, and pediatric obesity is more prevalent than any of the other childhood eating problems covered in this book, with the possible exception of the subclinical feeding problems discussed in Chapter 5. Like the childhood feeding disorders discussed in other chapters, pediatric obesity evolves from the complex interaction of biological and environmental variables and can be responsive to biobehavioral intervention. The excesses of caloric intake that contribute to pediatric obesity are seldom, if ever, conspicuous. Hyperphagia does occur in pediatric populations but with much less frequency than obesity. Hyperphagia of organic origin appears to be less amenable to behavioral intervention than psychogenic hyperphagia.

REFERENCES

Achenbach, T.M. (1988). *Child Behavior Checklist for Ages 2–3* (Rev. ed.). Burlington, VT: Author.

Agras, W.S., Berkowitz, R.I., Hammer, L.D., & Kraemer, H.C. (1988). Relationships between the eating behaviors of parents and their 18-month-old children: A laboratory study. *International Journal of Eating Disorders, 7,* 461–468.

Agras, W.S., Kraemer, H.C., Berkowitz, R.I., & Hammer, L.D. (1990). Influence of early feeding style on adiposity at 6 years of age. *Journal of Pediatrics, 116,* 805–809.

Agras, W.S., Kraemer, H.C., Berkowitz, R.I., Korner, A.F., & Hammer, L.D. (1987). Does a vigorous feeding style influence early development of adiposity? *Journal of Pediatrics, 110,* 799–804.

American Psychiatric Association. (1987). *Diagnostic and statistical manual of mental disorders* (3rd ed., rev.). Washington, DC: Author.

American Psychiatric Association. (1994). *Diagnostic and statistical manual of mental disorders* (4th ed.). Washington, DC: Author.

Aragona, J., Cassaday, J., & Drabman, R.S. (1975). Treating overweight children through parental training and contingency contracting. *Journal of Applied Behavior Analysis, 8,* 269–278.

Baker, R.C., & Kirschenbaum, D.S. (1993). Self-monitoring may be necessary for successful weight control. *Behavior Therapy, 24,* 377–394.

Berkowitz, R.I., Agras, W., Korner, A.F., Kraemer, H.C., & Zeanah, C.H. (1985). Physical activity and adiposity: A longitudinal study from birth to childhood. *Journal of Pediatrics, 106,* 734–738.

Birch, L.L., McPhee, L., Sullivan, S., & Johnson, S. (1989). Conditioned meal initiation in children. *Appetite, 13,* 105–113.

Bouchard, C., & Perusse, L. (1993). Genetics of obesity. *Annual Review of Nutrition, 13,* 337–354.

Brownell, K.D. (1994, December 15). Get slim with higher taxes [Editorial]. *The New York Times,* p. A29.

Brownell, K.D., Kelman, J.H., & Stunkard, A.J. (1983). Treatment of obese children with and without their mothers: Changes in weight and blood pressure. *Pediatrics, 71,* 515–523.

Brownell, K.D., & Wadden, T.A. (1991). The heterogeneity of obesity: Fitting treatments to individuals. *Behavior Therapy, 22,* 153–177.

Brownell, K.D., & Wadden, T.A. (1992). Etiology and treatment of obesity: Understanding a serious, prevalent, and refractory disorder. *Journal of Consulting and Clinical Psychology, 60,* 505–517.

Burkhart, J.E., Fox, R.A., & Rotatori, A.F. (1988). Obesity in the developmentally disabled. In D.C. Russo & J.H. Kedesdy (Eds.), *Behavioral medicine with the developmentally disabled* (pp. 239–263). New York: Plenum.

Cassidy, S.B. (1984). Prader-Willi syndrome. *Current Problems in Pediatrics, 14,* 1–55.

Charney, E. (1993). The overweight child. In R. Dershewitz (Ed.), *Ambulatory pediatric care* (pp. 853–856). Philadelphia: J.B. Lippincott.

Crocker, R. (1993). Childhood obesity. In P.M. Queen & C.E. Lang (Eds.), *Handbook of pediatric nutrition* (pp. 560–572). Rockville, MD: Aspen Publishers.

Davies, P.S., Gregory, J., & White, A. (1995). Physical activity and body fatness in pre-school children. *International Journal of Obesity, 19,* 6–10.

Davies, P.S., & Joughin, C. (1993). Using stable isotopes to assess reduced physical activity of individuals with Prader-Willi syndrome. *American Journal of Mental Retardation, 98,* 349–353.

Demb, J.M. (1991). Reported hyperphagia in foster children. *Child Abuse & Neglect, 15,* 77–88.

Dietz, W.H. (1983). Childhood obesity: Susceptibility, cause, and management. *Journal of Pediatrics, 103,* 676–686.

Dietz, W.H. (1984). Obesity in infancy. In R.B. Howard & H.S. Winter (Eds.), *Nutrition and feeding of infants and toddlers* (pp. 297–307) Boston: Little, Brown.

Dietz, W.H. (1986). Prevention of childhood obesity. *Pediatric Clinics of North America, 33,* 823–833.

Dietz, W.H. (1987). Nutrition and obesity. In R.J. Grand, J.L. Sutphen, & W.H. Dietz (Eds.), *Pediatric nutrition* (pp. 525–538). Boston: Butterworths.

Dietz, W.H., & Gortmaker, S.L. (1985). Do we fatten our children at the TV set? Obesity and television viewing in children and adolescents. *Pediatrics, 75,* 807–812.

Dietz, W.H., & Robinson, T.N. (1993). Assessment and treatment of childhood obesity. *Pediatrics in Review, 14,* 337–344.

DiPietro, L., Mossberg, H., & Stunkard, A.J. (1994). A 40-year history of overweight children in Stockholm: Life-time overweight, morbidity, and mortality. *International Journal of Obesity, 18,* 585–590.

Drabman, R.S., Hammer, L.D., & Jarvie, G.J. (1977). Eating styles of obese and nonobese black and white children in a natural setting. *Addictive Behaviors, 2,* 83–86.

Epstein, L.H. (1990). Behavioral treatment of obesity. In E.M. Stricker (Ed.), *Neurobiology of food and fluid intake: Handbook of behavioral neurobiology* (Vol. 10, pp. 61–73). New York: Plenum.

Epstein, L.H., McCurley, J., Valoski, A., & Wing, R.R. (1990). Growth in obese children treated for obesity. *American Journal of Diseases of Children, 144,* 1360–1364.

Epstein, L.H., Valoski, A., Koeske, R., & Wing, R.R. (1986). Family-based behavioral weight control in obese young children. *Journal of the American Dietetic Association, 86,* 481–484.

Epstein, L.H., Valoski, A., Wing, R.R., & McCurley, J. (1994). Ten-year outcomes of behavioral family-based treatment for childhood obesity. *Health Psychology, 13,* 373–383.

Epstein, L.H., Wing, R.R., Koeske, R., Ossip, D., & Beck, S. (1982). A comparison of lifestyle change and programmed aerobic exercise on weight and fitness changes in obese children. *Behavior Therapy, 13,* 651–665.

Epstein, L.H., Wing, R.R., Koeske, R., & Valoski, A. (1985). A comparison of lifestyle exercise, aerobic exercise and calisthenics on weight loss in obese children. *Behavior Therapy, 16,* 345–356.

Epstein, L.H., Wing, R.R., & Valoski, A. (1985). Childhood obesity. *Pediatric Clinics of North America, 32,* 363–379.

Epstein, L.H., Wing, R.R., Woodall, K., Penner, B.C., Kress, M.J., & Koeske, R. (1985). Effects of family-based behavioral treatment on obese 5- to 8-year-old children. *Behavior Therapy, 16,* 205–212.

Figueroa-Colon, R., vonAlmen, K., Franklin, F.A., Schuftan, C., & Suskind, R.M. (1993). Comparison of two hypocaloric diets in obese children. *American Journal of Diseases of Children, 147,* 160–166.

Foreyt, J.P., & Cousins, J.H. (1989). Obesity. In E.J. Mash & R.A. Barkley (Eds.), *Treatment of childhood disorders* (pp. 405–422). New York: Guilford Press.

Foreyt, J.P., & Goodrick, G.K. (1988). Childhood obesity. In E.J. Mash & L.G. Terdal (Eds.), *Behavioral assessment of childhood disorders* (2nd ed., pp. 528–551). New York: Guilford Press.

Ganley, R.M. (1989). Emotion and eating in obesity: A review of the literature. *International Journal of Eating Disorders, 8,* 343–361.

Garn, S.M., & Clark, D.C. (1976). Trends in fatness and the origins of obesity. *Pediatrics, 56,* 443–456.

Goldstein, D.J., & Potvin, J.H. (1994). Long-term weight loss: The effect of pharmacologic agents. *American Journal of Nutrition, 60,* 647–657.

Gortmaker, S.L., Dietz, W.H., Sobol, A.M., & Wehler, C.A. (1987). Increasing pediatric obesity in the United States. *American Journal of Diseases of Children, 141,* 535–540.

Gortmaker, S.L., Must, A., Perrin, J.M., Sobol, A.M., & Dietz, W.H. (1993). Social and economic consequences of overweight in adolescence and young adulthood. *New England Journal of Medicine, 329,* 1008–1012.

Greeno, C.G., & Wing, R.R. (1994). Stress-induced eating. *Psychological Bulletin, 115,* 444–464.

Guy-Grand, B. (1992). Long-term pharmacological treatment of obesity. In T.A. Wadden & T.B. VanItallie (Eds.), *Treatment of the seriously obese patient* (pp. 478–495). New York: Guilford Press.

Haddock, C.K., Shadish, W.R., Klesges, R.C., & Stein, R.J. (1994). Treatments for childhood and adolescent obesity. *Annals of Behavioral Medicine, 16,* 235–244.

Hammer, L.D., Kraemer, H.C., Wilson, D.M., Ritter, P.L., & Dornbusch, S.M. (1991). Standardized percentile curves of body-mass index for children and adolescents. *American Journal of Diseases of Children, 145,* 259–263.

Hardy, S.C., & Kleinman, R.E. (1994). Fat and cholesterol in the diet of infants and young children: Implications for growth, development, and long-term health. *Journal of Pediatrics, 125,* S69–S77.

Harper, L.V., & Sanders, K.M. (1975). The effect of adults' eating on young children's acceptance of unfamiliar foods. *Journal of Experimental Child Psychology, 20,* 206–214.

Holm, V., & Pipes, P. (1976). Food and children with Prader-Willi syndrome. *American Journal of Diseases of Children, 130,* 1063–1067.

Israel, A.C. (1990). Childhood obesity. In A.S. Bellack, M. Hersen, & A.E. Kazdin (Eds.), *International handbook of behavior modification and therapy* (2nd ed., pp. 819–830). New York: Plenum.

Johnson, S.L., & Birch, L.L. (1994). Parents' and children's adiposity and eating style. *Pediatrics, 94,* 653–661.

Keesey, R.E. (1986). A set-point theory of obesity. In K.D. Brownell & J.P. Foreyt (Eds.), *Handbook of eating disorders: Physiology, psychology, and treatment of obesity, anorexia, and bulimia* (pp. 63–87). New York: Basic Books.

Kennedy, E., & Goldberg, J. (1995). What are American children eating? Implications for public policy. *Nutrition Reviews, 53,* 111–126.

Kinston, W., Loader, P., & Miller, L. (1988). Talking to families about obesity: A controlled study. *International Journal of Eating Disorders, 7,* 261–275.

Klesges, R.C., Coates, T.J., Brown, G., Sturgeon-Tillisch, J., Moldenhauer-Klesges, L., Holzer, B., Woolfrey, J., & Vollmer, J. (1983). Parental influences on children's eating behavior and relative weight. *Journal of Applied Behavior Analysis, 16,* 371–378.

Klesges, R.C., Eck, L.H., & Ray, J.A. (1995). Who underreports dietary intake in a dietary recall? Evidence from the Second National Health and Nutrition Examination Survey. *Journal of Consulting and Clinical Psychology, 63,* 438–444.

Klesges, R.C., Shelton, M.L., & Klesges, L.M. (1993). Effects of television on metabolic rate: Potential implications for childhood obesity. *Pediatrics, 91,* 281–285.

Kraemer, H.C., Berkowitz, R.I., & Hammer, L.D. (1990). Methodological difficulties in studies of obesity: I. Measurement issues. *Annals of Behavioral Medicine, 12,* 112–118.

Kral, J.G. (1992). Surgical treatment of obesity. In T.A. Wadden & T.B. VanItallie (Eds.), *Treatment of the seriously obese patient* (pp. 496–506). New York: Guilford Press.

Kuczmarski, R.J. (1992). Prevalence of overweight and weight gain in the United States. *American Journal of Clinical Nutrition, 55,* 495S–502S.

Kuczmarski, R.J., Flegal, K.M., Campbell, S.M., & Johnson, C.L. (1994). Increasing prevalence of overweight among U.S. adults. *Journal of the American Medical Association, 272,* 205–211.

Kumanyika, S. (1993). Ethnicity and obesity development in children. *Annals of the New York Academy of Sciences, 699,* 81–92.

Lifshitz, F., & Moses, N. (1989). Growth failure: A complication of dietary treatment of hypercholesterolemia. *American Journal of Diseases of Children, 143,* 537–542.

Logue, A.W. (1991). *The psychology of eating and drinking* (2nd ed.). San Francisco: W.H. Freeman.

Mallick, M.J. (1983). Health hazards of obesity and weight control in children: A review of the literature. *American Journal of Public Health, 73,* 78–82.

Manson, J.E., Willett, W.C., Stampfer, M.J., Colditz, G.A., Hunter, D.J., Hankinson, S.E., Hennekens, C.H., & Speizer, F.E. (1995). Body weight and mortality among women. *New England Journal of Medicine, 333,* 677–685.

National Task Force on the Prevention and Treatment of Obesity. (1996). Long-term pharmacotherapy in the management of obesity. *Journal of the American Medical Association, 276,* 1907–1915.

Nielsen Media Research. (1990). *1990 Nielsen Report on Television.* New York: Author.

Page, T. (1988). Clinical-research issues in the treatment of obesity in the developmentally disabled. In D.C. Russo & J.H. Kedesdy (Eds.), *Behavioral medicine with the developmentally disabled* (pp. 265–272). New York: Plenum.

Pisacano, J.C., Lichter, H., Ritter, J., & Siegal, A.P. (1978). An attempt at prevention of obesity in infancy. *Pediatrics, 61,* 360–364.

Pi-Sunyer, F.X. (1991). Health implications of obesity. *American Journal of Clinical Nutrition, 53,* 1595S–1603S.

Robinson, T.N., Hammer, L.D., Killen, J.D., Kraemer, H.C., Wilson, D.M., Hayward, C., & Taylor, C.B. (1993). Does television viewing increase obesity and reduce physical activity? Cross-sectional and longitudinal analyses among adolescent girls. *Pediatrics, 91,* 273–280.

Saris, W.H. (1993). The role of exercise in the dietary treatment of obesity. *International Journal of Obesity, 17,* S17–S21

Sjostrom, L. (1980). Fat cells and body weight. In A.J. Stunkard (Ed.), *Obesity* (pp. 72–100). Philadelphia: W.B. Saunders.

Skorzewska, A., Lal, S., Waserman, J., & Guyda, H. (1989). Abnormal food-seeking behavior after surgery for craniopharyngioma. *Neuropsychobiology, 21,* 17–20.

Sobal, J., & Stunkard, A.J. (1989). Socioeconomic status and obesity: A review of the literature. *Psychological Bulletin, 105,* 260–275.

Strauss, C.C., Smith, K., Frame, C., & Forehand, R. (1985). Personal and interpersonal characteristics associated with childhood obesity. *Journal of Pediatric Psychology, 10,* 337–343.

Stunkard, A.J. (1992). An overview of current treatments for obesity. In T.A. Wadden & T.B. VanItallie (Eds.), *Treatment of the seriously obese patient* (pp. 33–43). New York: Guilford Press.

Stunkard, A.J., Harris, J.R., Pedersen, N.L., & McClearn, G.E. (1990). A separated twin study of the body mass index. *New England Journal of Medicine, 322,* 1483–1487.

Stunkard, A.J., Sorenson, T.I.A., Hanis, C., Teasdale, T.W., Chakraborty, R., Schull, W.J., & Schulsinger, F. (1986). An adoption study of human obesity. *New England Journal of Medicine, 314,* 193–198.

Troiano, R.P., Flegal, K.M., Kuczmarski, R.J., Campbell, S.M., & Johnson, C.L. (1995). Overweight prevalence and trends for children and adolescents. *Archives of Pediatric and Adolescent Medicine, 149,* 1085–1091.

Varni, J.W., & Banis, H.T. (1985). Behavior therapy techniques applied to eating, exercise, and diet modification in childhood obesity. *Journal of Developmental and Behavioral Pediatrics, 6,* 367–372.

Wadden, T.A., & Bartlett, S.J. (1992). Very low calorie diets: An overview and appraisal. In T.A. Wadden & T.B. VanItallie (Eds.), *Treatment of the seriously obese patient* (pp. 44–79). New York: Guilford Press.

Waxman, M., & Stunkard, A.J. (1980). Caloric intake and expenditure of obese boys. *Journal of Pediatrics, 96,* 187–193.

Wilson, G.T. (1993). Relation of dieting and voluntary weight loss to psychological functioning and binge-eating. *Annals of Internal Medicine, 119,* 727–730.

Wolf, A.M., & Colditz, G.A. (1996). The social and economic effects of body weight in the United States. *American Journal of Clinical Nutrition, 63,* 466S–469S.

Wong, N.D., Hei, T.K., Qaqundah, P.Y., Davidson, D.M., Bassin, S.L., & Gold, K.V. (1992). Television viewing and pediatric hypercholesterolemia. *Pediatrics, 90,* 75–79.

Wooley, S.C., & Garner, D.M. (1994). Dietary treatments for obesity are ineffective. *British Medical Journal, 309,* 655–656.

Woolston, J.L. (1991). *Eating and growth disorders in infants and children.* Beverly Hills: Sage Publications.

Zipf, W.B., & Bernston, G.G. (1987). Characteristics of abnormal food-intake patterns in children with Prader-Willi syndrome and study of effects of naloxone. *American Journal of Clinical Nutrition, 46,* 277–281.

Epilogue

The preceding chapters emphasize the importance of using empirical research as a guide to clinical practice with children with feeding disorders. The quantity and quality of research available to the practitioner are, however, quite uneven. As would be expected, feeding problems associated with significant health risks (e.g., failure to thrive [FTT], pediatric obesity) have generated more research than feeding disorders that are apparently medically benign (e.g., mild selectivity) or very rare (e.g., psychogenic hyperphagia). Expanding the current knowledge base relevant to children's feeding problems is an essential prerequisite to the further development of the field. Of equal importance is ensuring that additions and improvements to the knowledge base are translated into clinical practice.

There are several areas in which the need for additional research is especially salient. First, much remains to be learned about the emergence and persistence of many early childhood feeding problems. Prevalence studies with representative samples and clear diagnostic criteria, as exemplified by the studies of children with nonorganic FTT in London by Skuse and colleagues (Skuse, Reilly, & Wolke, 1994) and the studies of children with food refusal in Sweden by Dahl and colleagues (e.g., Dahl & Sundelin, 1986), merit replication in the United States. Similar epidemiological investigations of pica and rumination in healthy children would be useful, as would studies of the prevalence of selectivity in special populations, such as children with specific chronic illnesses (e.g., bronchopulmonary dysplasia). Additional longitudinal studies would contribute to our understanding of the persistence of feeding problems in infancy and early childhood (e.g., Dahl & Sundelin, 1992; Marchi & Cohen, 1990). Carefully designed prevalence and persistence studies also would provide a firmer basis for the differentiation of clinical feeding problems from subclinical feeding problems and,

379

thereby, would help determine the degree of intervention necessary to remedy the problem. Also needed are descriptive studies of typical parent management techniques and culturally specific variations in parenting techniques for dealing with common feeding problems.

Second, there is very little research on the primary prevention of childhood feeding problems. Evaluation of the efficacy of anticipatory guidance during well-child health visits and related strategies such as bibliographic and other public education efforts is needed. It is not known, for example, whether children whose parents receive anticipatory guidance about feeding issues develop fewer feeding problems than those who do not or whether more discussion of feeding problems during health care surveillance visits would yield benefits. The increasing prevalence of pediatric obesity since the 1960s would suggest that the guidance provided during routine health care surveillance visits is, in many cases, insufficient.

Third, some childhood feeding disorders appear to be amenable to subtype classification, but there has been little research to validate proposed classification schemes. For example, subtypes of FTT (e.g., Chatoor, Dickson, Schaeffer, & Egan, 1985), as well as subtypes of rumination (e.g., Mayes, Humphrey, Handford, & Mitchell, 1988), have been proposed. Empirical validation of these clinically derived subtypes would set the stage for research to evaluate the efficacy of differential intervention strategies with different feeding problem subtypes.

Fourth, basic scientific research in areas such as gustation, olfaction, and appetite regulation (to cite a few relevant areas) is too rarely integrated with clinical research on childhood feeding disorders. For example, it is widely known that there are genetic differences in taste perception (Duffy & Bartoshuk, 1996); to what extent these differences contribute to selective eating or to other childhood feeding problems is unknown. Basic experimental research to evaluate venerable, but untested, etiological hypotheses (e.g., the critical period hypothesis) also would be valuable.

Fifth, some childhood feeding disorders (e.g., rumination, extreme food refusal, psychogenic hyperphagia) are "low-incidence, high-intensity disorders," meaning that the children present with relatively rare but clinically significant feeding disorders. Much of the intervention research on these disorders relies on case studies or single-subject experimental designs. Greater emphasis on multicenter collaboration would provide larger, potentially more representative, samples of children, which would allow for stronger empirical testing of intervention effects. An example of such a collaboration is a 5-year project funded by the National Institutes of

Health to evaluate feeding intervention outcomes for children with cystic fibrosis (Stark et al., 1996). Researchers at two sites in the United States are comparing the efficacy of nutrition education alone to nutrition education plus behavioral parent training for increasing food intake in children.

Sixth, the changing economics of health care delivery in the 1990s has necessitated a shift in emphasis from inpatient to outpatient feeding interventions and from the use of professional therapists to reliance on parents as therapists. Little is known about efficient methods of teaching feeding interventions to lay caregivers, which strategies are more acceptable to parents (Ahearn, Kerwin, Eicher, Shantz, & Swearingin, 1996), or how proficient caregivers need to be to facilitate meaningful change in child feeding patterns. Very few studies (Stark et al., 1996; Turner, Sanders, & Wall, 1994) have implemented controlled comparisons of intervention protocols delivered in outpatient settings with parents as primary therapists. Further research is vital to ascertain both the effectiveness and the limitations of caregivers as therapists for their children's feeding disorders.

Bringing an increasing knowledge base to bear on clinical practice is as important as increasing the knowledge base itself. There are many potential obstacles to applying research to clinical practice. These obstacles include 1) institutional and professional barriers to interdisciplinary collaboration, 2) health care economic constraints on providing the often labor-intensive interventions that may be required to ameliorate severe feeding disorders, and 3) the low priority of prevention (as compared with treatment or intervention) in the competition for health care dollars. The first issue can begin to be addressed through greater emphasis on interdisciplinary training for professionals likely to encounter children with feeding disorders. Advocacy at the level of the health care institution (e.g., the tertiary care hospital) to support collaboration among diverse professionals, as well as advocacy at the public policy level to secure the necessary resources for children with feeding disorders and their families, is needed to address the first and second issues. With regard to the third issue, prevention has been advocated as the most efficacious approach for reducing many adverse health-related conditions, yet prevailing policies for funding health care in the United States discourage families' access to services until diagnosable problems arise. Prevention-oriented research is costly in terms of time, numbers of participants, and money; as a result, few guidelines are available regarding how to establish effective preventive services. Even in the area of obesity, in which the research is more extensive than in other areas of feeding disorders, little is known

382 ■ ■ ■ Epilogue

about how to successfully prevent overweight in children. Prevention studies with various feeding disorders may be able to take advantage of advances in other areas (e.g., smoking, drug abuse, heart disease) regarding promising prevention strategies.

Many of the issues that complicate research on pediatric feeding problems also make clinical work in the area challenging. The influence of multiple, interacting, etiological variables can produce unique, often puzzling, constellations of clinical features in different children, rendering feeding disorders both intellectually stimulating and humbling to clinicians. Clinical wisdom in this field depends on the continued pursuit of a scientist–practitioner approach, informed by the diverse perspectives of colleagues in multiple disciplines, the personal experience of parents, and mindful observation of the evolving intricacies of child behavior.

REFERENCES

Ahearn, W.H., Kerwin, M.E., Eicher, P.S., Shantz, J., & Swearingin, W. (1996). An alternating treatments comparison of two intensive interventions for food refusal. *Journal of Applied Behavior Analysis, 29*, 321–332.

Chatoor, I., Dickson, L., Schaeffer, S., & Egan, J. (1985). A developmental classification of feeding disorders associated with failure to thrive: Diagnosis and treatment. In D. Drotar (Ed.), *New directions in failure to thrive* (pp. 235–258). New York: Plenum.

Dahl, M., & Sundelin, C. (1986). Early feeding problems in an affluent society: I. Categories and clinical signs. *Acta Paediatrica Scandinavia, 75*, 370–379.

Dahl, M., & Sundelin, C. (1992). Feeding problems in an affluent society. Follow-up at four years of age in children with early refusal to eat. *Acta Paediatrica, 81*, 575–579.

Duffy, V.B., & Bartoshuk, L.M. (1996). Sensory factors in feeding. In E.D. Capaldi (Ed.), *Why we eat what we eat* (pp. 145–171). Washington, DC: American Psychological Association.

Marchi, M., & Cohen, P. (1990). Early childhood eating behaviors and adolescent eating disorders. *Journal of the American Academy of Child and Adolescent Psychiatry, 29*, 112–117.

Mayes, S.D., Humphrey, F.J., Handford, H.A., & Mitchell, J.F. (1988). Rumination disorder: Differential diagnosis. *Journal of the American Academy of Child and Adolescent Psychiatry, 27*, 300–302.

Skuse, D., Reilly, S., & Wolke, D. (1994). Psychosocial adversity and growth during infancy. *European Journal of Clinical Nutrition, 48*, S113–S130.

Stark, L.J., Spieth, L., Opipari, L., Quittner, A.L., Jelalian, E., Lapey, A., Khaw, K.T., Higgins, L., Duggan, C.P., & Stallings, V.A. (1996, October). *The efficacy of behavioral intervention: Parent training vs. nutrition education.* Paper presented at the North American Cystic Fibrosis Conference, Orlando, FL.

Turner, K.M., Sanders, M.R., & Wall, C.R. (1994). Behavioral parent training versus dietary education in the treatment of children with persistent feeding difficulties. *Behaviour Change, 11*, 244–258.

Index

Page numbers followed by *t* or *f* indicate tables or figures, respectively.